# STABILITY, SPORT AND PERFORMANCE MOVEMENT

## PRACTICAL BIOMECHANICS AND SYSTEMATIC TRAINING FOR MOVEMENT EFFICACY AND INJURY PREVENTION, SECOND EDITION

JOANNE ELPHINSTON

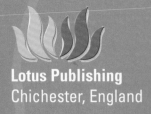

**Lotus Publishing**
Chichester, England

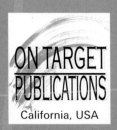

ON TARGET
PUBLICATIONS
California, USA

First published in 2008 by
**Lotus Publishing**
Apple Tree Cottage, Inlands Road, Chichester, PO18 8RJ and
**North Atlantic Books**
P.O. Box 12327, Berkeley, California 94712.

This second edition published in 2013 by **Lotus Publishing** and
**On Target Publications**
PO Box 1335, Aptos, California 95001.

**Anatomical Illustrations** Amanda Williams
**Technique Photographs** Joanne Elphinston/CMD
**Sportsperson Photographs** Getty Images
**Cover Design** Richard Evans
**Text Design** Simon Hempsell
**Printed and Bound** in England by Cubiquity Media

**Disclaimer**

The information in this book has been presented with care on the basis of the author's professional experience and the available research. The programmes are designed for healthy individuals with normal levels of fitness unless under the supervision of a health professional. The author is not liable for misuse or misunderstanding of the material herein, nor any injury which may be incurred while pursuing the programmes provided.

**British Library Cataloguing-in-Publication Data**
A CIP record for this book is available from the British Library
ISBN 978 1 905367 42 9

**The Library of Congress has cataloged the first edition as follows:**
Elphinston, Joanne.
  Stability, Sport, and Performance Movement: great technique without injury / joanne elphinston.
  p. cm.
Includes bibliographical references and index.
ISBN 978-1-55643-746-5
  1. Sports--Physiological aspects. 2. Movement therapy. 3. Human mechanics. 4. Sports injuries. I. Title.
RC1235.E47 2008
612'.044--dc22
          2008013790 3

# Contents

# Preface to the Second Edition

Much has changed since 2008 when the first edition of this book in English emerged. At that time misunderstandings about stability, particularly the distortion of the "core" concept, and conflict between professions were a major stimulus for my writing.

Fast-forward four years, and the term "functional" is suffering a similar fate to core before it. If an exercise is deemed functional, it is thought to be superior to something else deemed non-functional. Integrated global body movement tasks are relevant, beneficial and ideally transferable, especially when designed to be appropriate to the individual's sport or occupation. However, in my clinical and consultancy work, I meet many people who have been trained functionally at a relatively high loading, but lack the fundamental foundations to gain optimal benefit from these tasks, and thus still struggle with their original injury or technical barrier.

**Sometimes in our effort to be functional, we skip the steps that actually create the potential for functionality.** These include recalibrating habitual activation patterns; releasing inappropriate tension; restoring available mobility; enhancing proprioception and engaging self-awareness. It may be that in order to achieve these foundations, an exercise may not grossly look like a functional exercise, yet it actively enables the body to relinquish its normal tension patterns and establish sustainable force management responses.

A simple change in tempo may reveal and address underlying control problems. Temporary load reduction in an optimal position may unlock a person's coping strategy and improve their timing and coordination. It may be that the person needs increased sensory input to enable them to feel body relationships in order for them to find a new strategy. The task involved may then appear to be non-functional, but is in fact a necessary motor learning step on the way to integrated, effective movement. It may be the ignition key that starts the movement engine.

It is time to look forward once more, recognising that stability and functional training are simply steps towards a goal of *movement efficacy* in athletic development. Although often seen as the coach's domain, anyone involved in athletic training can influence the athlete's ability to transcend the building blocks of strength, power, stability or whatever other training modes they might use, working towards an end goal of fluent, confident, unrestricted movement.

My terminology has shifted slightly since the last edition. While the 2008 text still stands, there is more to be discussed about forces and how we view them in order to build function-appropriate programmes. Where I once needed to limit my discussion to stability, now we can speak more openly of movement efficacy, the concept of moving beautifully.

Moving beautifully is open to anyone. I am grateful to the non-athletes who bought the first edition to learn about themselves and wrote to tell me their favourite concepts and techniques. For those in the training industry who seek much higher-loaded exercises, there are many fine authors to choose from whose expertise lies in fitter/harder/stronger. This book, however, has emerged from my experience with athletes who have tried to wallpaper over the cracks with strength and power work, but whose repeated injuries or performance plateaus have been overcome with seemingly small, quiet techniques which have nevertheless provided the keys to unlocking their barriers and blocks.

This leads me to an important point. Earlier in my career, I thought that I was identifying a deficit and then addressing what was missing with my programmes. These days, I realise that I mostly help people to *get out of their own way*. Movement issues, especially those to do with control, are commonly seen as arising from a fundamental lack of something. I have increasingly found that many people already have much of what they need to move much better than they do, but are locking themselves out of fluent movement through tension, effort, habit and beliefs.

A diamond can only be exposed by peeling away the rock that encases it. Then it can be polished to reveal its full potential. So it is with many of my clients – releasing their habitual blocks as a first priority allows their potential to emerge, and change to happen remarkably quickly. If we release what we do not need, and develop progressively, the body finds new resources. If we master this, then we can apply increased loading as an enhancement to a system that knows how to manage forces and express movement effectively.

I also meet many athletes who have more power than they can use because they have rigorously been trained in horizontal and vertical lines. They hold themselves so prescriptively in form that they lose the timing, fine-tuning and elastic potential that bring an organic, fluent and even explosive quality to their movement. This is a misapplication of the control concept. Control should enable movement, not restrict it. These athletes often need to be given permission to "move with the handbrake off".

The less concrete elements that I describe here fall into the realms of skill. We have become an information dominant culture, and in many sectors knowledge is now routinely mistaken for skill. Master practitioners understand that we need to assimilate and interpret the scientific research while meeting the practical challenges of coaching, training and rehabilitating human beings. We also need simple ways to understand and communicate about movement – to practically translate the science in way that is meaningful.

In edition one, I made a commitment to straightforward language, and in this new edition I have maintained this while adding new information which I hope will be both helpful and enjoyable. Some of you will read the whole book, others will dip into certain chapters. Most concepts are best explained in simple terms, so I have tried to remove the language barrier between athlete, coach and medical professional where possible in order to help you to communicate with each other.

These past four years since the first edition have been abundantly filled with continuing exploration and development, stimulated by the specific needs and interests of groups as disparate as professional footballers and dancers, musicians and golfers, skiers and Pilates teachers, coaches and children. Through the inception of JEMS (Joanne Elphinston Movement Systems), a vibrant community of like-minded professionals is also developing, and I thank each and every one of these individuals for their enthusiasm and passion for movement and the approach.

I hope you enjoy using the new content as much as I have enjoyed developing and communicating it.

Joanne Elphinston
May 2013

# Acknowledgments

Although I had intended to write this book at some stage, it may not have come about when it did had it not been commissioned by SISU Idrottsböcker of Stockholm and guided into life by Catarina Arfwidsson for the Swedish sports community. For the first two years of its life it existed only in Swedish, until Jon Hutchings of Lotus Publishing had the vision to produce it in English. It was Jon who persuaded me to undertake this second edition.

There are many people without whom this book would never have been written. The athletes who have challenged me to look for solutions, and who have taken responsibility for themselves and their training; the coaches who have applied the principles with their athletes and upheld my belief in raising the bar for coach education; the sports scientists who have been willing to share in the multidisciplinary process, and the physiotherapists and other sports professionals who have so kindly shared their enthusiasm for simple specific concepts and who have spurred me on with their support.

There are some individuals who must be thanked personally. Allan Uhlmann, Sarah Hardman, Heather Watson, Jackie Zaslona, Susie Morel, Jo Racle, Jenny Manners and Liz Blenkinsop kindly read and shared their thoughts on the text.

Danielle Nichols, Rob Ahmun, Kent Fyrth, Nick Jones and Leah Cox gave their time to be models and for this I am very grateful. Jo Thomas-Kemp of Esporta Cardiff very kindly lent her support by making space available for photography.

Finally, I must thank my husband, Kent Fyrth, without whose unfaltering support I could not do what I do.

# Introduction

In every sport there are athletes who represent true technical excellence. We recognise them instinctively, as their efficiency is expressed through the beauty of their movement and the effortlessness with which they seem to perform. This technical mastery requires a physical structure that supports the sport's biomechanics, the neuromuscular coordination to correctly sequence the movement, the psychological skills to focus effort without unnecessary tension and the physiology to sustain the movement pattern until the event is completed.

With its ability to move through multiple planes in complex combinations, the body is capable of extraordinary movement diversity. This makes possible an enormous range of sporting endeavours, but versatility can become the greatest challenge to technical proficiency. It permits unwanted movements, which then provoke increased muscle tension to try to control them. It allows deviation from the most effective line of motion, compromising efficiency. It allows variability in joint angles, timing and movement sequencing which gives us many movement options but can also amplify control problems under conditions of increased complexity, fatigue, speed, agility, endurance or technical demand.

In closed skill sports such as swimming, pole vaulting or sprint kayak, performance depends upon an ability to accurately reproduce a movement with minimal variation. These athletes hone their movement skill to progressively narrow the window of variability. This does not limit their adaptability however. Their fundamental technical consistency allows them to make small but accurate adjustments if their environment requires it in order to deliver their best performance.

In open skill sports such as tennis, football and alpine skiing, athletes must be able to move in a variety of ways and adapt to rapidly changing situations, but still produce accurate and effective movement by controlling the forces acting on them. Their challenge is to widen the diversity of their skills but to control their variability. They aim to develop more movement options with reliable results.

Even at world-class level we can observe differences in movement economy and control. Some athletes compensate for their technical limitations by maximising other assets, such as an astounding natural physiology or a combination of strength and determination. They may achieve success, but using this method is somewhat like taking a jigsaw puzzle with a missing piece and trying to make up for it by making the other pieces bigger. You may cover the space, but the picture will not be as coherent as it might have been with the missing piece in place. The question is not how athletic success was achieved, but how much more might have been possible with all systems optimised.

The building blocks of stability, mobility, posture, body awareness, symmetry and balance provide the foundation for sporting movement development and injury resistance. These elements work in combination to ensure that physical restrictions, imbalances and inefficient muscle recruitment patterns do not hold you back from meeting your technical movement goals. The right muscles firing at the right time in the right sequence can increase your chance of achieving your physical potential.

## It's Not All About the Core

The purpose of this book is to promote the foundations for effective movement, rather than to solely develop core stability. Core stability has been transformed from a training concept into an industry in its own right, and great claims are made for its potential effects despite a lack of consistent evidence in the scientific literature to support them. Part of the problem is that it has become isolated from the context of integrated functional body movement.

When stability is perceived to be a separate fitness marker like speed or power, athletes start to look for exercise regimens that activate more core. Some professionals advocate instability activities such as Swiss Ball exercise and others argue in favour of Olympic lifts for developing core stability. Both in fact stimulate the trunk in different ways and for different purposes. Research to determine the amount of trunk activity involved in different activities sometimes compares loaded with unloaded activities. Unsurprisingly, researchers find that there is more activity in the trunk when the body is loaded [37]. This is then taken as evidence that the loading approach is more effective.

If our objective is movement efficiency, then more is not necessarily desirable. Certainly if you are squatting with a heavy weight, you will require an increase in trunk activity to support your spine against that resistance. You will be training a response to a predictable, loaded, symmetrical movement, and this may be appropriate to certain specific sporting demands. However, you will not have trained for unpredictability, change of direction, control through different motions or at the low levels of continuous muscle activity needed to optimise whole body movement over extended periods. These conditions require a different set of neuromuscular responses. It is a matter of what is appropriate for your functional requirements.

Core stability cannot independently optimise movement availability and control. The moving body in sport requires a complex sequence of activation and timing appropriate to the activity that you are performing. This sequence is known as a *functional motor pattern* and it requires an interplay between your musculoskeletal system and your nervous system from the soles of your feet through your whole body to your head.

# The JEMS Approach

Joanne Elphinston Movement Systems (JEMS) has evolved over many years of performance consultancy and teaching to meet the needs of a diverse array of athletes and the professionals who support them. These people have challenged me to find ways to communicate concepts in a way that is meaningful to them, and which lend a new perspective to their existing training methods while identifying and integrating any missing elements. These methods are now passed on through a variety of JEMS educational seminars and through resources such as this book. Where they appear in the text, key JEMS principles are highlighted in orange.

JEMS has been used with international-level athletes in disciplines as diverse as swimming, badminton, gymnastics, karate, judo, cycling, football, weightlifting, basketball, athletics, snow sports, golf, equestrian sports and tennis. However, it works just as well for weekend warriors and people who just want to enjoy their sport and develop their own sporting movement.

The programme presented in Part Two develops functional motor patterns by integrating control concepts with posture, balance, mobility and neuromuscular control to provide you with a physical platform for fluent, trainable movement. Once you have this movement, you can train to make it faster, stronger and more powerful.

There are top athletes who have all of this working naturally. There are others who don't realise that there are elements that could be improved because no one has ever looked. There are many who are unaware that they have lost elements due to injury, and wonder why they just can't seem to make a successful comeback. Then there are those of us who are just trying to find the natural athlete within ourselves.

The JEMS approach is not a purely orthopaedic/structural programme. Motor learning is more than muscle contractions, and often the key to unlocking a body response requires a sensory opportunity, a change in loading or an alternative position for an athlete to experience change and gain new understanding.

The early stages of the programme use the Swiss Ball as it is one of the simplest tools for providing clear sensory feedback, modifying load on the body and facilitating low-threshold autoresponses. It is not, however, the only equipment that can be used to stimulate control! TRX, red cords, kettlebells and all manner of equipment can stimulate movement efficacy responses when used appropriately. Conversely, they can also create movement dysfunction when used without sufficient insight.

Almost anything can be used to develop movement efficacy if the principles are understood – it is not so much the tool but the skill involved that is key.

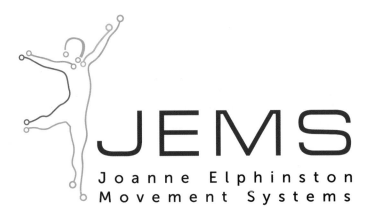

# How to Use This Book

Although it is helpful to have ideas for what to do, it is even better when you understand why. In Part One, Foundations and Fundamentals, Chapters 1 to 4 explore the relationship between movement and stability, introducing new concepts and examining existing models. Here we establish a foundation for this approach and set the scene for the functional assessment of Chapter 5 and the exercises laid out in Part Two, Developing Fluent Control.

Chapters 6 to 12 of Part Two involve active application of the programme. They contain a library of exercises. Two important themes have guided their structure:

1. Movement efficacy, which involves the interplay between multiple elements. An effective programme should therefore contain a variety of stimuli which support and enhance each other. Each exercise chapter contains complementary elements for improving control, balance, mobility, awareness and neuromuscular coordination so that the programme has balance.

2. Systematic progression, which is key for an effective programme. Each of the four chapters therefore builds upon the previous one, either introducing greater skill or load elements. Many of the exercises will be familiar. Understanding why you are doing them, what they should look like, how they should progress and what you can use as alternatives is what makes the difference.

> Pay attention to the small things. The key seed movements that unlock or prepare the body for the big motions often reside within them.

Moving well doesn't have to be complicated. The principles are based in science, but in practice you need to know what to look for, what it means and how to fix it if it isn't what you are after. That is what this book is all about.

## A note on language and expression

This text is a practical resource written as simply as possible in order to establish a common language between athletes, coaches, sports scientists and medical professionals working in sport. It was written to be a bridge so that we all can make ourselves understood to one another. The different readerships would normally be addressed in separate publications but it would have taken away the opportunity for those who are interested in a bigger picture to see how different perspectives fit together. Switches between the athlete's perspective and that of the medical, science or coaching professional will be recognisable in the book but should enhance rather than detract from its usefulness.

Appendix 1 (p.357) provides a glossary of terms for those needing help with the language of anatomy and movement.

# Part One
## Foundations and Fundamentals

# 1 | Force, Flow and Functional Force Management

Forces in Motion
Control Zones
Functional Force Management Strategies
Movement Initiation and Force Transmission
Direction of Movement Impulse

Functional force management is a method for conceptualising the ways through which we support and facilitate controlled, efficient motion. I developed this approach for communicating about forces in order to overcome the confusion and conflict that many people perceive between some of the common control methodologies and the biomechanics and behaviours of normal movement.

The work on movement impulse comes from meeting the practical coaching and clinical challenges brought by my own clients, and I have found it useful both in identifying issues and in addressing them. I hope you will too.

# Forces in Motion

Body movement involves a constant flow of forces. Every motion demands that we create force and control force. The degree to which we are able to do this effectively and efficiently will influence our technical proficiency and our resistance to injury. This is functional force management (FFM). It is the key to our capacity for physical *expression* through qualities such as power, speed or balance, and for physical *conservation*, or protection, through strategies such as shock absorption and force sharing to divert pressure from body structures.

There are four key elements to FFM:

1. How effectively force is generated and directed,

2. How effectively forces are transmitted throughout the body,

3. How effectively forces are dispersed or shared across the structures of the body, and

4. How effectively force is dispersed or released from the body.

These four factors will directly influence your technique, your performance and your ability to minimise injury risk.

Conceptualising movement through the generation and transmission of force allows us to appreciate the biomechanical interactions throughout the body, and the integration necessary for fluency and efficiency. It also gives us a means for understanding movement breakdown in a practical way.

# Control Zones

There are several basic principles for understanding force management. The first of these is the zone concept. The body can be divided into three primary zones. These can be described as power zones, control zones or force management zones with equal accuracy. For the purposes of this book, we will call them *control zones*.

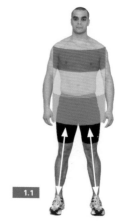

1.1

Connection between control zones is essential for force management, and each control zone must be capable of moving independently against adjacent control zones whilst maintaining this connection.

## The Lower Control Zone

The lower control zone (LCZ) supports and carries everything above it, and its major component is the pelvis. However, reflexes from the feet are instrumental in driving pelvic muscle activation. This will be investigated in more detail later but for the moment it means that the feet must be considered in lower zone performance.

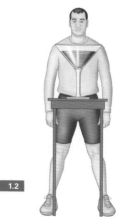

1.2

The lower control zone does not just provide support for the control zones above it. It also disperses forces down through the legs which otherwise would have to be managed elsewhere in the body, most commonly the spine and the knees. This is effective vertical force management, and is the mechanism for shock absorption. In landing from a jump for example, smooth, coordinated hip and knee bending keeps vertical forces flowing down and out (fig. 1.3).

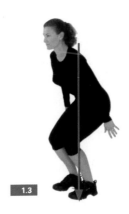

1.3

If the athlete blocks their motion at the hip and knee by over-contracting the muscles around them, the pelvis stops moving downwards and the force from above crashes into the lower back. This can cause a buckling effect in the spine and, over time, lower back pain. The athlete may alternatively react to vertical force by collapsing inwards at the knees in an attempt to divert the load. This deviation from the vertical increases stress at the knees and ankles, and can cause a variety of injuries.

FFM in the lower control zone also involves the fundamental behaviours of propulsion, momentum control, support and balance. These will be further investigated in Chapter 3.

## The Central Control Zone

The central control zone (CCZ) is what is commonly thought of as the core, and includes both the deep and superficial muscles of the trunk. One of its functions is the protection of the spinal structures; however, it is also the fundamental connector and communicator between the upper and lower control zones. As such, it is critical for the transmission of forces between these control zones for efficient movement.

The performance of the central control zone is highly dependent upon the lower control zone's ability to carry, support and position it, regardless of whether the athlete competes on their feet or sitting on their pelvis, e.g. equestrian/kayak/rowing. If the lower control zone is tilted sideways, forward or backward, for example, the central control zone must adapt in order to remain vertical – it does not float in isolation. Too frequently, attempts to correct the spinal posture are focused firmly on the abdominal muscles. However, the spine can only be positioned where the pelvis places it, and often it is the lower control zone that needs to be addressed. Any isolated core training will need to be integrated with lower control zone work in order to achieve functional transference.

## The Upper Control Zone

The upper control zone (UCZ) encompasses the scapulae, chest and shoulders, and again its position is heavily influenced by the control zones that support it. Shoulder positional problems often arise from a lower control zone force issue or an inefficient central control zone.

For example, a sideways tilted pelvis due to lower control zone problems can provoke a counterbalancing response from the upper control zone, such as dropping or raising a shoulder. Central control zone problems may show up as a spine that collapses into flexion, extension or side-bending under load, which in turn disconnects the shoulders from the support of the trunk. Posturally, positionally and functionally, the shoulders are dependent upon the quality of support and connection beneath them. In Chapter 3, we investigate the many specific force management strategies involved with the upper control zone.

## Clipboard Notes: A Control Zone Disconnection Story

An elite judo athlete was suffering from severe neck pain, with which he had struggled for two years. He had received various forms of soft tissue and joint treatment in that time, as well as a specific neck-strengthening regimen, but the symptoms did not respond.

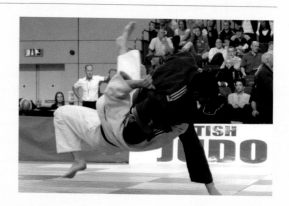

Looking at him from a FFM perspective, the athlete did everything with his shoulders raised, from basic standing posture through his strength and conditioning and into competition. This is quite frequently seen in asthmatics, and indeed, this athlete had asthma. He was unaware that he was constantly elevating his shoulders – he just thought that he was standing tall.

Judo is a whole-body sport – the athlete needs force production capability and support from the ground up. Raising the shoulders effectively unplugs the upper control zone from the lower and central control zones, isolating the arms from the power and control potential of the lower body (figs 1.5a–b). Unable to access his central and lower control zones, the athlete needed to find an alternative solution to anchor his upper control zone. The only available solution was to raise his shoulders, stabilising his arms through muscular connections to the neck. Every time he wanted to create force with his arms, his neck would take the load.

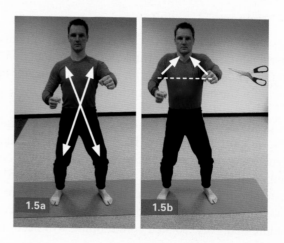

To address this, the athlete was guided to experience the difference in the sensation of effort, neck stress and control when his shoulders were raised, compared to when they were released to settle into his upper control zone (mid chest level). This was referred to as his "power zone". By working in his power zone when managing force through his arms, he felt more connected through his feet into the ground. This was the result of triple zone connection and the sharing of forces through the body. If allowed to work above his power zone, he lost connection and aggravated his neck pain.

Always working in his power zone and never above it was this athlete's main cue across his entire training programme, and his neck pain reduced surprisingly quickly despite the simplicity of the solution.

# Functional Force Management Strategies

Strategies for managing forces are dictated by the task being performed, and in many sports a number of different strategies will be used at different times. This will vary the muscle actions and control zone interactions required.

## Zone Stacking

*Zone stacking* connects and maintains adjacent control zones in a relatively consistent positional relationship. When achieved through efficient muscle coordination, the muscle activity used for zone stacking can be increased or decreased to meet the demands of the task, but the trunk position itself is maintained with very little change in muscle length. Zone stacking creates a sustainable, secure central pillar to support the effort of the limbs as they exert force, while allowing transmission of force through the body.

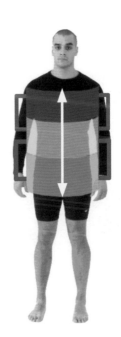

For example, a freestyle swimmer will use zone stacking to connect all three control zones for force generation, and to achieve the most effective line in the water. Freestyle swimming requires a longitudinal rotation, or body roll, and for this the swimmer's control zones need to maintain a consistent positional relationship. If the control zones rotate or side-bend against each other, efficiency will be lost.

The rower pictured below is using zone stacking to protect his spine and effectively transfer forces from his feet through his body and out through his hands.

Cycling is also an example of a zone stacking sport. If all three control zones maintain a consistent and secure relationship, they create a platform to contain forces between foot and hip for greatest force transmission through the pedal. The force will be directed from a secure centre out through the legs. Zone stacking also promotes efficient rotation around an axis, as used in hammer (fig. 1.8) or discus throwing and gymnastics. The important thing to remember about zone stacking is that it is not compressive. The zones are connected but the trunk maintains its length.

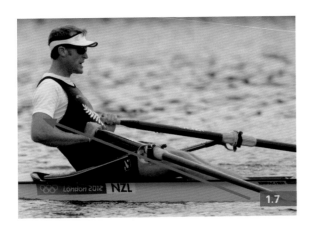

1.7

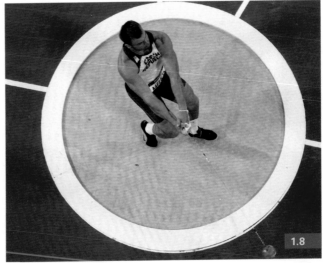

1.8

## Suit of Armour (Compression) Strategy

Zone stacking is often confused with the *suit of armour strategy*. Suit of armour is a compression strategy that involves stiffening the large trunk muscles. It is primarily a protective behaviour which constrains the shoulders and hips, and locks the trunk to the pelvis using high muscle force. In terms of force flow, the impulse is compressive and directed centrally into the body (fig. 1.9). In essence, it halts force transmission through the body and eliminates independent motion between control zones. This strategy is extremely useful when withstanding an impact such as a rugby tackle, for example.

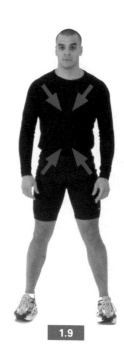

1.9

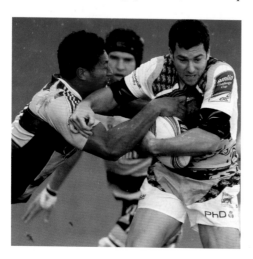

The suit of armour may also be fleetingly utilised in some sports, for example during a track cycling start, when the torso must be strongly controlled against very high forces from the legs. This behaviour, however, has a high energy cost, and is not a strategy to use continuously. Neither is it helpful when fluent, sustainable, dynamic movement is necessary because its role is to restrict and constrain motion.

### Training Note

Road cyclists and triathletes need to be clear about the difference between these two strategies. Those who pull back on the handlebars to stabilise their trunk set up the suit of armour, creating abdominal compression which can interfere with rib expansion for breathing and with smooth hip motion. Encouraging them to imagine the impulse to release and lengthen their hands away from their tailbones often brings about rapid improvements in the sense of effort and smoothness of motion over long distances.

Likewise, the rugby player cannot train only for the tackle; the modern player must be fast and agile no matter what position they play in. The suit of armour is only one of several trunk strategies that they must utilise.

## Elastic Support Strategy

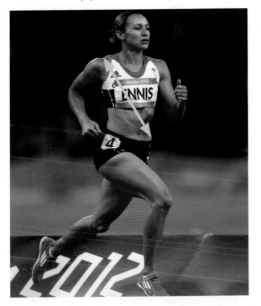

The next possibility is the *elastic support strategy*, which allows unrestricted movement in the limbs, and creates a mechanism for efficiently transferring force from the lower control zone to the upper control zone and back again.

Elastic support works through several mechanisms. For example, running utilises *diagonal elastic support*, a constant diagonal stretch and release created by counter body rotation. This is extremely efficient biomechanically, allowing the effort of the upper control zone to transfer to the lower control zone and vice versa. Force flows continuously up and down through alternating diagonals across the body. This mechanism also shares forces over a large area, which helps to avoid excessive stress on any one area or structure in the body.

The impulse of diagonal elastic support is shown in this runner. The central control zone connects and transmits while upper and lower control zones counter-rotate.

The same principle of elastic connection can be seen in this baseball player. The diagonal stretch sets up a force pathway from the foot in the lower control zone all the way to the upper control zone and out through the hand.

A well-functioning central control zone is critical in connecting and integrating the upper and lower control zones, but it is important to note that in an example such as this, the force is not generated in the core, as is so often quoted, and it is certainly not generated by the arm, which is at the end of the kinetic chain. The force impulse is generated in the lower control zone and channelled all the way through the body by the forward drive and rotation of the motion.

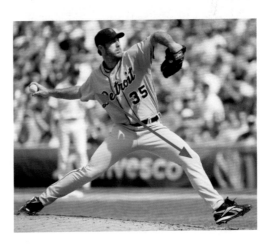

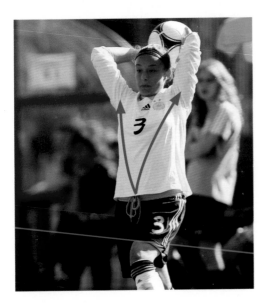

Elastic support does not only have to be diagonal: in figure 1.13 we can see that the pelvis connects through the central control zone to the upper control zone into both arms. The force impulse is up and out. This is *linear elastic support*. If the abdominal wall is lax and the force flow is halted by a disconnected central control zone, the upper control zone is left unsupported to generate the force.

1.13 The impulse of symmetrical upward force flow in linear elastic support. All three control zones are connected.

---

**Training Note**

The Greyhound (Chapter 6) is a classic foundation exercise relevant for both diagonal and linear elastic support. It is a low load exercise in its first stages, which allows an athlete to release an inappropriate suit of armour pattern and make the deeper connections necessary to establish effective elastic support by stretching fully into the hip and shoulder range.

---

Elastic support is also utilised in a spiral motion. Sports such as tennis and golf depend upon *spiral elastic support* to create power through force transmission up through the body and out through the hands, and in football, down and out through the foot when kicking. The athlete must maintain a connection between the control zones, but to access this form of force transfer he must at the same time be able to move the chest and pelvis independently of each other to create spiral tension.

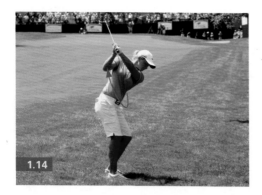
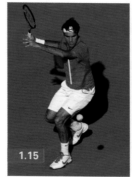
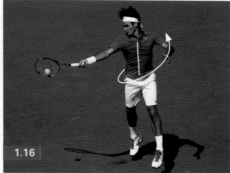

In golf, this creates the so-called 'X Factor', the differential between the shoulder and pelvis angle at the height of the backswing which sets up the spiral elastic support (fig. 1.14). In a different application of the same principle, these tennis photographs depict the coiling of the springs to generate power in the lower control zone by bending at the hips and knees, followed by the transfer of force from the legs as it spirals through the pelvis, up through the central control zone and out through the arm (figs 1.15–1.16).

## Neuromuscular Response Strategy

A discussion of FFM must also include the *neuromuscular response strategy*. This is the body's ability to cope with the unexpected, to be able to respond instantly to an external challenge, to minimise potential body stress, and to regain control and balance. It is a stabilising response that must be instant, adaptable and, above all, not rigid, in order to cope successfully with the unpredictable. We look at some examples of neuromuscular response tasks in Chapter 9.

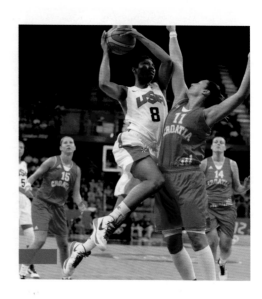

## Training Note

With the rise in popularity of core training has come a corresponding array of biomechanical problems due to a lack of consideration for task-specific training. It is not unusual for a runner, golfer or basketball player to be given high-force trunk strengthening exercises appropriate to the suit of armour strategy. The underpinning idea for this is that increased trunk strength will provide the necessary support and power for performance. However, these athletes consequently lose the functional mobility for efficient sports-specific motion, having trained the zones to maintain a fixed but compressed relationship.

In runners, this is often expressed through lack of hip and shoulder mobility and decreased counter-rotation. In golfers, a diminished X Factor will lead to a decrease in potential power, leading to compensation strategies that manifest as swing technique problems. The basketball player might become strong, but is too slow to activate the necessary neuromuscular protective mechanisms that will save their knees or back from the effects of a poor landing.

Central control zone training may appropriately be made up of a mixture of elements and may have aspects of each different strategy, but ultimately the training you choose for the central control zone should reflect what the body actually needs to do.

## Clipboard Notes

A pentathlete presented with back issues and performance problems. Her trunk conditioning programme comprised many classic variations involving high-force trunk flexion and rotation, but nothing to train her control in a neutral trunk position. They simply focused on general concentric (shortening) strength of her abdominal muscles. Her sports, swimming, running, shooting, fencing and riding, all require excellent control in a neutral (non-flexed) spinal position, often with the trunk muscles at a consistent length and without excessive tension. When her programme was adjusted to include a variety of exercises that addressed body awareness and control of a neutral spine, she made rapid improvements across all of her sports.

As we have now seen, effective force transfer during movement requires that the control zones maintain their connection with each other, even though they may move in relationship to each other. In the later discussion on stability, we will see that any movement of the limbs requires force management from the muscles that connect them to the central skeleton, so the legs are never trained without attention to the trunk, and the arms are never trained without establishing the foundation support from the control zones beneath them.

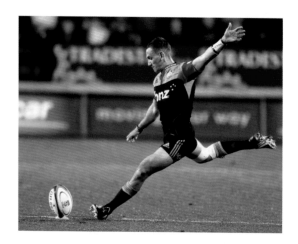

The three control zones in connection while allowing freedom of motion.

## Blocking of Force Transmission

One of the primary errors in the core stability approach is an emphasis on the control zones staying in a fixed relationship in order to maintain connection. While this is relevant for some sports, the idea of keeping the ribs and pelvis the same distance apart at all times interferes with normal biomechanics to a significant degree and is a misapplication of the connection concept. It is perfectly possible, and indeed essential, for the positional relationships between the control zones to change. This is achieved through the mechanism of *lengthening*.

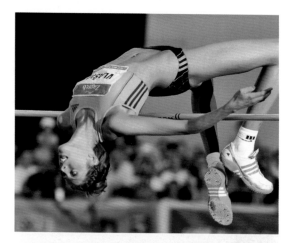

### Key Point

Lengthening is expansion, and expansion is the impulse of poise, self-assurance and positive controlled movement. Inappropriate shortening is the impulse of self-protection and coping, and is frequently seen when control is inadequate or confidence low.

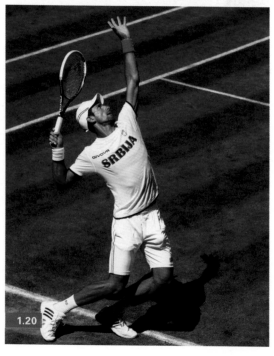

Some of the misunderstanding has arisen from people mistaking lengthening for disconnection. If the person simply lets go of their mid section and buckles into back extension, they create spinal compression instead of trunk lengthening. The impulse is down and in at the back, instead of up and out through the whole trunk.

Figure 1.20 illustrates trunk lengthening all the way from the left hip and through the rib cage to achieve full arm

1.20

elevation. If this athlete was asked to keep his ribs and pelvis at a constant distance, he would be unable to attain his service position and would need to compensate further in his spine. Those athletes who do not lengthen must get their movement from somewhere, and this is frequently produced from excessive spinal extension or side-bending. They are then prescribed more core work to control this, but it is often not specific to the action required.

Common trunk training options include crunches, which involve a strong trunk shortening action, or planks, which train the control zones to maintain a consistent relationship at a relatively high degree of tension. Both may be of value to a tennis player, but he will also need to work on deep control to achieve the connection necessary to allow his body to expand and lengthen into the full range required for optimal technique.

---

### Personal Investigation: The Top Shelf Test

Standing evenly through both feet, imagine that you need to reach a can of beans on the top shelf of your kitchen cupboard. Maintain the distance between your ribs and pelvis by placing your thumb on the bottom of your ribs and the fingers of the same hand on the pelvis and see what happens as you reach up with your other arm. Feels odd doesn't it? It also feels as though you cannot reach that can.

This time reach up naturally. Did you notice that to really reach, your ribs moved away from your pelvis? You are lengthening. It is not dangerous or dysfunctional. It is what is necessary to stretch fully through your arm. It only becomes a problem if you disconnect your control zones.

---

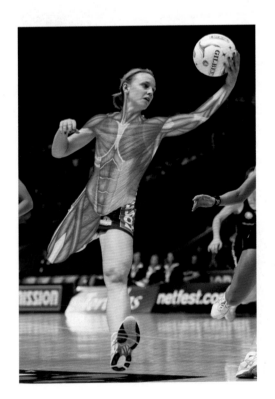

## How can we stay connected, yet achieve lengthening?

The answer lies in our anatomy. Our bodies are made up of an extraordinary network of relationships between muscles linked through a matrix of connective tissue, the fascia. These myofascial relationships span multiple joints and create connections across the zones. If trained appropriately, they allow for the functional expansion needed in many contexts, including overhead sports, gymnastics and dance.

Optimising these myofascial relationships requires the balancing of tensions across the myofascial line of action. This involves the coordination and timing of the muscles, and a number of biomechanical factors which we will consider over the next two chapters.

## Movement Initiation and Force Transmission

Which part of the body first initiates the movement? This will determine whether you can actually access the muscles you have trained.

The source of movement initiation will bias the flow and direction of forces throughout the movement, so it is critical to ensure that it is starting in the right place. Often it is in the very first instant, the intention to move, in which technique is lost.

Sports involving the upper limbs, such as throwing sports, grappling sports and paddle sports often provoke the initiation error of beginning the movement in the arm instead of generating the impulse from the lower and central control zones. Not only does this cause major technical errors, it also amplifies stress on upper body structures and cuts off the possibility of force sharing over a large surface area. Injury and lack of performance go hand in hand.

In cross-country skiers, the double poling technique frequently causes back and shoulder problems if the motion is initiated from the spine and upper body. This causes the skier to use excessive pulling of the body forward through the poles, instead of engaging the powerful lower body to help push it over the snow.

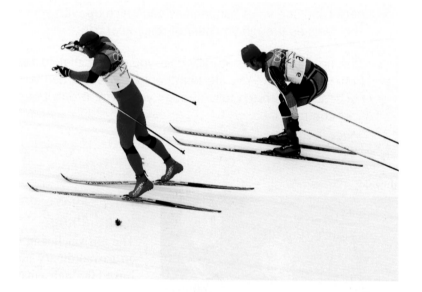

Strong engagement from the feet through to the hips for forward propulsion of the body.

In all of these scenarios, this fractional timing and coordination issue means that no matter how strong or stable the central and lower control zones are, they cannot get involved in time to support the arm, leading to reduced power and increased incidence of shoulder, elbow, wrist and neck problems, not to mention wasted training time.

### Key Point

A timing or sequencing problem can often appear as weakness or poor activation. Strengthening a muscle does not guarantee that it will improve its function during movement. Having the right body part in the right place at the right time allows a muscle to activate appropriately.

Inappropriate preparatory reactions which are triggered by the impulse to move are a closely related phenomenon. The body uses a feedforward mechanism to prepare for movement, which means that muscles necessary for support activate fractionally before the movement actually occurs. Muscles such as transversus abdominis (TrA), which is explored more fully in Chapter 3, have been shown to behave in this way. However, habit, stress and injury can cause inappropriate muscles to act in a preparatory manner.

The easiest way to see this is from a standing start when the athlete is not moving. Watch only the very beginning of the movement. What happened first? Raising the shoulders is a very common preparatory response. This disconnects the upper control zone from the rest of the body, again leaving it vulnerable and inefficient. Another response is a rapid tightening and shortening of the spine, locking it into extension and blocking rotational forces from flowing up and down. This is frequently, although not exclusively, seen in runners.

In athletes with groin pain, it is interesting to observe many who prepare for or initiate movement with rapid, high-force adductor muscle contraction. If this is the case, it is unsurprising that the area becomes vulnerable to breakdown – the body needs a new first response if it is to overcome the overload.

Initiation issues contribute greatly to force management problems, and are addressed through increased sensory awareness, relaxation and timing drills.

## Direction of Movement Impulse

An understanding of the planes of movement (Chapter 2) can help to identify errors in the direction of movement impulse. For example, some children naturally throw a ball effectively, initiating movement from the lower control zone and transferring it up through the body to the hand through rotation; here the transverse plane is used. Others initiate from the arm, which tends to create an ineffective forward-tipping impulse from the body; in this instance, the sagittal plane is used. The site of initiation and the direction of impulse are therefore closely connected.

Athletes and particularly runners are often cued to "stay up". While the intention behind the cue may be appropriate, there are many ways for an athlete to physically interpret it. A common error is tilting the chin upwards and excessively lifting the sternum, which in turn rotates the rib cage upwards at the front, with a consequent locking down at the back into spinal extension. The resulting tension creates the effect of running with the handbrake on. Mechanically this posture disconnects the upper control zone from the lower control zone, blocking spinal rotation and sacrificing technique and power. In terms of the overall movement impulse, the runner looks as though they are fighting through a backward impulse instead of generating a strong, unrestricted forward impulse as they run.

### Key Point

Gain an impression of movement impulse direction when observing movement. Significant changes in performance and muscle action can occur through a well-worded cue to alter the athlete's sensation and understanding of motion direction.

## Chapter Summary

To generate power and minimise stress on body structures, force must be allowed to transmit effectively through the body across large surface areas.

This means that:

- the control zones remain connected but able to move independently against each other.

- the planes used are appropriate.

- the movement is initiated from the right area.

- the direction of movement impulse is correct.

Having considered movement in its most general and global senses, we can start to become more specific about how optimal movement is brought about. Many variables contribute to FFM, and one of these is stability. However, the application of stability principles can either support or interfere with an athlete's FFM, and as such, it is important to understand the factors involved.

# 2 | Exploring the Stability Concept

The concept of stability can mean different things to the athlete, the coach, the sports scientist and the sports medicine professional.

It may be used to describe how the whole body produces movement, directs force, or reacts to load challenges. This can be termed *functional stability*. Simply put, this is *your body's ability to meet the load and control demands of the required task*. It includes the controlled, sequenced relationships between moving body parts, and the planes and proportions in which they move. It also includes your neuromuscular responses and reactions, and overall movement efficiency. For the coach and the athlete, this meaning corresponds closely to sporting *technique*.

"Core stability" has been defined as the capacity for the trunk to support, control and withstand the forces acting upon it, so that the body structures can perform in their "safest, strongest and most efficient positions" [26]. For fitness professionals in many sporting programmes, this is addressed as part of athlete *conditioning*. Links between core stability deficits and increased risk of injury have been identified [73, 136], but it is important to note that core stability contributes to, but cannot fully account for, overall functional stability, which is the result of multiple interrelated factors. This may be why research has found little direct correlation between core stability training and performance enhancement [122], but has found support for programmes which may include core stability principles as part of a broader neuromuscular programme [93, 124, 70, 111].

Core stability is sometimes confused with *core strength*, where these central muscles are trained with high-load exercises to produce and withstand large force demands safely, as would be relevant in the suit of armour (compression) strategy. For some athletes, core strength is extremely important, but for others this type of training will have little positive effect.

A rugby player will need high core strength in order to withstand sudden impacts and the physical pressure of other players, whereas a triathlete will need a continuous but lower level of stabilising muscle activity to support optimal biomechanics for long periods. Core strength builds muscular potential, but core stability is the result of being able to effectively utilise it.

Stability can also refer to the integrity of the joints and the specific muscles that ensure that joint movement is controlled within safe structural limits. For physiotherapists and other sports medicine professionals, this meaning relates to *motor control*.

The term stability can be applied in all of these ways, and they are all important and interrelated in the context of injury prevention as well as performance in sporting movement. To be stable across all of the above categories, you must be firing the right muscles in the right sequence so that your forces are sent in the most efficient direction. This is a *functional motor pattern*, which encompasses timing, proportion and sequencing of muscles in a chain of activation. Your joints are being moved in the appropriate order by the most suitable muscles. You are also able to optimally control the forces acting upon you.

## Pillars of Functional Stability

The functional motor pattern is one of a collection of interdependent characteristics that form the *pillars of functional stability*. These are the fundamental components that must be in place in order to train for optimally efficient movement.

**FUNCTIONAL MOBILITY:** the ability to move through the full necessary range of motion required by the sport under dynamic conditions.

**BALANCE:** the ability to organise the body over its support point quickly and accurately.

**POSTURE:** the neuromusculoskeletal relationships that optimise joint motion and muscular action, trigger automatic stabilising activity, and minimise structural stress on the body.

**OPTIMAL FUNCTIONAL MOTOR PATTERN:** the timing, proportion and sequencing of muscle activation.

**NEUROMUSCULAR RESPONSE AND CONTROL:** the unconscious, automatic activation of joint stabilising muscles to prepare for the impulse to move, or respond to rapid, sudden or unexpected body control challenges or loading [71].

**MOVEMENT SYMMETRY:** the balance of movement and counter-movement around a controlled central axis in the body.

Understanding these concepts can help you to structure your programme in a way that ensures tha the motion and control necessary to move well. They prepare the foundations from which you can effectively develop:

• speed

• power

• strength

• agility

• flexibility

• injury resistance

The entire training programme is therefore influenced by the concept of functional stability.

## Functional Stability in Sport

**In the human body, the term stability describes how effectively a body manages forces.** The body must *produce* force in order to move, and therefore must manage the biomechanical stresses it produces within itself.

A footballer must balance himself perfectly over his stance limb and maintain a firm and supportive hip and trunk in order to strike the ball accurately and powerfully with his other leg. Without this stable foundation, the force generated by the kicking leg affects the positioning of the player's pelvis and spine, causing stress on the groin muscles and on joints of the lower back, as well as decreasing power and accuracy. Similarly, a tennis player with a weak or poorly coordinated trunk will compensate for the loss of this firm supportive foundation when playing a forehand by overusing their shoulder muscles, affecting their timing and movement patterns, losing power and risking injury.

The body must also *withstand* forces imposed by its environment. A good swimmer uses the resistance of the water to generate an effective pull, but without sufficient trunk and shoulder stability that same resistance can force the shoulder into a poor position, leading to biomechanical inefficiency and often shoulder injury. The ground reaction forces pushing up through the foot of a runner as it strikes the ground should help to propel them forward, but without a stable pelvis these forces can instead cause a vertical collapse in joints from the foot to the hip. An ice hockey player must withstand a direct blow from an opponent, and a shot putter must overcome gravity in order to project the shot up and away. All of these external elements exert forces upon the body and will require an athlete to respond and adapt to control them.

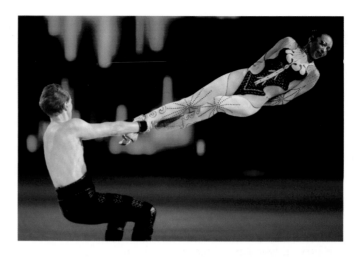

Controlling against external forces. Strong compressive connection between the control zones as the male skater exerts high-force trunk control to manage the long lever of his partner. The female skater maintains an elongated body but must strictly maintain the control zones in a consistent positional relationship.

Stability in this context is the athlete's ability to utilise the body's structures in the safest, most efficient positional relationships for the functional demands imposed upon them.

The key words here are *efficiency* and *safety*. The concept of *efficiency* sits at the heart of sports training. Ideally, an athlete should be able to produce the best result for his or her effort investment. For example, when novice golfers try to drive the ball, they generate a great deal of muscle activity but are unable to consistently focus the forces that they generate into the most effective pattern of movement. The relationship between effort and outcome is skewed towards effort. This is inefficiency. When professionals perform the same activity, their greater skill results in a longer, straighter drive, but the level of muscular activity, or effort investment, is less. They do not use what they do not need. The professional is more efficient.

The same effect can be observed in any sport. Those who truly excel manage to minimise the impression of effort when compared with the result or outcome. They are able to channel their effort into the most effective line of force. They are *efficient*. In simple terms, champions are not people who make difficult things look difficult. They are people who make difficult things look easy.

Functional stability can influence technical performance by increasing biomechanical efficiency. By increasing biomechanical efficiency, we can achieve better results for our effort. In certain circumstances this may influence physiological efficiency, although the precise relationship is yet to be clearly defined [3, 62].

The other key word in our definition is safety. Insufficient stability alters biomechanics, which can lead to injury for a variety of reasons. Athletes in multidirectional sports can sustain acute injuries because they are unable to balance and control their body mass in response to sudden acceleration, deceleration or change of direction [6]. Endurance athletes with biomechanical inefficiency can develop overuse injuries as they try to overcome a performance plateau by training harder and longer to compensate for it. There is a limit to how far determination and training volume can compensate for functional inefficiency without the body breaking down.

Functional stability can reduce injury risk by minimising musculoskeletal stress, managing forces and increasing balance and control.

# How Can Functional Stability Influence Movement?

## Directional Limitation

The principle of movement direction limitation is at the heart of technical training, and functional stability training directly targets this.

To actively move a limb, a muscle must contract, and there must be a secure or stable point for that muscle to pull from if it is to fulfil its function effectively. If it does not have a stable point to pull from, it will lose efficiency, i.e. take more effort to achieve the same outcome.

For example, a force applied to a secure structure (fig. 2.2a) will produce a result that corresponds to the effort, and the skateboard will speed away from the wall. The only direction of movement in the system is away from the wall.

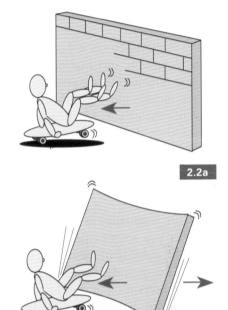

2.2a

If force is applied against a semi-stable surface (fig. 2.2b) the result will not be so positive: the effort is the same but force is lost as the surface gives against the pressure. There are two opposing directions of movement involved. Applying this knowledge, if you wanted to push another person over, you would want to make yourself into a secure structure, so that the force of your push went entirely forward.

2.2b

If you are unbalanced, part of your effort will go forward, but the resistance you encounter in the other person's weight will push you slightly backward. If the stable point is lost, an extra direction of movement is introduced into the system and force is lost. In a contact sport such as ice hockey, this is an important principle to know.

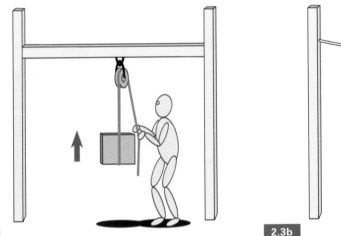

2.3a

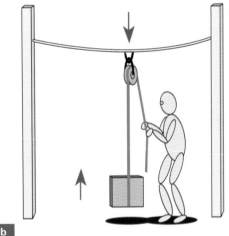

2.3b

Now imagine two pulley systems. The first has a pulley fixed to a horizontal beam (fig. 2.3a). The second has a pulley attached to a firm bungee cord instead of the horizontal beam (fig. 2.3b). Both offer some level of support for the pulley. However, pulling the weight over the fixed beam involves one direction of movement: the weight towards the beam. When pulling against the bungee cord, two directions are involved: the weight towards the bungee and the bungee towards the weight. The bungee cord cannot provide sufficient stability for the force to be efficiently transferred to the weight.

If we apply this understanding to the body, imagine the action of muscle pulling on bone. If the origin of the muscle is secure, or stable, the muscle shortens to pull the bone towards it. The insertion of the muscle moves towards the origin. There is one direction of movement in the system (fig. 2.4a).

If the support point is not secure, it gives under the load of the muscle pulling, just like the bungee cord (fig. 2.4b). Instead of one direction of movement, we now have two: the origin of the muscle moving towards the insertion and the insertion towards the origin. The bone will still move, and the muscle is working just as hard, but the result is a weaker movement. By losing stability, efficiency is lost. There are many people wasting time in gyms because they don't apply this principle to lifting weights.

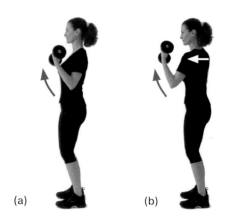

2.4 (a) A secure shoulder bicep curl, and (b) a bicep curl with loss of the shoulder as a fixed point.

A secure foundation is therefore needed to support an efficient muscle contraction. This principle applies whether you are moving your thumb or your whole body. The control of each segment of the body builds upon the stability of the next in the chain, so the hand's stability depends on a stable wrist, elbow, shoulder joint, then shoulder blade, then trunk. The trunk is supporting the entire chain, and is responsible for the greatest proportion of stability. The trunk must in turn be supported by a stable pelvis in order to cope with this demand. If any one of the links in the chain is compromised, an additional and unwanted direction of movement can appear.

In summary, to benefit most from a muscle contraction, you must create a secure point for the muscle to pull from. In a dynamic movement, the secure point may move relative to other body parts, but should not collapse towards the insertion of the contracting muscle.

## Managing the Planes of Movement

Efficient movement maintains motion in the most direct plane for the required task. Some sports, such as Olympic weightlifting and cycling are predominantly uniplanar, i.e. they are most effective when the gross movement is limited to one plane. Multidirectional sports such as tennis and football require control in multiple planes.

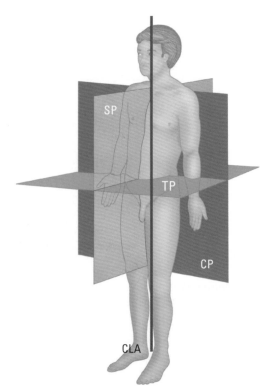

Sagittal plane (SP), transverse plane (TP), coronal plane (CP) and the central longitudinal axis (CLA).

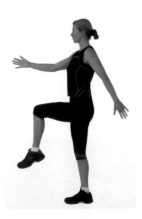

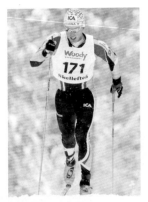

The *sagittal* plane is the forward and backward plane. Running, classic Nordic skiing and cycling represent sagittal limb movement. Allowing the spine to absorb the motion of a horse when sitting to the trot, or performing a series of back flips as a gymnast, demonstrates spinal sagittal motion. The movements of the sagittal plane are flexion (forward motion in the trunk, bending in the limbs) and extension (backward motion in the trunk, straightening in the limbs).

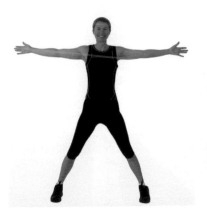

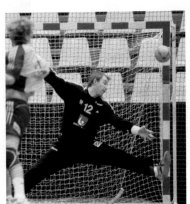

The *coronal* plane is the side movement plane. A gymnast's spine must side-bend to allow his legs to swing over the pommel, and a volleyball player may need to adjust her arms sideways to block a spike effectively. A defensive player in handball may have his arms out from his sides to block a pass, or he may need to change direction sideways quickly, moving his legs apart. The movements of the coronal plane are abduction (moving limbs away from the body), adduction (moving the limbs towards the body) and side-bending (in the spine or pelvis).

The *transverse* plane is the rotational movement plane. The rotation of the pelvis and trunk in a golf swing or a tennis forehand occur within this plane, as does a sprint canoe paddler's stroke or a discus thrower's wind-up.

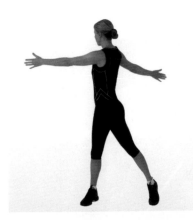

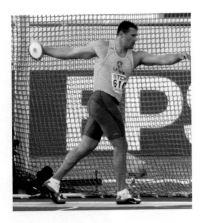

Whether they are mostly sagittal, coronal, rotational or multidirectional, all sports require control of a *central longitudinal axis* (CLA), also referred to as the central axis, to achieve their most efficient movement. In practice, this central axis is not a rigid position: it is the sense of a firm but flexible central reference point that supports movement of the torso and limbs. Imagine a firm, thick metal cable passing vertically through the top of your head and down through the middle of your body. This cable would form an axis for your shoulders, thorax and pelvis to smoothly rotate around, but still enable you to move easily in all directions.

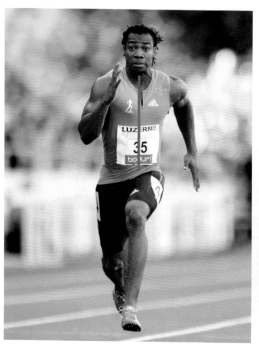 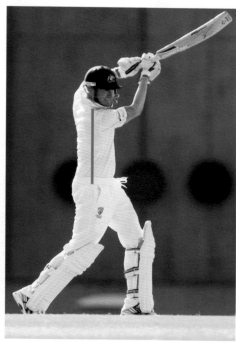

The CLA is not just for movement in vertical positions – it applies at any angle depending upon the activity. It makes it possible for gyroscopic motion in diving, gymnastics and free-style skiing (below), and for balanced, controlled motion in dynamic, multidirectional sports, such as squash.

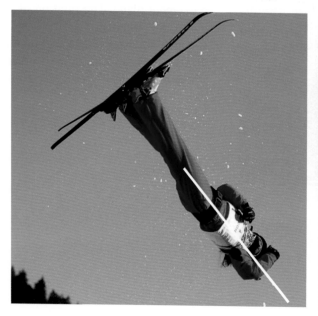 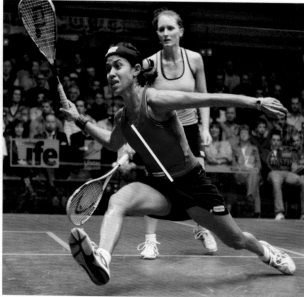

To achieve a stable CLA, the pelvic stabiliser muscles must provide a secure platform to support the trunk, and a deep stabilising muscle system works to support each segment of the spine. If the CLA is not stable, it will buckle under load in a forward, backward or sideways direction, causing postural and movement deviations and control problems.

If the axis buckles in the sagittal plane (figs 2.13, 2.14), the pelvis tilts either forward or backward and the trunk is placed in a position of weakness. If the axis buckles in the coronal plane (fig. 2.15), the pelvis and trunk will tilt sideways, once again placing their supporting musculature in a position of weakness and compressing the joints on one side.

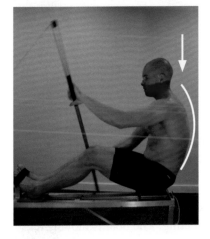

2.13 Collapse of the central axis in the sagittal plane. The slumped posture demonstrates a collapse into spinal flexion. The spine appears bowed. This is a poor position from which to generate rotational force.

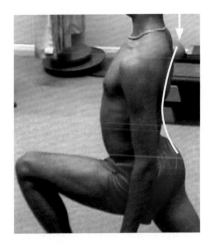

2.14 The arched position of the spine in this lunge demonstrates a collapse into spinal extension.

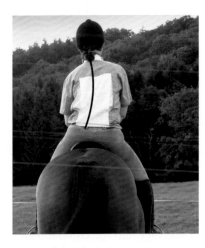

2.15 Collapse of the central axis in the coronal plane. One hip is higher and the spine is buckled sideways, concave on the left.

## Key Point

If the central axis collapses, rotational movement will be restricted due to joint compression on the concave side of the collapse, and soft tissue tension on the convex side. Performing stretches to increase trunk rotation will not transfer effectively to sporting movement unless you work on stabilising your central axis.

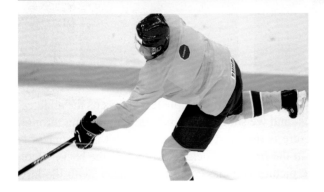

This ice hockey player has a firm central axis, forward tilted but not bent. He then rotates around this axis.

## The CLA and the Sharing of Forces

A secure CLA is often the key factor in force sharing.

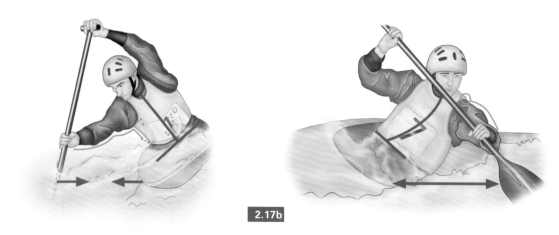

2.17a    2.17b

In fig. 2.17a, the paddler is maintaining a firm CLA, which supports a consistent connected relationship between his upper and lower body. In doing so, he is able to share his forces from the hand all the way up the arm and down the trunk to the pelvis. He is able to move the boat effectively and maintain its connection through his body to the paddle.

In fig. 2.17b, the paddler is losing the inside edge of the boat and the pelvis is drifting sideways. The CLA is collapsing into the coronal plane and the upper and lower body are disconnecting. The boat is moving away from the paddle, and the forces transfer from the hand to the shoulder, but at this point can go no further. The forces amplify in the shoulder, creating a high injury risk over time.

## The CLA and Force Transmission

If the CLA collapses, it can effectively block body integration between the zones and halt force transmission.

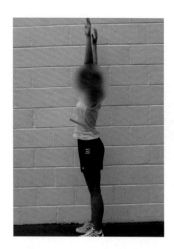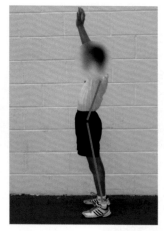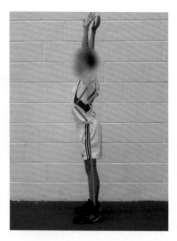

The child athletes above are all performing the Double Arm Raise test. This simple test shows us the athletes' natural strategy for managing the motion of arms on trunk, and we should see a natural lengthening through the body to accompany full shoulder range. The left picture is the most subtle strategy but nevertheless is significant. The athlete is upwardly rotating her rib cage at the front and locking it down at the back, which breaks her connection just above waist level. The centre picture is a classic child's strategy, with the hips sagging forward, breaking the connection at the pelvis. The picture on the right has a double break – one at the hip and again with upward rotation of the rib cage. In each case, the CLA has buckled in the sagittal plane, and the potential for accessing the most effective myofascial connections is lost. Top priority for these children is to establish a sound CLA and be able to move their limbs freely without compromising it.

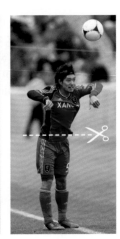

Here, the footballer has locked his lower spine into extension (backward bend), compressing it in the sagittal plane and pulling his hips back. This disconnects his lower and central control zones from his upper control zone, leaving him with only his arms to create force.

## Introducing Unnecessary Planes

Technical errors are often spotted as unwanted movements, but we can be more specific by identifying unwanted planes. The most common occurrences of unwanted planar movement occur when the central axis collapses sideways into the coronal plane. For example, running is primarily a sagittal and transverse plane activity (the legs move in a forward-backward direction while the shoulders and pelvis rotate around the central axis), but athletes can be observed diverting forces into the coronal plane when their feet hit the ground, collapsing at the pelvis so that it tilts sideways on impact, allowing their knee to deviate inwards, rolling their foot and ankle into excessive pronation, or tipping their shoulders from side to side. Forces that should be directed at moving forward are seeping sideways costing the runner here propulsive potential and ultimately speed.

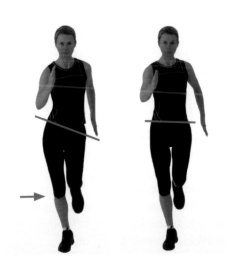

A sprint kayak paddler who does not have sufficient pelvic rotation will divert his movement into the coronal plane, causing the boat to tip from side to side while excessively side-bending in the spine.

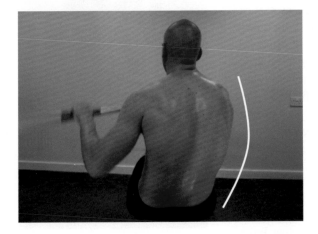
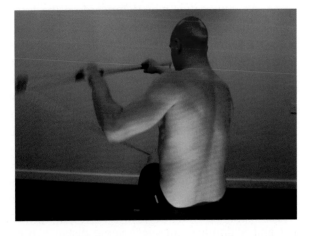

2.21 (a) shows a collapse of the central axis into the coronal plane. Side-to-side movement will be greater than rotational movement; (b) demonstrates a firmer central axis, with rotation as the primary motion.

A golfer with poor rotational mobility or inadequate trunk and pelvic control will try to gain swing motion by shifting their weight sideways into the coronal plane as they take their club head back.

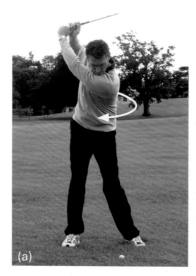
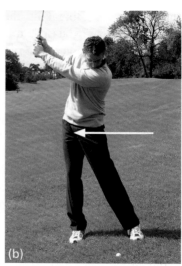

2.22 (a) shows the golfer rotating his pelvis and shoulders. In (b), he fails to rotate adequately. He must find another plane to move in, and so shifts his hips sideways into the coronal plane.

The planar concept of motion occurs at two levels: local (individual joint motion) and global (total direction of motion). We will be working mainly with the global concept within this book; however it is useful to be aware that small joint movements contribute to the efficiency of global movements.

## Rotating Through the Kinetic Chain

The *kinetic chain* is the series of joint relationships that make up a movement. From a global perspective, walking and running are largely sagittal movements, with the arms and legs moving in a forward and backward direction for a total movement direction objective of forward motion. However, if we take a more mechanical perspective, walking and running are in fact rotational activities. As you take weight onto one leg, the bones of your ankles, shins and thighs rotate to lock the joints in order to support weight, and then unlock as the leg swings through for another step. There is therefore a continuous alternating locking and unlocking action going on.

There is also a continuous rotation/counter-rotation action occurring. As you step forward with your left foot, your pelvis on the left also moves forward. In doing this, your pelvis is effectively rotating to the right relative to your shoulders. This motion drives rotation of the spine. As your pelvis moves forward on the left, your chest moves forward on the right, bringing your right shoulder forward. Your spine is *counter-rotating* so that the shoulders and pelvis move in opposite directions. This natural motion allows us to use the impulse created when our feet strike the ground to propel us forward, driving smooth, efficient gait [23]. It is so critical to walking and running efficiency that is has been called the *spinal engine* [34]. Degree and speed of pelvic and shoulder rotation are among the factors that have been linked to running economy [3].

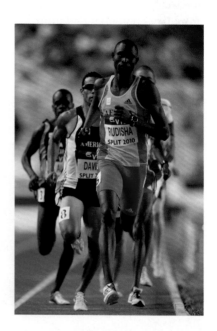

The CLA in action: Note the relaxed rotation through the torso.

This counter-rotation action also dissipates the load on your spine as your foot strikes the ground. In doing so, it can reduce joint stress. From a mechanical perspective, it also changes the demands on the leg and abdominal muscles. Some distance running coaches have misunderstood the core stability concept and train their runners to keep their pelvis and shoulders parallel and facing forward as they run. In doing so, they increase load on the propulsive leg muscles, decrease stride length and compromise shock absorption in the athlete's joints.

Without counter-rotation of the pelvis and shoulders (or more accurately, the thorax) in both directions, your body will find another plane in which to move. This is most commonly the coronal plane. Instead of the shoulders and hips looking relatively level and the head position reasonably consistent, they appear to tip or rock from side to side in response to leg movement. From a global perspective, instead of energy being directed forward, it is being dissipated sideways.

Athletes with rotational restrictions can complain of movement limitations that don't immediately seem to be related. Runners with a stride length difference will often present complaining of a short hamstring on one side, when in fact the difference is caused by an asymmetry in pelvic rotation. If the pelvis does not advance as the foot swings through, the foot will fall short. The hamstring is simply the site where the compensation is perceived.

A runner may alternatively complain that one shoulder is stiff or that the arm does not swing freely, yet no mobility restriction can be found in the shoulder. When observed carefully, their movement indicates an asymmetry in rotation of the thorax (upper body). If the athlete's upper body is blocked from rotating in one direction, their perception is that their arm swing is uneven. If they further compensate for lack of rotation by collapsing into side bending on that side, they will drop the elbow and restrict its excursion back and forth, despite the availability of shoulder motion.

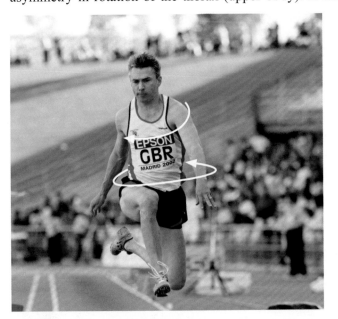

Becoming more aware of your natural rotational movement can improve your symmetry, but specific movements can also help to pinpoint specific areas of decreased rotation. Rotational exercises for the foot and lower leg, hip, pelvis, thorax and trunk are included in Chapters 4, 6, 7 and 9.

2.24 Counter body rotation for effective propulsion. Note the degree of trunk rotation around the CLA.

## Key Principle: Forces Always Need to Go Somewhere

1. If there is insufficient mobility available in a certain plane, the body may need to accommodate forces in another plane. You need sufficient *movement* in all involved joints to perform your technique effectively.

2. If your body does not have sufficient stability in a certain plane, it can divert forces to another plane. This appears as unwanted motion. You need sufficient *control* of all involved joints.

## Personal Investigation

Which is your predominant walking plane? We often don't notice how we walk, but we are aware that some people are more efficient walkers than others. Some people can walk quickly with little effort, but some of us tire after a short period of walking faster than usual.

### Observation exercise

Start by walking normally. Look at yourself as you walk towards a mirror: does your head stay balanced in the centre of your movement or does it move from side to side? Look at your shoulders: do they stay level or do they tip from side to side? They may only tip to one side. Is your stride length the same on both sides?

### Awareness exercise

Start by walking normally. If there is visible side-to-side movement, your global objective of forward (sagittal) motion is being compromised by diverting movement into the coronal plane. Your effort is not going in the direction you want it to! This is usually caused by decreased rotation of the pelvis and shoulders, which you can investigate as follows.

Place your hands on your pelvis and note that as your foot moves forward so does the pelvis on that side. Does your pelvis move forward the same distance on both sides? Take some time to examine this, especially if running is part of your sport.

Allow your arms to swing freely now, and notice that your shoulders move forward and backward as you walk. If you imagine a line across your chest from shoulder to shoulder, you will notice that it is not just your shoulders but your whole chest and rib complex rotating from left to right. Do you rotate the same distance in both directions?

Did you notice that as your pelvis rotates forward on one side, the shoulder moves forward on the opposite side? This is called *counter body rotation*, and it is the driving force for efficient walking and running.

If you have found a difference between the sides, can you invite it to become more even just through awareness? Rather than forcing one side to move more, think about relaxing to *allow it* to move more. As your pelvic rotation becomes more even, does your stride length change?

## Training Note

To improve your connection and mobility in rotation, try Thigh Slides, Knee Creepers and Counter Body Rotation in Chapter 6.

## Collapse Within the Same Plane

Functional stability problems can also appear as collapse within the same plane. This occurs most commonly when the CLA collapses into the sagittal plane.

A footballer throwing in from the sideline can collapse within the sagittal plane by taking his trunk into an excessive backward bend as he moves the ball over his head, losing control of his lower back and decreasing the power of his throw. A volleyball player landing from a jump may fail to absorb the landing force through her hips and knees, causing her lower back to buckle under the impact. A cross-country skier may not have sufficient stability to maintain a consistent trunk position against the strong movement of his arms as he pulls through with them, and this shows up as a wave-like up and down motion in the spine.

In the lower body, collapse within the same plane leads to longer foot contact times on the ground and decreased power. Endurance runners or sprinters who appear to sit down on foot strike, or jumpers who drop their hips too far on take-off, will find their performance reduced if this happens.

Imagine your legs are filled with pressurised air. You will bounce off the ground each time your foot hits it. However, if a small puncture appears, air starts to escape and your leg starts to buckle on impact with the ground. It may buckle in the same plane, or it may buckle sideways. The more it buckles, the more effort it is to push off again. In your legs, your muscles work in partnership to provide the same support as the imaginary air. If the muscles supporting your joints react too slowly, or are in fact the wrong ones for the job, they will permit too much bending in response to load, increasing foot contact times. The most likely area to have a "puncture" is the pelvis and hip.

---

**Personal Investigation**

For most sports, there is a predominant plane and possibly a number of plane variations in the limbs at different times. In your sport, which are the main planes of movement? They could be forward-backward (sagittal), side (coronal) or rotational (transverse) movements. For many sports, a number of planes will be used.

To work out the planes used in a movement, first identify a start position for the trunk and legs. From that point, work out which direction the legs will move, which way the pelvis will move, and which way the trunk will move.

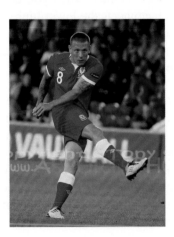

Example: To kick a football, an axis is formed from the stance foot up through the trunk. Once this axis is secure, the trunk movement is largely rotational, with the pelvis and shoulders rotating in opposite directions.

**Relevant exercise:** Rotational Leg Swing (Chapter 6).

In freestyle swimming, the whole body should rotate cleanly around the central axis so that the positional relationship between the chest and the pelvis will not markedly change. The major rotation does not occur within the body itself. The motion of the kick is primarily sagittal. The arm motion combines all three planes.

**Relevant exercise:** Over the Top (Chapter 7) develops a strong axis for the body to rotate around.

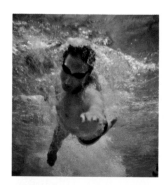

In skiing, the hips and knees must absorb landings in the sagittal plane, but the trunk and pelvis use rotation and side-bending on turns.

**Relevant exercise**: Medicine Ball Square Rotation (Chapter 7) emphasises lower body alignment against upper body movement.

Think of something about your technique that you would like to improve. Is there a plane that you are not controlling? Are you dropping into a less effective plane?

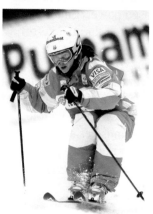

## Securing Your Limbs

Your arms and legs do not attach directly to your trunk. Instead, they attach to bony girdles, and it is through these that forces transfer between limbs and trunk. For forces to transfer between the limbs and the trunk, they must pass through the shoulder girdle or pelvic girdle.

The only bony attachment securing the shoulder girdle, and therefore the arm to the spine, is where your clavicle (collarbone) attaches to your sternum (breastbone). This is a tiny attachment when you consider the loads that we expect our arms to bear. Similarly, the pelvic girdle, which connects the lower limbs to the trunk, only has bony attachments between the fifth lumbar vertebra and the sacrum. Once again, considering the forces that we expect the legs to produce, this is a very small area. Clearly, bony attachments alone cannot secure the limbs. There must be a high degree of muscular support to enable us to function.

For the most effective support, the forces from the limbs are ideally transferred through the girdles to the trunk over *large* surface areas via multiple myofascial attachments to the central skeleton. The broad structure and interconnections of the stabilising muscles make them perfectly suited to the job. However, when structure or function are compromised, alternative patterns are used to secure the arms and legs. Unfortunately these emphasise muscles that are not suited to stabilising and controlling joints. They may transfer the forces to small surface areas, which focuses loads on body tissues that are not designed to tolerate them repeatedly or for extended periods of time. Their action may also pull their attachment points towards each other, changing the body's posture and compromising breathing patterns and muscular lines of pull.

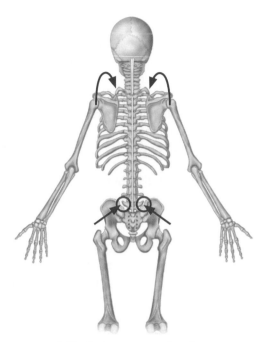

2.28 Skeleton, posterior view.

The shoulder girdle comprises the scapulae (shoulder blades) and the clavicles (collarbones) (see page 89). The shoulder girdle's only direct bony attachment to the axial (central) skeleton is at the sternoclavicular joint.

The pelvic girdle is made up of the triangular shaped sacrum at the bottom of the spine, with an innominate either side. The pelvic girdle's only bony attachment to the lumbar spine is at the two intervertebral joints between the fifth lumbar vertebra and the sacrum. Note the size of these attachment points, and then consider the size of the muscles acting on the girdles and the forces that athletes need to transfer through these girdles to the trunk. A considerable muscular network will be necessary to secure and support the pelvis and the shoulders.

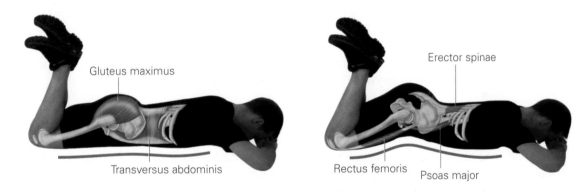

2.29 Prone hamstring curl. (a) When the broad, corset-like deep abdominal muscles work in partnership with the large gluteal muscles, the pelvis is stabilised by spreading the force across a large surface area of the trunk. (b) When the hip flexors and back extensor muscles are used to stabilise the pelvis, it is held in place with relatively narrow muscles that attach directly to the spine, and the force is focused on a smaller, more vulnerable area.

*Stability* achieves secure attachments for muscles to contract against, eliminates unnecessary movements so that force is focused in the most effective direction, and activates muscles that are physiologically designed to work at low cost for long periods. In doing these things, it can influence speed, power, strength, flexibility and agility. *Functional stability* combines stability concepts with functional mobility, balance, posture and symmetry to provide movement control relevant to the requirements of an individual sport.

Stability must not be achieved at the expense of force transmission. A very strong core that does not allow independent rotational motion of the thorax, for example, would be performance diminishing, not performance enhancing, in many sports. It would however enhance performance in a sport like hammer throw, where the body must maintain a highly consistent relationship between the central and lower control zones.

# Optimal Performance Vs. High-Level Compensation

*"The human being has a particularly deep attachment to his movement habits since he created them himself"* (Alon, R. 1996).

Every athlete has a movement objective. Whether it is to move faster, jump higher, or lift a heavier weight in training, they will try to find a way to meet that objective. If an athlete has a deficit in strength, flexibility, coordination, balance, stability or perception, they will unconsciously try to find a way to achieve their movement objective, even if their method is not biomechanically ideal. This is known as *compensation*.

Compensation will cause deviation from a technical ideal, and can be dramatically obvious or very subtle. Even high-performance athletes compensate, and it is challenging for the coach to evaluate the root cause of the compensation and formulate a strategy to overcome it.

The problem with compensation is that while it initially appears to allow the athlete to perform a certain task, it rarely yields optimally efficient performance over time. This is seen even in high-performance athletes. Many athletic performance plateaus are associated with compensatory movement strategies that cannot support further development. The athlete may have demonstrated great potential or even achieved success at an early stage, but a loss of form or persistent barrier to improvement is eventually reached if the compensatory strategies are not addressed.

Compensation can alter the stress ratios on different body structures. This can lead to overuse injuries, such as tendonitis, or even contribute to traumatic injuries where the athlete has been unable to control the forces that are acting on his or her body.

An athlete can cope quite successfully by compensating as long as their ability to compensate always meets or exceeds the degree or duration of physical loading upon their body.

## Ability to compensate > physical/functional loading ➡ trainable system is intact

If the functional loading on the body exceeds its ability to compensate, injury can occur. Increasing the training load, setting new goals, or trying to find that extra tiny percentage when it counts in a competition, can be just enough to overload the system.

## Physical/functional load > ability to compensate ➡ trainable system is impaired (injury/plateau)

Being injury-free in the present doesn't guarantee that all is well for the future. Sometimes it seems that the body is coping well, but after years of unbalanced forces, a body structure breaks down and resists healing. Basic testing as outlined in Chapter 5 can help to identify the control problem that led to the breakdown. If the issue is not addressed, the injury tends to recur or persist.

Compensation alters the movement pattern of the athlete away from the ideal movement strategy for his or her structure and sport. Compensation for a physical shortcoming causes a movement *dysfunction*. A movement dysfunction is an inefficient strategy to meet a physical demand. *In coaching language, a movement dysfunction is synonymous with poor technique.*

Sometimes compensation is confused with personal style. We all have different physical characteristics, and this can produce variations in the overall appearance of a movement. Many athletes with highly distinctive movement are successful, as they use the movement strategies that best suit their physical make-up. Despite this, the successful athlete who is relatively injury resistant will demonstrate fundamentally sound movement and control strategies, which are consistent with normal biomechanics, joint control and muscular patterning.

Differentiating personal style from compensation is not easy when looking at the athlete performing their sport. Isolating and examining the elements of control can help to make that distinction. The testing section in Chapter 5 focuses on the fundamental building blocks of control that support efficient movement. These should be consistent from athlete to athlete. There is no personal style involved.

## Clipboard Notes

An elite male triathlete returned from an international championship with a right quadriceps injury which was failing to heal. When examined, he displayed exceptionally poor trunk and pelvic control, poor balance and fixing patterns of excessive muscular activity from his feet to his neck during all movements. On the treadmill, he ran with his trunk tipped to one side, and when asked to perform a simple Standing or Seated Knee Lift, he used so much extra trunk muscle activity to stabilise himself that he could not inflate his lungs fully. Technically he had made few improvements over the previous years, but had nevertheless enjoyed success at national level.

The athlete was overusing his right quadriceps as part of a compensation pattern for poor stability and balance. He used them even in movements where the quadriceps would not normally play a major role. The muscle could not heal as it was being constantly overused. The stability and balance deficits also prevented him from improving his running technique.

This athlete needed to:

1. Secure his central longitudinal axis in order to maintain symmetry and decrease uneven loading.

2. Integrate better trunk and pelvic stability into his movement.

3. Re-establish normal breathing mechanics.

4. Re-establish normal balance reactions.

The athlete was given remedial exercises to address the problems, but needed to start at extremely low levels in order to activate the correct neuromuscular patterns. This is common in elite athletes who have repeated their existing movement patterns many thousands of times.

Gradually the athlete was able to progress, and detected a difference in his running technique. A session on transference of the new principles and patterns to cycling demonstrated that with correct patterning, his power output could be maintained with less effort. The athlete also achieved greater speeds at lower heart rates than he had previously, demonstrating an interesting relationship between his physiology and his biomechanics.

Stability is often implicated when movement dysfunctions appear, but stability problems can be the result of other movement-altering issues, not just the cause.

# What Can Cause Movement Dysfunction?

## Primary Loss of Stability

Stability can be divided into structural and functional categories. *Structural instability* occurs when a body structure fails, usually as a result of direct trauma. Anterior cruciate ligament ruptures of the knee and lateral ligament ruptures at the ankle are common injuries. In the presence of structural instability, control of the injured joint itself is affected, but balance, stability, muscle patterning and whole-body control are also usually altered. Even with surgery, a functional stability programme will have an important role to play in the athlete's rehabilitation.

In the case of *functional instability,* the structures are sound but the athlete is unable to consistently control and produce forces without compensating. Functional stability training will incorporate balance, proprioception, muscle patterning and control to address this type of problem. Any athlete who is repeatedly injured should be screened for functional instability to identify control problems affecting the area of injury. Control problems are rarely confined to one body area, so whole-body movements should be examined.

## Poor Postural Awareness

Stability can help maintain an efficient posture but, paradoxically, poor posture can make it hard to activate postural stabilisers. Some athletes do not understand what an efficient postural position feels like, as it does not come naturally to them. There may be several reasons for an athlete to adopt a less than ideal posture:

1. They may not have the flexibility to achieve the best position. For example, a young sprint kayak paddler whose tight hamstrings pull his back into a slumped position.

2. They may not have the right muscles activating to maintain their posture. For example, a swimmer who has trained her abdominals with trunk curls but has not trained the abdominal muscles that maintain a secure posture in the water when the trunk is straight.

3. They may have insufficient body awareness. Even when corrected, they cannot feel when they change their position and return to their normal posture.

If an athlete cannot change their posture while actually performing their sport, they need to be trained in less complex ways first. It may be that they need to practice postural awareness in simple tasks such as those provided in Chapter 6, or that joint mobility and control need to be restored to make it possible to change posture when the body is moving. The tests in Chapter 5 should help to identify these issues. Reinforcing postural principles in all aspects of training, including flexibility, strength and conditioning, will help to develop postural awareness.

## Loss of Range of Motion

If range of motion (ROM) is restricted, whether because of joint stiffness, muscle tightness or motor patterning, it is likely that the body will have to compensate to fulfil performance objectives.

For example, a common response to restricted shoulder flexion is excessive extension of the lumbar spine, which gives the false impression that the limb is achieving adequate range. If not corrected, this movement dysfunction will be very difficult to dislodge as it becomes integrated into the nervous system of the athlete. This particular pattern is often associated with lower back pain in sports that require good shoulder flexibility. Trunk stability training will not relieve lower back pain in this athlete, nor will it improve their form unless it is combined with techniques to restore normal shoulder joint motion.

This compensation pattern can be seen in many young swimmers and gymnasts as they perform their warm-up and stretches, and if the coach is not attentive to form, the pattern will persist. Coaches in charge of young athletes should be aware that loss of specific flexibility can occur during growth spurts, and this ROM can be very difficult to recover.

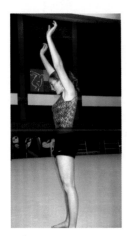

The concept of *relative flexibility* explains this phenomenon [101]. For most of us, some structures in our bodies have more give than others, that is, they are more flexible. This is not always a good thing – structures that tend to move more readily become vulnerable to increased strain and eventual injury, especially when their contribution is not part of the normal movement pattern for the activity.

The gymnast here is demonstrating poor shoulder mobility with her lumbar spine in a neutral position. In her sport, she must be able to hold another gymnast over her head. To do this, the load must be supported directly over her body. Due to her poor shoulder mobility, the only way that she can bring her arms directly over her head is to arch her spine into a deep extension curve. This can result in spinal stress fractures, as it did with this athlete. Stability training will only prevent further injury if the shoulder mobility is restored.

## Training Tip

Exercises which combine shoulder mobility with trunk control are ideal for training a healthy movement pattern. The Floor Press in Chapter 6 should be a staple exercise in young athletes.

## Key Principle

For the movement to be functional it must first be available.

## Functional Rigidity

If an athlete's joints move normally when tested passively, but they don't use that available motion as part of their technique, it may be that they are displaying *functional rigidity*. This often develops as an athlete tries to cope with a higher balance or stability challenge than they can adequately control. Instead of using functional stability, which allows them to move fluently while still in control, the athlete creates a false stability by increasing their general muscle activity to partially immobilise a series of joints. This locks body parts into place but doesn't allow the athlete to move freely and subtly.

This will be a big disadvantage in sports where swift reactions and fine adjustments are necessary, such as in alpine skiing or equestrian events. In sports that require larger movements of the limbs such as tennis, it will cause difficulties in movement sequencing, changes in joint alignment or loss of balance. If the situation is allowed to continue, the athlete loses body awareness in the area, making technical improvement extremely difficult.

## Clipboard Notes

A junior alpine skiing squad was functionally assessed to establish whether there were links between technical problems on the slopes and their physical characteristics. In all of the skiers who had difficulty making right turns, functional rigidity of the left foot was found, along with left pelvic stability problems and decreased ability to actively change the pressure under the sole of the left foot with subtlety.

The body depends upon accurate information coming from the foot in order to know how to balance itself. A rigid foot cannot feed back accurately, as it is effectively immobilised. In order to cope on the slopes without having good-quality information coming from the foot, the skiers were using a compensatory but inefficient technique to keep their balance and control. They made their leg more rigid and did not transfer their weight effectively.

In this situation, the first priority is to establish the athlete's ability to create and detect small pressure changes. Restoration of awareness in the area is a part of this process. Stability activities which link the foot to the hip and activate the pelvic stabilisers in response to weight transference can then be added in combination with balance training. Finally, sports-specific warm-up drills involving foot pressure changes and weight transference are performed on skis prior to hitting the slopes.

## Personal Investigation

Stand on both feet and feel the surface of the floor under your soles. Shift your weight onto one leg: has the muscle tension in the foot you are standing on changed? Now close your eyes while standing on that foot, and to challenge yourself even more, move your arms in any direction.

Do you feel the tension in your foot increase as the balance challenge increases? Some people increase it so much that the foot becomes completely rigid, which means that it is not in such good contact with the floor. When this happens, the foot cannot transmit accurate information to you to help you to balance. It also increases tension elsewhere in the body, which can restrict mobility.

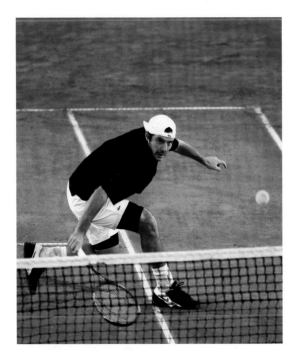

## Ineffective Momentum Control Strategies

Speed is sometimes developed without attention to whether the athlete can control their own momentum. If the athlete can't control momentum, their change of direction will be clumsy and slow, or they will be poorly balanced to perform an action.

Depending upon the sport, forward, backward, sideways or rotational momentum may need to be controlled. A tennis player may be very quick to accelerate to a drop shot over the net, but will need to control his forward momentum to set up the shot. A footballer may be quick off his right foot to move left, but when he tries to move right off his left foot, his trunk momentarily continues to tip away from the new direction of movement, slowing him down. A basketball player may receive a ball in the air and turn his body to land facing a different direction, but injures his knee as he fails to control his rotation.

## Poor Balance

Poor balance is surprisingly common, even in elite athletes and dancers, and has been linked to injury risk [133]. Balance requires an interplay between sensory information from your vision, your sensitive inner ear structures and feedback from your body. Over-dependence upon vision is common, but if this is the athlete's primary balance mechanism, the quality of sensory feedback from the body is often found to be lacking.

Testing an athlete's responses with their eyes closed is sometimes thought to be non-functional as the athlete would not have them closed when competing. This is overly simplistic. In examples such as an unexpected change in terrain while cross-country running, difficult lighting or vision-obscuring costuming for a dancer, a team or ball sport that demands head and eye movement to track play, or any multidirectional sport needing sudden responses and reactions, vision is not enough to maintain dynamic balance. Speedy automatic communication from the body is required to maintain equilibrium, and closing the eyes forces the body to access these feedback systems.

Routine functional testing of international sprinters, badminton players, golfers and contemporary dancers, frequently reveals that many of them cannot carry out simple balance tasks. Many of these athletes were unable to complete even simple tests with their eyes distracted. To compensate, they increased the muscle tension in their body, which decreased their mobility and affected their technique.

Balance is not only a problem in standing. In dressage riders and kayak paddlers, significant differences in balance between left and right sides when standing have been noted to correlate with technical problems when seated. The simple sensory communication test (SSCT) in Chapter 5 highlights the willingness of the body to orientate itself over each side in balance. If the body is unwilling to orientate itself over one side, or exhibits a range of compensatory strategies when weightbearing on that side, these habits are usually evident in sitting as well. Although superficially a standing test does not seem functional for a seated sport, it turns out that it is exceptionally relevant when considering the neurological processes involved. This is therefore an appropriate test of the athlete's function.

## Fatigue

Even sound movement patterns can be eroded in the presence of fatigue. Athletes may test very well on functional movement screening, yet continue to struggle in training or competition because they do not have sufficient endurance to maintain their motor control.

This effect on functional control may be caused by both local muscular fatigue and global physiological fatigue. Studies have shown that bursts of high-intensity global exercise can negatively influence knee kinematics [16, 40, 99].

### Clipboard Notes

A professional footballer presented to the clinic with a lower limb problem that tended to present towards the end of a game. His performance was sound during standard functional control testing, however bearing in mind his history of late onset of symptoms, he was then asked to perform a burst of intense global body movement to induce a fatigue effect. His post-fatigue testing revealed consistent weight transference and coordination problems on one side which had not been evident on initial testing.

### Clinical Tip

If an athlete's problem is most evident towards the end of an event, consider fatigue as a factor. You may need to pre-fatigue them to provoke their movement issues when testing.

## Lack of Coordination and Movement Patterning

The sequencing of movement may cause a movement dysfunction. This can be seen in any dynamic sport, but very obvious examples can be found in sports such as tennis, hammer throwing, judo or golf, where coordination and timing of pelvic and shoulder rotational movement is critical for force production.

Perception is linked to patterning problems. In all of these sports, the athlete may perceive that the most important element is the arm movement. They therefore focus on this body part and it is moved earlier in the sequence than it should be, closing down the real source of power generation which is in the pelvis and trunk.

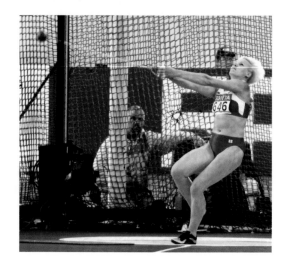

Champion hammer thrower demonstrating sound trunk and pelvic alignment. Her power is produced with rapid, whole-body rotation, and the arms are used only as the end of the movement chain.

## Timing Problems

Sometimes poor stability is associated with timing problems or slow reaction times. If this is the case, stability training needs to be done in conjunction with technical modification. Here, two netball players demonstrate jumps. Their sport requires that they must catch overhead, be able to turn in the air and pass the ball before landing. In (a) the player is taking off too late, and is therefore having to catch the ball behind her head, causing a weak spinal position. In (b) the player has good timing and takes off earlier, allowing her to achieve a stronger spinal position.

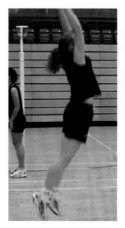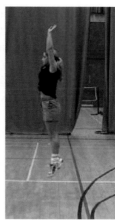

Two netball players demonstrate jumps; (a) the player is taking off too late, (b) the player has good timing and takes off earlier.

## Not Understanding the Movement Required

This is a communication issue between the coach and the athlete. It is not unusual for the athlete to be instructed to perform a movement or skill in a certain way, but the cue that makes sense to the coach may mean something different to the athlete. The athlete therefore performs the action as best they can, but may choose movement strategies that resemble, but do not replicate, the action. This is often seen when athletes are trying to learn weightlifting. The neuromuscular pattern may not be working effectively due to a misunderstanding regarding body position and muscle action.

### Clipboard Notes

A power lifter injured his back while attempting a deadlift. When questioned on what he thought the movement should be, he said he had been told to strongly push his hips forward as he lifted. He therefore tried to quickly thrust his pelvis forward and throw his shoulders backward, overloading the spinal structures.

Once the athlete understood the role of the gluteal muscles in straightening his hips, he was able to access them along with his deep spinal stabilisers as part of the movement. His lifting action changed from a forward thrust of the pelvis under the spine (forward impulse) to a strong hip extension movement (upward impulse). Both techniques straightened the hip, but the new technique increased the action of the powerful gluteal muscles and decreased the pressure on the small spinal structures. The athlete began lifting safely and powerfully, moving past his performance plateau and regularly improving his personal bests.

## Inappropriate Training Design

Injuries and performance plateaus may arise from training practices that are unsuitable for the capabilities of the athlete. There are many training programmes devised, based on an idea of what the athlete should be able to achieve rather than what they actually can achieve under control. When this disparity occurs, the athlete must compensate to manage the training demands, and this leads to tissue breakdown or failure to progress. Monitoring how an athlete performs a task rather than just whether he or she completes it will help to prevent errors like this.

### Clipboard Notes

A high-jumper was experiencing performance deterioration, and although her coach had worked out a periodised programme based on her competition schedule, nothing seemed to be working. Observation of the athlete performing bounding drills explained the problem. This athlete demonstrated poor pelvic stability even in static drills. The overload of bounding was causing a collapse of her joints and was switching off the very muscles that she was trying to train.

The problem was easily overcome. The high-jumper's programme was modified so that power work was initially done off both legs while her pelvic stability developed adequately to cope with single leg work. The correct muscle pathways were activated so that she could start to absorb and produce forces more effectively. The performance plateau was overcome by focusing on the quality of the athlete's movement, and this was achieved by initially reducing the level of training difficulty instead of increasing it.

## Stress

Stress is an emotional and psychological response which can immediately be reflected in the body. Stress-induced changes in muscle activation can appear as extremely subtle movement dysfunction, and it may take a highly skilled evaluation to detect it. Stress may compromise shock absorption, available range of motion, movement patterning and fluency, and under the demand of high-level training and competition, can lead to pain and compromised performance. The diaphragm is a key part of the trunk stability mechanism [47], so stress-induced changes in breathing pattern can influence trunk stability.

An athlete can tighten up under pressure, or unconsciously guard their movement as a result of a past injury. They might feel insufficiently physically prepared, or over-think their technique, knowing exactly what should be happening (as though in a textbook) but lacking the insight to tell if it is actually happening in their own body. Stability may appear to be the primary problem, and indirectly it may be. However, if stress is the trigger mechanism for the breakdown in the movement pattern, remedial stability work must be combined with management of environmental factors, stress management techniques and establishing awareness in the athlete of the link between their tension and their movement.

## Towards a Model of Movement Efficacy

Stability, then, is only one of many elements contributing to an athlete's overall movement efficacy, and stability itself is dependent upon many factors. Sometimes the body must sacrifice stability to overcome some other barrier to function. The reason for movement testing is to ensure that we address the cause and not just the outcome of this compensation.

The model below is by no means exhaustive; however, it illustrates some of the interrelated factors that can be involved in effective movement. The inner circle represents the key seed factors within the individual. The outer boxes are examples of how these must interact with the function itself. Each factor can influence any other on the diagram, and any of them can be used to affect or improve another.

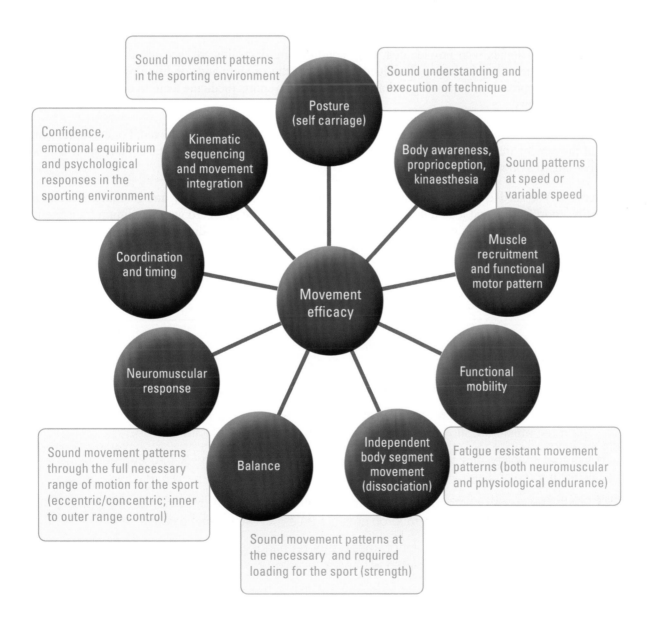

## Movement Efficacy Principles in the Training Programme

For body control and movement efficacy training to have an impact upon athletic performance, several steps should be implemented. An assessment of functional body movement will establish a baseline from which to work. By doing this, you can identify specific weaknesses and structure a programme to accurately target problems. This is more effective than performing general core exercises that might miss the main issues. (Assessment methods are described in Chapter 5.)

Relate the test findings to technique. Test findings usually relate to technical problems, and this establishes the relevance of the stability training. What needs to improve? It could be any number of things, including body alignment and dynamic posture, foot contact times, ability to turn quickly, ability to resist an opponent, coordination of the upper and lower body, or the ability to be balanced but mobile.

If you or the athlete you are working with has a technical problem, ask yourself what they would need to make improvement possible. Examples of this could be better leg alignment, more body rotation, improved weight transference, a more strongly connected arm, greater hip strength or improved flexibility.

Involve any professionals who provide coaching, conditioning or healthcare, because the findings will be relevant to all of them. The findings will influence design of the strength and conditioning programme, give the coach a new approach to improving technique, and help the sports medicine team to understand possible mechanisms of injury.

Relate the demands of the sport to the level of stability training that needs to be achieved. For example, which planes of movement are involved, what are the speed and endurance demands, is it a contact sport and is it an open or closed skill sport?

Be systematic. You need to activate the correct muscle groups to gain basic stability, and gradually increase the complexity, coordination and load until you meet the demands of the sport. To gain maximum transference, the same principles should be emphasised in all aspects of training, including the warm-up, strength and agility training, sports-specific drills and the sports movement itself.

Chapter 3 will explain the basic anatomy of stability so that you can familiarise yourself with the muscles involved and their relevance to sporting performance.

---

### Chapter Summary

- Stability helps you to create and control force for more effective movement.

- We have choices in the muscle patterns that we use, but our habits are not necessarily the most efficient option.

- Without stability, the joints can buckle within the same plane, or into another plane, leaking force and amplifying pressure on body structures.

- Poor stability can contribute to movement dysfunctions but it may not be the primary issue. Sometimes body control problems are an effect rather than a cause.

- If our movement habits cannot meet the demands of training, we compensate. Compensation is often associated with poor technique.

- Multiple factors, including body awareness, balance, breathing, posture and mobility, all contribute to functional stability and movement efficacy.

# 3 | The Anatomy of Stability

Many of my clients have been told that "poor stability" is the root of their problems. This is not sufficient information to determine what the problem actually is, and what to do about it. If an athlete does not appear to have adequate control, we need to ask "in what way?", "when?" and "while doing what?" Understanding force management allows us to see that movement is made up of a series of strategies and behaviours which can be teased apart in order to be more specific in our programmes. Being able to analyse movement in this way helps my clients to make meaningful connections between their movement habits and their sport.

This chapter deals with the behaviour of muscles in functional and dysfunctional relationships. A deeper understanding of the anatomy and relationships of the muscles you will be activating may help you to interpret your own observations and assess movement with greater insight. Depending upon your interests and level of involvement in sport, you may wish to pursue the subject in greater depth, or you may feel that this is a chapter to dip into when a question arises.

# Stabilisers and Mobilisers

To produce a movement, muscles must work in coordinated patterns or chains. Within these patterns some muscles are ideally designed to provide support and others to produce force. They have specific physiological and neuromuscular characteristics and therefore different roles. To better understand the roles of different muscles within a functional movement pattern, muscles can be grouped according to their behaviour and structure. These groupings provide general guidelines that help to interpret movement and plan training programmes. The most basic model is that of stabilisers and mobilisers [5,14], which is summarised in the diagram below.

A movement needs a firm foundation, and a muscle group called the *local stabilisers* provides the most fundamental level of joint support. Think of these as **joint controllers**. The *global stabilisers* provide control of the moving parts throughout the motion and also produce force. Think of these as **movement controllers**. The *global mobilisers* are the **movement producers**. This grouping does not exclude mobilisers from having a stabilising role, however based on structural characteristics and behaviour, their movement-producing role is most relevant when considering training implications.

The bottom of the pyramid supports the other muscular actions, yet it is least attended to in training. When considering the functions of muscles, it is clear that any movement will involve the interplay of stabilisers and mobilisers, so it is important to train patterns rather than muscles. If a muscle is not activating correctly, the pattern will be distorted. If this is the case, it is most likely to be a stabiliser that is the missing link. A muscle that is not firing as part of the pattern must be stimulated to activate and then reintegrated into the pattern. Trying to compensate with other muscles will not promote smooth, efficient movement.

Global mobilisers
Movement

Global stabilisers
Force production/control
through motion

Local stabilisers
Joint control (foundations)

## The Local System

Much current research on local stabilisers focuses on control of the lower spine, but there is a growing body of research into the behaviour of local stabilisers in the knee [7, 85], shoulder [79, 88] and neck [61]. In the public domain, the most familiar of the local stabilisers is transversus abdominis (TrA), a deep abdominal muscle.

Local stabilising muscles provide a foundation for movement, just as a solid foundation supports a house. When you generate the impulse to move, they become active just prior to the movement in order to support the body's structures and provide a stable platform for the movement. This is called a *feedforward response*.

When functioning normally, they activate regardless of the direction in which you want to move [44], and they continue to work throughout the whole movement. Local stabilisers do not change length greatly when they contract. They are usually positioned to spread closely over a joint, so they are ideally suited to controlling joint position but not for producing a wide range of motion. Because of these characteristics, local stabilisers maintain joints in the safest and most suitable position to support muscular forces, and provide a secure axis for movement.

Despite their crucial role in efficient movement and joint protection, the local stabilisers can switch off for a variety of reasons. Pain can inhibit the function of these muscles, and even when the pain resolves, they can remain switched off [46, 42]. Even fear of pain can alter their function [89]. Without local stabilisers functioning as part of the normal neuromuscular pattern for movement, other muscles in the system alter their roles to compensate for them.

These larger *global* muscles normally produce force or movement and are not designed to maintain safe and secure joint position. Nor are they physiologically suited to the sustained activity required in a stabilising role. The ongoing inhibition of local stabilisers therefore leads to chronic biomechanical problems, and an athlete can end up in a frustrating injury cycle or performance plateau as a result.

Even without injury, the local stabilisers can switch off. Athletes will commonly use the movement and force-producing global muscles as stabilisers in order to cope with a training demand beyond their true biomechanical and neuromuscular capabilities. This can occur in response to excessive loading, skill demand or training volume. The underlying reason for this altered pattern may be neuromuscular, physiological or psychological, but it can be avoided if sound sports-specific profiling is provided and good communication between coach, sports science and medical personnel is established.

## Clipboard Notes

A judo athlete arrived at the clinic with laxity and pain in her right knee. She had undergone surgical reconstruction of the knee several years previously and continued to struggle with it. She was in full training and had been given a heavy resistance programme in order to gain the necessary weight to fight in her chosen category. Despite adherence to the resistance programme provided by sports science personnel, the quadriceps on the painful side did not respond to strengthening exercises and remained atrophied.

The local stabiliser for the knee is the medial quadricep, vastus medialis, which in this athlete was inhibited, or switched off. She had poor pelvic control, and could not prevent her knee from falling inwards, out of the sagittal and into the coronal plane. Her stabilisation strategy was global muscle dominant, not just in her lower limb but also in her trunk and upper body. Her pectorals, upper trapezius, rectus abdominis, hip flexors, superficial spinal muscles and hamstrings were all working constantly to stabilise as well as create movement. Her local stabiliser system, including her lower abdominals, deep spinal muscles, scapular stabilising muscles and deep neck muscles, were all underactive.

The athlete's resistance programme was aimed at gaining muscle mass, so the athlete was using poor patterns to push heavy weights. This reinforced the patterns, and the athlete started to experience neck and lower back pain in addition to her knee problems due to her inability to manage forces efficiently.

The athlete's weights programme was temporarily suspended in order to activate her local stability system, and then reintroduced as quickly as possible with modifications to enable her to learn more efficient technical patterns. To the athlete's surprise, low-load, partial bodyweight activities for her quadriceps activated her inhibited medial quadriceps muscles, and her thigh circumference increased. Slightly lower resistance with better patterning throughout her programme reduced musculoskeletal stress and increased functional strength.

Throughout the programme, the amount of resistance was monitored against the athlete's ability to use her entire system without compensating. Instead of focusing on strength in individual muscles, it prioritised strengthening muscle relationships to develop effective force production.

Despite a structural instability in the knee, the athlete's functional stability improved and she was able to compete and secure a medal at international tournament level.

## The Global System

The global system can be divided into the global stabilisers and the global mobilisers. *Global stabilisers* usually have broad attachments and are suited to controlling joints throughout a movement. Unlike local stabilisers, they do change length and therefore can create force. If working in their correct role in the neuromuscular pattern, these muscles can be very powerful. Muscles such as gluteus maximus (GMax) and the external oblique abdominals are examples of global stabilisers.

The *global mobilisers* have a predominance of fast twitch muscle fibres and are designed to produce movement. The local muscles activate tonically to provide continuous support, but the global mobilisers behave phasically, that is their activity, being task and movement dependent, is an on/off behaviour. As more research is published, muscles in this category are being found to have specific stabiliser roles. However, with their relatively long muscle fibres, superficial placement, ability to build tension quickly, and greater susceptibility to fatigue, the mobilisers are considered to be *action muscles*.

## Models for Muscles

Despite the best efforts of scientists, the body resists most attempts to definitively categorise its systems. The stabiliser/mobiliser model is helpful to understand broad movement control principles, but in practice some muscles defy categorisation by having dual roles, acting as mobilisers and stabilisers under different conditions.

For many years, muscles have been grouped according to their predominant fibre type. Muscles that behave tonically have a larger proportion of slow twitch, or Type I fibres. They are fatigue resistant and work at low load, and so are suited to supporting the body against gravity. Muscles with greater proportions of fast twitch, or Type II fibres are considered to be phasic, although this is further classified into whether the fibres are Type IIa (which are less fatigueable) or Type IIb (which are more fatigueable).

As research progresses, it is becoming clear that muscles do not always behave in such clearly defined ways. Muscles that have been thought to operate exclusively tonically have been found to modulate their activity phasically under certain conditions. TrA and the diaphragm, both predominantly tonic muscles, have been found to display phasic characteristics at faster running speeds [118].

Due to these new discoveries about the behaviour and physiology of muscles, the model we will use is based on movement. For practical purposes in most training environments, remember that each movement is made up of muscles that *create motion* and muscles that *control motion*. To allow smooth, powerful movement, there needs to be a balance between the local and global systems. Positioned closely over joints, the local stabilisers have short lines of pull, which are ideal for controlling joints, but produce insufficient force to create and control movement. Global stabilisers have long lines of pull over more than one joint, so they are effective for producing and controlling movement. When both sets of muscles are working together, stability and mobility are achieved.

An athlete with *stability dysfunction* may try to achieve joint control by using large global muscles such as the external abdominal obliques, rectus abdominis, latissimus dorsi, the erector spinae and hamstrings. Because these muscles cross more than one joint, their line of pull produces a compressive force which can be helpful to stabilise against high forces when contracting in partnership with other muscles. However, if the local stabiliser system is not working effectively to secure each joint segment against the next, this long line of pull can contribute to joint buckling. Buckling produces unwanted and poorly controlled joint motion, leading to technical control problems and eventually injury (fig. 3.2).

As global muscles commonly cross more than one joint, an increase in their stabilising activity causes problems in differentiating movement from one body part to another. The ability to move body parts independently of one another is called *dissociation*, and every sport needs this to some degree. For example, to hit an effective drive, a golfer must be able to rotate his pelvis slightly before his trunk begins to rotate in order to effectively use his trunk muscles to create power in his swing-through. If he is unable to separate the motion of his pelvis from the motion in his thorax because he is bracing his trunk using his global abdominal muscles, he will either lose power or start overusing another body part, such as the arms.

Imagine a flatwater kayak paddler who overuses her external oblique abdominals to stabilise her trunk and maintain her posture as she paddles. The primary trunk action for this sport is rotation. She needs the obliques to be able to lengthen and shorten alternately to produce torque, but instead the paddler works them continuously in the same range to keep her trunk secure. The continuous action of these global muscles impairs the paddler's breathing by pulling on her lower ribs and decreasing rib expansion. Her trunk mobility is also decreased as is the power in her stroke, which she tries to compensate for with increased upper body effort. The paddler needs to re-establish a pattern where her local stabilisers secure her central longitudinal axis (CLA) and her external obliques produce force.

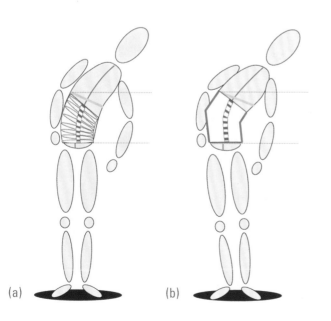

The global stabiliser muscles do not always over-activate. Sometimes their activity is poorly timed or inadequate for the task, leading to a failure to control a joint through motion. This can easily be observed watching people climb the stairs. Without the gluteal group controlling the femur, the knee moves inwards as the person transfers their weight onto that leg.

3.2 (a) Deep stabiliser system providing segmental joint control of the spine. The action of strong superficial global muscles will not buckle the spine as they create force; (b) without adequate deep stabiliser action, the long global muscles cause segmental buckling as they create force due to their long line of pull over multiple joints.

(a)    (b)

Ultimately, the interplay between local and global muscles should lead to smooth efficient movement. To ensure a sound movement pattern, the quality of a movement should be emphasised in all aspects of training. In other words, pay as much attention to *how well* you perform the movement as you do to any other measure of a good training session. If you perform the movement accurately, you have a better chance of stimulating the correct pattern.

Some athletes ignore this principle. For example, an endurance athlete's exceptional cardiovascular endurance may significantly outstrip their technique and their ability to cope with repetitive musculoskeletal loading. They nevertheless continue to prioritise their physiology over their biomechanics in training. Instead of addressing their weaknesses, they try to squeeze a tiny improvement out of a cardiovascular system that is already operating at maximum capacity. These athletes will commonly break down, or peak early, and then fail to meet their projected potential as they progress to higher levels of competition.

## Movement Control and Muscle Action in the Three Zones

### 1 The Central Control Zone: The Trunk

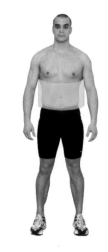

For pelvic stability and segmental stability in the spine, the local stabilisers **transversus abdominis** (TrA) and multifidus need to be functioning normally in partnership with the internal abdominal obliques, the diaphragm and pelvic floor. Between them, they represent the roof, floor and walls of your deep trunk stabilising system shown opposite. In addition to their direct stabilising action via their musculoskeletal attachments, these muscles coordinate their activity to create and control a balloon of pressure within the abdominal cavity. This pressure, known as *intra-abdominal pressure*, contributes to trunk stability in response to movement [45]. Breathing patterns, pelvic floor control and trunk stability are therefore intimately connected.

Wrapping around the trunk, TrA connects the front and back and upper and lower halves of the body. Through these connections, it plays a role in supporting the functional movement of the upper and lower limbs as well as stabilising the spine. With its extensive attachments, TrA is able to disperse force across a large surface area, decreasing load on isolated body structures. TrA has attachments to the cartilages of the lower six ribs, and reaches down to the upper surfaces of the pelvis. It spans the trunk to connect into the thoracolumbar fascia, a thick connective tissue sheath with attachments to the individual vertebral segments of the spine, as well as the pelvis and ribs.

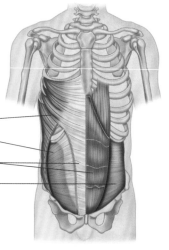

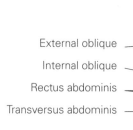

External oblique

Internal oblique

Rectus abdominis

Transversus abdominis

The thoracolumbar fascia helps to stabilise the trunk and pelvis when muscles connecting into it are tensioned [132]. Latissimus dorsi connects the upper limb to the **thoracolumbar fascia**, GMax connects the lower limb into the thoracolumbar fascia, the deep spinal stabiliser multifidus connects the spine into the thoracolumbar fascia along with TrA, and various other muscles including biceps femoris influence thoracolumbar fascial tension via attachments to ligaments that connect with it.

The upper and lower body are therefore anatomically integrated, with TrA and the thoracolumbar fascia providing a web to connect them centrally. It can be appreciated then that TrA is involved in supporting powerful upper limb actions, as well as influencing leg movement by helping to stabilise the pelvis on the spine and creating a firm foundation for the strong leg muscles to pull from.

## Transversus Abdominis Key Points

1. Local stabiliser.

2. Connects front–back and upper–lower parts of the body.

3. Large surface area.

4. Connects into thoracolumbar fascia.

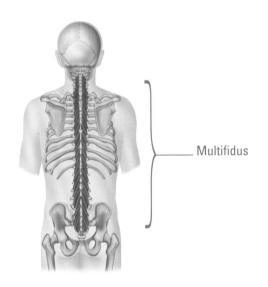

Multifidus

**Multifidus** muscles connect the individual segments of the spine in the cervical, thoracic and lumbar regions. Like TrA, multifidus reacts in anticipation of movement, providing close direct support to the vertebral segments and contributing to tension in the thoracolumbar fascia in preparation for load. Like TrA, multifidus activity can be delayed or absent in response to pain [42]. Multifidus is also involved in pelvic stability, so it should be considered in athletes with groin or pelvic pain.

The muscular pairing of **iliacus** and **psoas major**, collectively known as iliopsoas, is usually referred to as having a hip flexion action. However, psoas major, which has direct attachments to the segments of the spine, is now considered to have both local and global stabilising functions. The posterior portions of the muscle act as local stabilisers, securing each segment for firm spinal alignment, while the anterior portions are thought to have a more global stabiliser role [33].

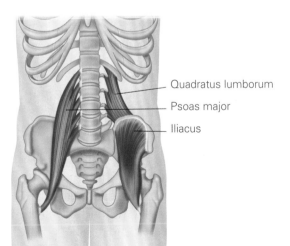

Quadratus lumborum

Psoas major

Iliacus

An athlete in a contact sport will need all of these deep muscles working to control the segments of their spine while the global muscles increase their bracing activity to control overall trunk movement. The effectiveness of this mechanism is further increased by co-activation of the diaphragm and pelvic floor, so that intra-abdominal pressure is momentarily higher to withstand an impact. Athletes will often unconsciously pause their breath at the moment of impact to maintain this internal pressure as an automatic stabilising response, and then release it a split second after impact. Protection of the spine using these stabilising effects depends upon the timing and activation of the local spinal stabilisers.

## Training Tip

Coordinated action of the deep stabilising muscles contributes to anti-buckling support for the spine. If you are running, for example, with gravity bearing down and ground reaction force pushing up, muscular support is needed around the segments of the spine to cope with vertical force. To begin training the spine for vertical force management, the simple task of Ball Bouncing (see Chapter 6) provides a repeated, low-load, vertical pulsed stimulus which teaches the trunk to support itself with coordination and timing. Rather than training a fixed contraction, the movement stimulus encourages a neuromuscular response to each pulse, encouraging timing and preparatory muscle behaviour.

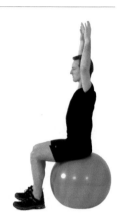

## Clipboard Notes

An elite female karate athlete presented for movement performance analysis. When asked what her training priorities were, she said that she needed more strength and power. To address this, she was lifting heavy weights in the gym, and in particular focusing on the bench press. When asked how she'd like to fight, however, she said that she wanted to be powerful and explosive, but quick, fluent and light.

On assessment, it was obvious that the athlete's central control was exceptionally poor, as was her pelvic coordination for driving quickly forward. She depended upon global muscles to provide stability, which made it hard for her to dissociate her movements. Her perception that she needed more upper body power was affecting how she was using her arms. Her movement was heavy and she was not meeting her potential for speed, despite the achievement of a European title as a junior.

The athlete was asked to perform the Wall Press (see Chapter 6). She primarily felt the load on her shoulders and arms, and even though she was capable of bench-pressing a substantial weight, felt that the Wall Press was an effort.

The athlete was then taught a simple postural cue, which established her central axis and activated her trunk stabilisers. Maintaining this position, she performed the Wall Press. She was surprised: her arms felt very little load. Instead she felt that the total body load was spread over her body so that nothing had to work too hard.

The notable aspect in this case was that the athlete performed the majority of her strength work in the gym with her trunk supported fully, but did very little to integrate this strength into a total body pattern. When her arms were loaded without trunk support, she lacked the functional motor pattern to support the body efficiently. Stimulating a pattern that activated her central control mechanisms redistributed the load to achieve greater total efficiency.

After this experience, the athlete was asked to perform punch and kick movements as she had in her initial evaluation, but this time was given a specific cue. She was asked to fight with the imagery of a helium balloon lifting her spine against gravity. This stabilised and lengthened her central axis and activated TrA, released the muscles across her shoulders allowing them to drop into a more effective position, and decreased the tension levels in global muscles around her trunk and hips. The result was fluent, swift striking from both arms and legs and the disappearance of the heavy movements that had previously characterised her fighting style.

The important thing to remember about the local stabilisers is that they should activate automatically just before a movement occurs, and work for long periods at low effort levels. They are a necessary foundation for safe, efficient technical movement, so they should not be neglected or overlooked.

Common problems with TrA and multifidus are an absence of activation as part of a neuromuscular pattern, or a lack of sufficient endurance of the neuromuscular pattern as a whole to keep supporting movement. Priorities are therefore to switch on an inhibited muscle and gradually increase its endurance within a total body pattern.

## The Neutral Spine

TrA and multifidus activity is necessary to support a *neutral spinal position*. The spine is not a straight structure, but instead has a gentle concave or inward curve (lordosis) in the cervical and lumbar regions and a convex or outward curve (kyphosis) in the thoracic region.

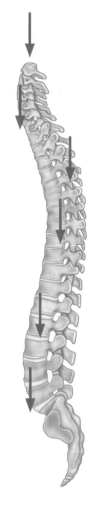

These curves allow the spine to share vertical load across many joints and decrease pressure on the discs which sit between each vertebra. The curves also allow for a certain amount of vertical shock absorption as we walk, run and jump or, if you are a rider, to absorb a horse's motion. If your spine was straight, the weight of your head would be transferred straight to the last disc in the spine, and this would break down quickly under the load.

The neutral spinal position decreases the need for global muscle stabilising activity to maintain an upright posture. Decreasing global stabilising strategies to maintain posture improves movement fluency and dissociation by reducing the stiffening effect over multiple joints. Good breathing patterns can be maintained and joint stresses are decreased.

The neutral spine: normal curves allow the spine to be mobile and share load evenly throughout the spine.

Athletes with poor local stabiliser activity in the trunk have difficulty controlling the neutral spine, and yet many sports depend upon this position for optimal technique, either in the sport itself or the training programme. Sporting examples of the sustained neutral spine are a freestyle swimmer, a weightlifter as they strongly drive up into a clean, a golfer in their address position, a gymnast in a handstand position, a dressage rider or a runner.

The spine does not have to be vertical to be neutral, and your hips can be at any angle, as long as the shoulder to pelvis relationship is maintained and the spinal curves are normal.

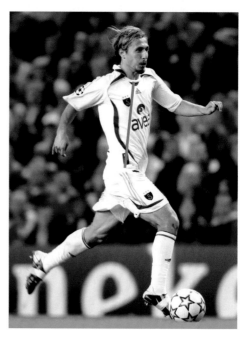

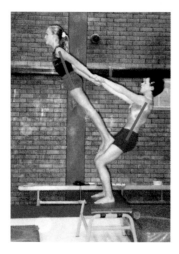

Learning to control a neutral spinal position helps you to establish your central longitudinal axis (CLA) and, as was discussed in Chapter 1, this axis is necessary for efficient rotational movement. It also prevents excessive joint compression which occurs when your CLA collapses.

If you consider the address position in golf, two common postural errors are seen below. Some golfers flex their spine, making it appear rounded (a). The CLA is bowed outwards, and if the golfer then rotates, he will increase the stress on his lumbar discs. Other golfers collapse their CLA inward, making it appear as if they are sticking their bottom out (b). This position closes the joints in the spine, and rotation causes further compression of the joints. Both postures are collapses of the CLA in the sagittal plane. A neutral spinal position (c) will disperse the load over multiple joints rather than focusing load on isolated structures.

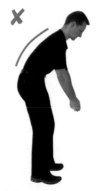
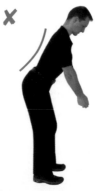
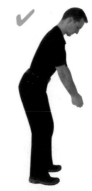

(a) flexed spine.     (b) extended spine.     (c) neutral spine.

Rotation will be strongest around a firm axis. This principle applies in sports that require rotation *within* the body, e.g. the golfer, the tennis player or the sprint kayak paddler, or for athletes who require rotation of the body in space, such as divers, gymnasts, hammer and discus throwers. Rotation around a firm CLA prevents the introduction of other planes of movement, maintaining technical movement and influencing consistency, accuracy, power and efficiency.

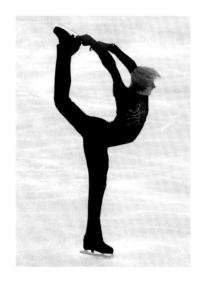

TrA and multifidus normally activate regardless of the spinal position you need in your sport, whether this involves forward, backward, side-bending or rotation movements. This makes sense: you need segmental spinal stability in all of these positions. Sports such as gymnastics require extreme spinal mobility, but TrA and multifidus must still support the joints throughout the full movement to make the movement optimally even and fluid. Although the overall position of the spine no longer looks neutral, each joint is supported within the range of motion for which it is structurally designed (see left).

Moving beyond this range increases stress on joint structures and injury risk. If TrA and multifidus are working effectively, they will support the joints in their normal physiological range even in these dramatic positions. This can only be safely achieved if the athlete maintains connection between their zones throughout their movement.

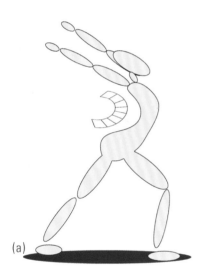
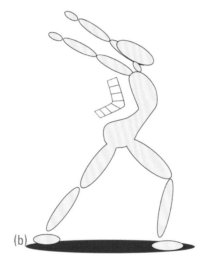

3.13 (a) Each spinal segment contributes evenly to the movement, giving the appearance of an even curve. Force is shared across many joints. (b) One spinal segment is moving more than the others, focusing forces in that area.

Collapse of the CLA in the *coronal* plane has been found to correlate with lower limb injury risk [136]. In addition to the segmental support provided by TrA, multifidus and psoas, the ability to minimise displacement of the axis in the coronal plane also involves the action of **quadratus lumborum** (see page 61). This muscle runs on either side of the spine from the iliac crest of the innominate (the upper margin of the pelvic bone) and the iliolumbar ligament (connecting the fifth lumbar vertebra to the innominate) to the lowest rib and transverse processes of upper four lumbar vertebrae. Its action is to side-bend the trunk, but also to withstand the trunk being pulled or pushed sideways in the opposite direction.

Stability of the CLA in the coronal plane is also dependent upon your pelvic control. If your pelvis tips from side to side due to weakness in the muscles around your hip, your spine will also have to bend sideways to keep you balanced, compromising your axis. Gluteus medius (GMed) is considered to have the most significant role in this control (see page 74), and weakness in other hip abductor muscles has also been linked to lower limb injury risk [73]. The hip and pelvic muscles will be further discussed in the lower control zone section of this chapter. Together, GMed and the quadratus lumborum on the opposite side are considered to be a functional pair for coronal plane control.

At low levels, any sideways deviation in simple tests such as the SSCT test in Chapter 5 indicates a lack of CLA control in the coronal plane, while at higher levels Push Jumps (see Chapter 5) can expose coronal plane control issues more dynamically.

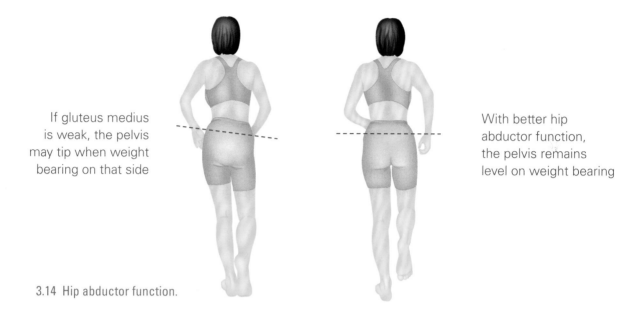

If gluteus medius is weak, the pelvis may tip when weight bearing on that side

With better hip abductor function, the pelvis remains level on weight bearing

3.14  Hip abductor function.

## The Anterior Chain

There is a variety of possible muscle pattern combinations for stabilising the trunk. If we look at the front (anterior) surface of the body and consider the relationship between the abdominal muscles as part of a functional chain, TrA and the internal obliques should work as local stabilisers, the external obliques as a global stabiliser and rectus abdominis as a mobiliser.

However, athletes often learn to use alternative patterns in order to compensate for poor local stabiliser activation. One of these patterns is the use of the external obliques, rectus abdominis and superficial hip flexors such as rectus femoris as the primary source of stability. This is not an effective method for stabilising the trunk, as these muscles do not offer segmental spinal control. They exert a compressive force over long lines of pull.

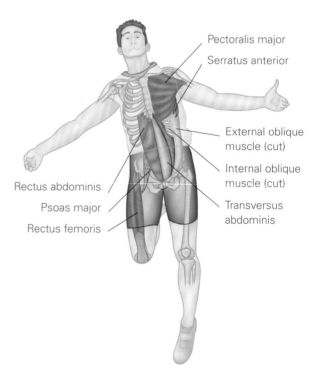

Pectoralis major

Serratus anterior

External oblique muscle (cut)

Internal oblique muscle (cut)

Rectus abdominis

Psoas major

Rectus femoris

Transversus abdominis

Ideally all of these anterior chain muscles should work in a coordinated fashion. A common compensatory pattern is the dominance of the red muscles, or red and yellow, with relative underactivity from the muscles marked in green.

Inappropriate action of the external obliques can decrease the mobility of the ribs by pulling them downwards towards the pelvis. Fixing the ribs in this way affects breathing patterns by preventing the lower part of the rib cage from expanding fully on inspiration. This will affect the potential for the large lower lobes of the lung to inflate fully, which in turn can influence the potential for oxygen and carbon dioxide exchange in this considerable area of the lungs.

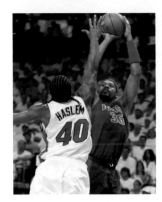

The compressive action of the external obliques on the ribs or the effect of rectus abdominis depressing the central rib cage can influence arm motion. As we investigated in Chapter 1, to fully reach upwards with your arm, your trunk needs to lengthen and the space between your ribs should slightly widen. If you are using compression to stabilise your trunk by activating the external obliques and rectus abdominis, this lengthening action will be blocked. If you then need to reach for a high ball in basketball (left), or stretch for a longer stroke in freestyle swimming, you will have to make a compromise. You can either maintain your trunk stability pattern and not reach so far, or you can lose your trunk stability in order to allow your trunk to lengthen. Either way, optimal performance is lost.

Overuse of the superficial hip flexors is common in dysfunctional trunk stability patterns, and they often pair with the superficial back muscles (the erector spinae) to compensate for poor local stabiliser and gluteal activation. The athlete with this pattern may stand with their pelvis tipped forward and an increased lordosis at the base of the spine. This combination of muscle actions produces a compressive or buckling force across a relatively small surface area of muscle attachment. This makes the spine vulnerable in all planes.

## Fascial Relationships and the Anterior Chain

Fascia is the continuous web of tissue that contains, shapes and connects the structures of our bodies, links individual muscles into functional relationships and makes it possible to share force and provide support across multiple body segments. These myofascial relationships can greatly increase our efficiency. However, coordination and regulation of muscle activity throughout the anterior chain will influence how well we can utilise them.

Some athletes are very dominant in their upper control zone but relatively disconnected from their central and lower control zones. They are tight and over-active in their pectorals, but lax in their deep abdominal musculature, so the balance of tension is inconsistent across the band of myofascial tissues crossing the front of their body. This can create vulnerability to injury of shoulders, the lower back and even the groin.

In a movement such as this gymnast demonstrates, where the shoulders must withstand multiples of bodyweight rapidly, a degree of spinal extension as the athlete activates both anterior and posterior chain muscles creates additional myofascial tension from the shoulders all the way down across the front of the trunk and into the thighs, creating a band of support that protects the spine and keeps the shoulders plugged in. If the athlete was lax in his abdominal wall, he would experience disconnection of upper and lower body instead of lengthening. His protective myofascial mechanism would be lost, and his shoulders and lower back would become vulnerable to injury.

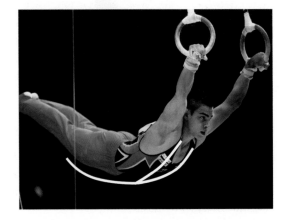

Myofascial connections support the body in all planes, and we use combinations of these to protect our joints, share and transmit forces, and store elastic energy in the contractile components – the muscles. The direction of movement impulse, the site of movement initiation, and the CLA, all have a part to play in this.

In figure 3.18, we see forces being generated in the sagittal plane. The buckling of the CLA into spinal extension disconnects the upper control zone from the rest of the body, blocking flow of force. The shoulder is relatively unsupported but must generate the majority of force. The athlete cannot access the support of her anterior chain myofascial structures.

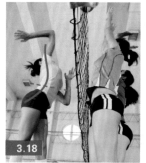 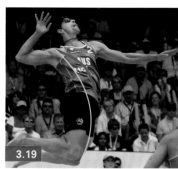

In contrast, the athlete in fig. 3.19 is spreading his forces between the sagittal and transverse planes. He engages and tensions his myofascial structures across the anterior chain both linearly and diagonally by extending his hips and flexing his knees, creating functional support for the shoulder. He also protects his spine from excessive backward bending by rotating his trunk.

## Relative Flexibility and the Central Control Zone

As discussed in Chapter 1, relative flexibility is the tendency of one body part to move more readily than another. In the case of shoulder inflexibility, the spine tends to give into extension, collapsing the CLA and requiring the lumbar curve to deepen in order to get the arms overhead.

---

**Personal Investigation**

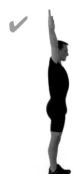 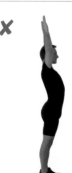 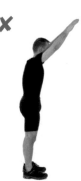

To investigate relative flexibility, stand next to a mirror so that you can see yourself from the side. Raise both arms so that they are straight above your head. Your hands should be directly vertically aligned with your feet. How easy was it to get your arms into this position? Did you maintain your pelvic position or did it slide forward? What happened to your weight? Is it centred or are you now standing with your weight in the front of your feet? Repeat the action, this time maintaining your weight in the centre of your feet and noticing your spinal shape in the mirror. Did you need to increase your spinal curve to allow your arms to raise all the way?

Repeat the action one more time. Be aware of the weight in the centre of your feet and see if you can maintain your spinal position while raising your arms.

Can your arms go as high? If not, it is likely that your shoulders are not as flexible as you thought! You were giving in your lumbar spine, as it is relatively more flexible.

---

The same phenomenon can occur when the hip is relatively less flexible than the spine. When an athlete needs to bend at the hip, the spine bends first, collapsing the CLA into flexion. There are different reasons for this, depending upon your body position. If you are trying to lift your knee or bring your thigh towards your trunk, poor hip mobility or hip flexion strength may cause you to bend your spine more readily.

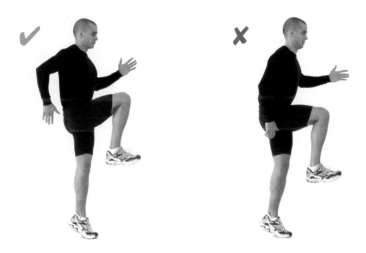

This can be seen when athletes perform high knee lifts poorly in their warm-ups, allowing their chest to sink towards their knee instead of bringing the knee towards their chest. It can also be observed in rowers, who may collapse into spinal flexion if their hips will not bend sufficiently. If you are in a closed chain situation such as squatting, you may bend your spine instead of your hips due to poor gluteal action in order to control the hip angle.

When there is a compensatory pattern in the anterior chain, the thoracic spine (from the point where your neck joins your trunk to the bottom of the rib cage) tends to be stiff and lacking normal mobility. The nerves supplying TrA emerge from the spinal cord at the level of the lower six thoracic vertebrae, and thoracic stiffness and TrA activation problems may be related.

Applying the relative flexibility concept, stiffness in one area will tend to cause excessive mobility in another so that the total amount of movement available remains roughly the same. When the thoracic spine is stiff, the cervical spine and lumbar spine will need greater motion to compensate which can lead to excessive motion and increased joint stress in these areas. If you do not restore thoracic mobility, training TrA will only help in situations where you do not need good spinal movement.

## Clipboard Notes

A professional surfer arrived at the clinic with lower back pain. He had been given exercises in the past for poor trunk stability, but he was not improving. This young man's thoracic spine was extremely stiff, and as total spinal mobility is necessary for surfing, he had to move excessively somewhere else in the spine in order to perform. The excessive motion took place in his lumbar spine.

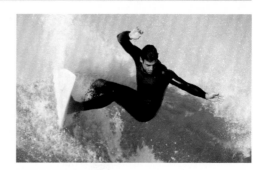

The surfer's TrA function was inhibited, and his external obliques were trying to provide primary stability as well as rotational control and rotational torque. Some of his thoracic stiffness may have been due to the overactivity of the external obliques. Muscle retraining alone could not solve this athlete's problem. Without normal thoracic mobility, his lumbar spine would continue to move excessively despite local stabiliser training. To improve his situation, he needed to combine mobility training with his stability exercises. By restoring mobility in his thoracic spine and activating TrA to work as the local stabiliser, the external obliques were released to work properly as a global stabiliser and torque producer. This allowed the surfer to return to his sport without pain.

### Key Points

- Local and global muscles must work together to maintain smooth, efficient movement and normal breathing mechanics.

- Breathing and trunk stability are interdependent.

- Local trunk stabilisers activate together to establish a secure CLA for efficient movement.

- Trunk stability can influence the performance of your arms and legs.

- The mobility of your joints can influence trunk stability.

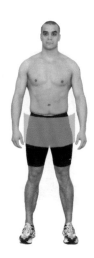

## ② The Lower Control Zone: The Pelvis

Control of the trunk greatly depends upon the security of the foundation that carries and supports it. We therefore need to look a little further down the chain to the group of muscles around the pelvis that primarily provide this support: the gluteals.

A large muscle with wide pelvic attachments, **gluteus maximus** (GMax) contributes to powerful hip extension for explosive activities like Olympic weightlifting, Nordic skiing, jumping and sprinting, as well as strong hip control as is needed for squatting, alpine skiing[43], uphill cycling[76] or a deep volley in tennis.

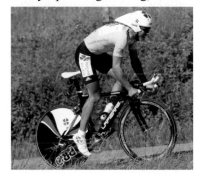

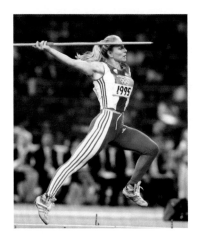

From a mechanical point of view, GMax performs key roles in controlling the relationship between thigh, pelvis and trunk. When the pelvis is stabilised but the foot is not fixed, GMax acts as an extensor of the hip, moving the thigh backward as in preparing to kick a ball. When the foot is fixed and the pelvis moves, as occurs in walking and running, GMax working concentrically (shortening while contracting) helps to propel the body forward over the fixed foot. Working eccentrically (lengthening while contracting) it controls the rate of hip bending as you lower your body mass, as should occur in a lunge or squat (fig. 3.26).

In partnership with **gluteus medius** (GMed) and **gluteus minimus** (GMin), GMax controls the alignment of the knee with respect to the pelvis and the ankle, and therefore influences the amount of stress on the knee structures. For example, in a step-up, GMax should contribute to controlling thigh rotation and vertical alignment of the knee with the hip and ankle, while powerfully straightening the hip to press the body upwards (fig. 3.27). The hip, knee and ankle should remain in line so that the motion occurs in only one plane.

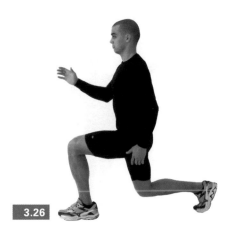

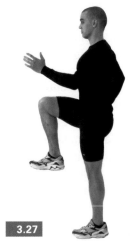

3.26 The lunge demonstrates eccentric action of GMax as the muscle is contracting as it lengthens to control the hip as it lowers.

3.27 GMax contracts concentrically to straighten the hip.

If the gluteal muscles are weak or underactive on walking or running, the knee moves inwards and the pelvis tips sideways (a coronal plane collapse). Under these conditions, the structures of the knee are put under abnormal strain due to poor alignment, and this can lead to pain at the front or inside of the knee. From a performance perspective, the additional planes of movement being introduced decrease the degree of force being applied in the most desirable direction.

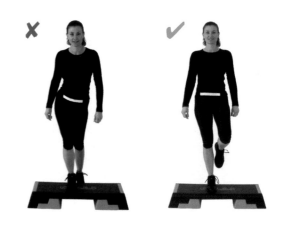

Free movement at the hip and spine depends on sound function at the sacroiliac joints of the pelvic girdle. These joints need a combination of muscles working in partnership to withstand the high forces that they must bear, and GMax plays a significant role in stabilising the sacroiliac joints by compressing the joint [52]. Like TrA, fibres of GMax attach into the thoracolumbar fascia. Via the thoracolumbar fascia, GMax forms a partnership with the latissimus dorsi muscle of the opposite side to form the posterior oblique myofascial sling.

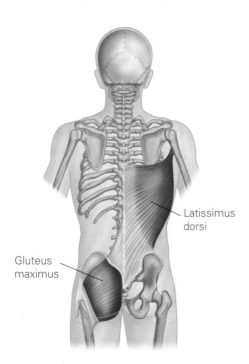

Latissimus dorsi

Gluteus maximus

The muscular components of myofascial slings store and release elastic energy, providing stability when they are under tension and increasing movement efficiency when releasing. By forming a diagonal connection across the pelvis and lumbar spine, the posterior oblique myofascial sling contributes to sacroiliac joint compression to help support the bodyweight. In any movement that involves rotation of the upper body on the lower body, e.g. walking, running or kayaking, the sling stores and releases energy to make the movements more economical.

Weakness or under-activity in GMax will predispose the sacroiliac joints to injury, and influence economy of movement by decreasing the effectiveness of the posterior oblique myofascial sling. If GMax is weak or underactive on one side, the body must compensate to protect itself from the high forces that impact on the sacroiliac joints. It may try to gain tension across the posterior oblique myofascial sling by increasing the activation of the opposing latissimus dorsi. If this happens, the trunk may tip to one side slightly, activation of the deep trunk stabilisers is affected, and it may appear that the shoulder is pulled down on that side (fig. 3.30).

These effects are easily seen in weightbearing movement such as a lunge, step-up or knee raise. When you spot the shoulder moving slightly downwards, you should check the function of the gluteals on the opposite side. If the shoulder is pulled down by latissimus dorsi action in this way, shoulder biomechanics will change and an injury can occur. GMax function should be tested in athletes with shoulder injuries to make sure that it has not contributed to the development of the problem.

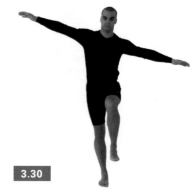

3.30

# The Posterior Chain

If we look at the lumbar spine, pelvis and hip region from the back, GMax is the central link in a vertical chain comprising the superficial back muscles (erector spinae), GMax and the hamstrings (fig. 3.31). These muscles should work in a coordinated partnership with the others in the chain, but if GMax is weak or uncoordinated, the proportion of activity from the other links in the chain will change, influencing movement coordination and timing [123]. These muscles are not suited to this increased workload, and can become chronically tight and susceptible to injury. Athletes who present with chronic hamstring tears or unusual levels of tightness in hamstrings and paraspinal muscles often exhibit poor GMax function on testing. Chronic groin strains can also be associated with poor GMax function.

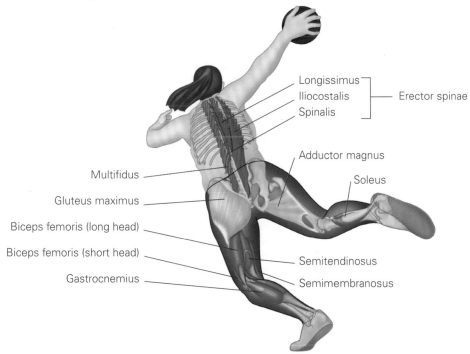

Longissimus ⎤
Iliocostalis ⎬— Erector spinae
Spinalis ⎦

Adductor magnus

Soleus

Multifidus

Gluteus maximus

Biceps femoris (long head)

Biceps femoris (short head)

Gastrocnemius

Semitendinosus

Semimembranosus

3.31 These muscles should work in coordinated patterns. However, in dysfunctional patterns, the muscles shown in red are often dominant, tight and overactive.

The largest of the inner thigh muscles, adductor magnus, has a role in extending the hip and supporting the thigh against the pelvis. Adductor magnus can increase its activity in an attempt to compensate for an underactive GMax, but this places abnormal strain on the muscle.

Problems with GMax can start from seemingly unrelated injuries. A back or sacroiliac joint injury can switch off the muscle, but so can an ankle sprain[9] or a past knee injury. The original injury may have healed and been forgotten about, but it may have switched off GMax without it being noticed. Even though there is no remaining pain in the area, the athlete's technique may have altered over time for no apparent reason and continue to resist improvement.

Posterior chain dysfunction also manifests itself in the anterior chain. It is not unusual to discover an athlete using hip flexor and quadriceps action to maintain postural control of the hip and pelvis despite the biomechanical disadvantage of this strategy. It is a common presentation associated with knee, hip, groin and back pain. In a squat, athletes with this pattern often feel painful and congested in the front of the hip. If the athlete presents with recurrent anterior thigh and hip issues, it is worth testing them using the pelvic control tests in Chapter 5 and addressing any deficits in posterior chain function.

## GMax Summary

| Athlete presents with: | What can it imply? | Likely finding |
|---|---|---|
| Tight/painful hamstrings or lumbar paraspinal muscles | Faulty posterior chain muscle activation pattern | GMax weakness or delayed timing on same side |
| Insufficient forward or upward power production from the legs | | |
| Pelvic position dropped when running | | |
| Tight/painful adductor magnus (inner thigh) | Faulty hip extension pattern: adductor magnus being over-used to extend the hip | GMax function decreased on same side |
| Asymmetrical body orientation | | |
| Better balance one side than the other | | |
| Excessively tight latissimus dorsi (remembering that the dominant arm will often be slightly less flexible than the non-dominant one) | Faulty posterior oblique myofascial sling | GMax function decreased on opposite side |

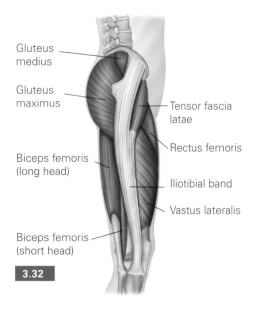

Gluteus medius

Gluteus maximus

Tensor fascia latae

Rectus femoris

Biceps femoris (long head)

Iliotibial band

Vastus lateralis

Biceps femoris (short head)

**3.32**

When acting as a stabiliser, the hip abductor GMed (fig. 3.32) helps to maintain a level pelvis when you bear more weight on one leg. This balances your trunk vertically with a minimum amount of postural muscle activity, which promotes good neuromuscular patterning in the trunk.

If walking normally, the spine should respond to the force of striking the ground with your foot by rotating and counter rotating around a vertical axis, which keeps the trunk centred over the pelvis. The primary plane is transverse (rotation). You can easily see this action as you walk by noting that your opposite foot and arm move forward at the same time, indicating that your shoulders and pelvis are rotating in the opposite direction.

If the hip abductors are weak, coronal plane movement becomes more evident. This can express itself in two ways. The pelvis may tip down on the opposite side to the stance leg, giving the appearance of a swagger on that side. This is known as a swagger, or *Trendelenburg gait* (fig. 3.33a). Alternatively, the individual will compensate by shifting their whole trunk excessively over the weak hip. This is known as a pendulum or *compensated Trendelenburg gait* (fig. 3.33b). The trunk is only centred over the pelvis for a short moment in the pendulum gait cycle, and appears more like a side-to-side movement which markedly decreases efficiency and increases the activity of the trunk side flexors, such as quadratus lumborum.

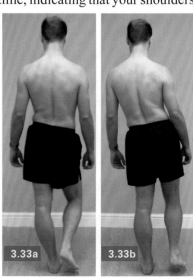

3.33a    3.33b

For athletes, the coronal plane movement that replaces efficient pelvic rotation around the CLA affects performance. It increases runners' foot contact time on the ground, making each stride cost more energy as their hip collapses slightly every time their foot strikes. In cyclists, it can be seen in excessive side-to-side trunk movement as they fail to keep a stable pelvis for the legs to push from. For footballers and basketball players, it shows up as difficulty changing directions and controlling sideways momentum, and in skiers, it will influence effective turning.

GMed weakness is associated with many common sports injuries. GMed's fundamental pelvic stabilisation role in weightbearing influences the entire kinetic chain, and weakness can be associated with a variety of painful presentations including the knee, sacroiliac joints and lower back. Shin pain in runners has also been linked to coronal plane collapse in the pelvis and loss of knee alignment [77].

Achilles tendinopathy in ballet dancers has been associated with increased internal rotation at the hip on taking off into a leap [69]. When GMed has been shown to be weak, hip abductor and external rotator strengthening has been shown to improve lower limb symptoms [64].

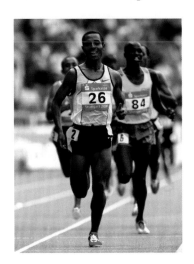

Effective hip abductor function maintains a level pelvis to support the trunk and the leg. When functioning normally, GMed works in partnership with other muscles; GMin, which lies deeper in the buttock, the adductor muscles of the inner thigh, and tensor fascia latae (TFL), a superficial outer thigh muscle which blends into the iliotibial band (ITB), to keep your pelvis level as you stand on one leg. If GMed is weak, then other muscles must increase their activity to compensate. TFL will become tensioned and overactive if GMed is not functioning properly, and this causes tightness in the long fibrous band down the outside of the thigh, the ITB.

A tight ITB interferes with normal knee and pelvic mechanics, and can cause pain around the patella, sacroiliac joint problems, nerve compression around the head of fibula causing pain on the outside of the knee, and even ankle pain due to altered biomechanics.

## Clinical Note

TFL has a role in hip abduction but it also can function as a flexor of the hip. In addition to testing for lateral pelvic control in stance, it may be necessary to test whether TFL is over-working as a hip flexor, which may create ITB tightness.

The Seated Knee Lift in Chapter 5 tests whether the trunk is stable enough to support a straight and coordinated hip flexion action. The knee should be lifted straight in line with the hip in the sagittal plane. If the Seated Knee Lift is effortful and the leg is pulled out of the sagittal plane, the loading on ITB may not primarily be from loading during stance, but may be caused by overuse due to a poor hip flexion pattern. In this case, a more effective hip flexion pattern should be trained.

Sometime it is not ITB acting as a flexor that is the problem, but a poor hip flexion action that places ITB in a stressful position. If, for example, a runner combines hip flexion with adduction as they bring their leg through, the advancing foot will meet the ground too far under the body. With the leg loaded and extending in an adducted position as the athlete passes their weight over the foot, ITB is placed repeatedly under tension. However, the problem is not solely a weightbearing issue: the foot must fall in a better position in the first place, so the athlete's strategy for bringing the leg through needs to be addressed.

Using movement testing, you will be able to identify whether the presentation is primarily a support problem which you will address with pelvic control work, or whether there is a hip flexion component, in which case you will add exercises to control and strengthen the relationship between the trunk and the flexing hip (see Chapter 5).

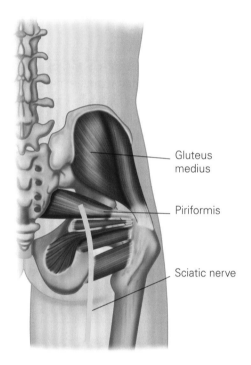

Gluteus medius

Piriformis

Sciatic nerve

The other common responder to GMed weakness is piriformis, a deep buttock muscle which crosses the sacroiliac joint. When overactive, piriformis interrupts normal pelvic and lower back mechanics and can cause sciatica and back pain.

An athlete may be able to balance on one leg but have difficulty maintaining a level pelvis and vertical trunk while still looking relaxed. Many use excessive global muscular activity to compensate for loss of deep postural stabiliser function, and this can be observed in excessive ankle and foot activity, fixing of the ribs with the obliques, pinning down of the chest with rectus abdominis, pulling the shoulder blades back and deepening of forward pelvic tilt. Because of this, GMed can influence breathing, posture, shoulder mobility, balance, power production around the hip and multidirectional agility.

3.35 The small piriformis muscle is not well suited to compensating for the larger GMed muscle.

## GMed Summary

| Athlete presents with: | What can it imply? | Likely finding |
|---|---|---|
| Swagger or pendulum gait | Faulty weightbearing strategy | GMed weakness / timing problem |
| Tight quadratus lumborum | Difficulty orientating the trunk vertically over the pelvis in gait, requiring overuse of side trunk muscles | GMed dysfunction either side |
| Tight piriformis | Faulty pelvic control on weightbearing requiring greater coronal plane control | GMed dysfunction same side |
| Tight ITB/lateral knee pain/kneecap pain | Faulty hip abduction or hip flexion strategy | Dysfunction of GMed or psoas, same side |

> ### Key Points
>
> • The gluteal group must activate effectively to produce the short foot contact times necessary for fast running.
>
> • The gluteal group is necessary for explosive lower body power.
>
> • For the trunk to perform well, it needs to be set on a secure pelvic foundation provided by the gluteal group.
>
> • Many common overuse injuries in the lower limb are associated with poor gluteal function.

## Functional Force Management and the Lower Control Zone

Lower control zone training becomes more specific once we move away from isolated muscle action and the basic elements of strength, stability and mobility to appreciate the lower control zone's primary movement roles and behaviours. These include:

- vertical force management
- support
- propulsion (forward, lateral and upward)
- momentum control
- neuromuscular response
- balance

## Vertical Force Management

Vertical force management is a measure of how effectively you are able to drop or raise your centre of gravity, and how well you manage forces that either push straight up or straight down on the body. Three key components are:

1. unlocking the hips (associated key movement: Vertical Hip Release)

2. dropping the centre of gravity (associated key movement: Natural Squat)

3. shock absorption (associated key movement: Jump Landings)

To perform any of the above components, the predominant direction of movement impulse for the pelvis is downwards. *Vertical hip release* is a small movement that unlocks the hips, fractionally lowering the centre of gravity while maintaining a vertical trunk. Although small, it is fundamental to much larger movements. The subtle action of unlocking the hips from the pelvis and lumbar spine releases tension in the hip flexors and lower back, and makes a spring action available in the hips. It creates a ready position so that the body is in balance and able to move in any direction. The movement is set up to allow for an efficient functional motor pattern, so the possibility for gluteal firing is made available.

GMax strengthening is not the key to restoring vertical hip release. The hip, pelvis and spine need to be in a positional relationship to enable the gluteals to fire, and this is set up in the very first few degrees of the movement, the *initiation phase*. It is very common to see athletes who are unable to bend their hips to even a small degree without excessive spinal involvement. They either couple hip flexion with back extension so that the pelvis is pushed backwards and the spine is compressed, or they drag their pelvis under into a posterior tilt, which consequently flexes the lumbar spine and prevents the hips from bending. Either way, the hip is unable to move independently without the spine being affected. They cannot lower their centre of gravity efficiently and they put their spine at risk.

If the initiation of the movement is tension free however, the lumbopelvic relationship is maintained and the posterior chain muscles can fire in coordination throughout the movement. Only then does strength come into play, as the muscles must be able to function both eccentrically and concentrically throughout whatever full range the activity requires.

## Personal Investigation: Vertical Hip Release

Stand quietly with feet hip-width apart. Soften your hips and knees and allow your pelvis to gently drop with your trunk vertical. It is not a big movement. Are your shoulders still aligned over your hips? They may have fallen either forward or backward without you realising. Where is the weight under your feet? Has it disappeared back towards your heels? If so, you will not have released your hips, and your body is not in balance.

Begin again, and find the centre of your feet. Maintaining your weight in this spot, soften the hips and knees again. You should find it easier to remain upright as your hips bend, and there should be little tension in your hips and knees.

## Clipboard Notes

1. A multidirectional sport coach decided to experiment with his players. To his great surprise, this small movement seemed to unlock the players, who began to move off the mark with increased fluency. The more relaxed position increased their dynamic possibilities by reducing muscular tension.

2. A keen hill walker who had experienced hip and knee pain had been taught the Vertical Hip Release as part of his rehabilitation. When making a descent down a mountain path, he noticed that his knees were starting to bother him. He remembered to unlock and slightly drop his hips, which rebalanced the load in his legs and relieved the symptoms.

The vertical hip release is a small movement which may be sufficient on its own for the task, such as delivery of certain shots in tennis and table tennis, or it sets up the muscle patterns for a larger motion. If a fast change of direction is needed for example, the athlete needs the ability to more deeply drop his or her centre of gravity. To do this well, the athlete first needs to be able to bend at the hips, knees and ankles freely, smoothly and in balance.

This is not possible when an athlete strongly couples hip flexion with back extension. This action locks the spine, tilts the pelvis forward and loads the hamstrings and quadriceps while discouraging gluteal activity. The pattern is frequently seen when athletes present with groin, hamstring and back problems. For gluteal exercises to transfer to function, the athlete needs to be able to independently bend the hips.

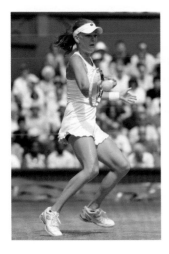
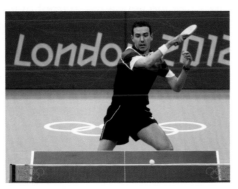

The hips are unlocked without the trunk being pulled from the vertical, allowing it to freely rotate.

**Training Tip**

It is often effective to use the Wall Squat (Chapter 6) as a way for the athlete to experience hip bending without back extension, as it a) interrupts their existing movement strategy by introducing a change in joint angle; b) increases sensory feedback to encourage body awareness, and c) reduces loading to encourage the body to release its fixed behaviour. Having interrupted their habitual pattern, this learning is immediately transferred to the Natural Squat, putting them into a functional position. The change can often be achieved within a single session, enabling a smooth progression into dynamic, full-range movements.

The Natural Squat drops the centre of gravity into a balanced position from where it is possible to move in any direction easily, smoothly and quickly.

The athlete first needs sufficient joint mobility in the hips, knees and ankles to perform the task. Then they need to be able to control their balance point. Athletes trained extensively in heavily weighted barbell squats may be able to move high loads at a prescribed rate with the feet in one place, but be unable to perform a quick, efficient Natural Squat action to drop their centre of gravity for agile, dynamic movement. A common error is associating a squat action with a balance point that is too far back. In addition to blocking dynamic motion off the mark, this also triggers excessive muscle activity around the ankle and the impression that the joints are stiff. These athletes need to be trained to effectively transfer their strength into dynamic motion.

The Natural Squat is the most direct method for dropping the centre of gravity. It involves accessing mid to outer range gluteals eccentrically at speed and being able to shift from eccentric to concentric muscle action rapidly at varying parts of the movement. During drills like Phase 4's Side Squat Tosses (see Chapter 9), the key sign that the hips are not being used fully is the inability to get the heel to the ground. Although some athletes do need ankle mobility restored to perform this properly, more frequently they need to train their dynamic balance point and gain outer range hip extensor control.

### Personal Investigation: Balance Point

First, in sitting, find your sitting bones with your hands. Get the hang of how they feel and where they are, and then stand up. Crossing your arms in front of you, place your feet hip-width apart. Feel the weight through your feet on the floor, noticing the pressure through your whole foot. Looking straight ahead, lower your sitting bones towards the floor by smoothly dropping through your hips and knees.

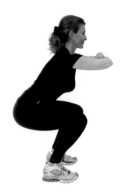

Experiment with the feeling of doing this with as little effort as possible, just dropping down as if "your strings have been cut" and bouncing back up as if off a trampoline.

For some people, this throws up the surprise realisation that if they stop trying so hard to control themselves, they actually take the handbrake off and move quite easily into range. For others, it flags up that they do not have a dynamic balance point. Most people find that they end up on their heels and are blocked by their ankles. If this is you, find the limit of your squat range, lift slightly from it, and play with changing your balance point between the back and the front of your feet.

You don't have to be stuck in your heels – whether you play football, handball or basketball, no one can move effectively with their weight back there. Find the balance point from which you feel as though you could move sideways, forwards or upwards if you choose to, but still be in balance. This point is further towards the middle of your foot.

Once you are able to do this, effective shock absorption in Jump Landings becomes easier. As with the Natural Squat and Vertical Hip Release, Jump Landings are sagittal plane activities. If you fail to bend the hips and knees in the sagittal plane, the body will find another plane to absorb the force of landing, so the knees fall inwards. Alternatively it may collapse through the trunk itself, shifting the forces up the spine in the sagittal plane. So, the pre-requisite for a good Jump Landing is a smooth Natural Squat which manages the forces in the lower body, followed by the neuromuscular coordination to prepare for the landing with appropriate muscle activity.

## Training Tip

Light, quick, repetitive springy pulsing motions through the legs in various parts of the Natural Squat range (shallow, medium and deep) help to train sagittal plane motion, progressing into light, soft jumps in various parts of the Natural Squat range. Keep a bouncy quality to the motion. Do not just practice the same depth every time – the body needs variability to best prepare for the widest range of possibilities.

### Variation to prepare for single-leg shock absorption: Lateral Pulses

Place one hand on your central chest and the other over your belly button. Perform the same light pulses as above, but smoothly move your whole body over one foot for several pulses, and then across over the other foot. Ensure that you maintain vertical alignment of your pelvis and chest – if the pelvis slips sideways beyond the chest, or your chest leads and moves beyond your pelvis, you will lose hip abductor function. These pulses can be performed at progressively deeper angles in the Natural Squat.

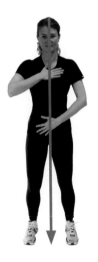 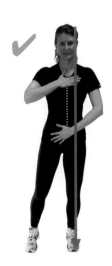 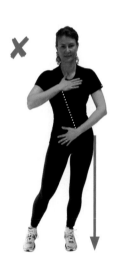 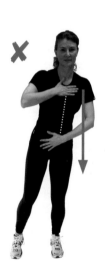

## Clipboard Notes

An international rugby player presented with low back pain associated with landing from a line out. He was a very tall, heavy and powerful athlete, and he was required to land from a considerable height as the jump is assisted by other players to achieve maximal height. He must then manage a huge vertical load on the landing.

On a very basic, low-level Jump Landing test, the player demonstrated exactly why he was struggling. Even with a small jump, he hit the ground and instantly braced his hips and knees, blocking his shock absorption. His spine consequently absorbed the vertical force, and jammed into a whiplash-like oscillation between extension and flexion. The player needed two key movement elements: to learn how to spill forces out through his legs by dropping his centre of gravity quickly through his lower control zone, and to learn how to prevent spinal buckling. Even on low-load activities, he could be observed spiking his intra-abdominal pressure with breath holding, indicating that although his suit of armour muscles were impressive, his deep control system was ineffective.

An athlete like this is often trained with high-load activities, and although these are relevant and necessary, they do need to be combined with training that ensures that the deep musculature around the spine is active and coordinated and that the force management around the area is effective. Although playing at international level, this athlete needed to:

- Learn Phase 1 trunk exercises to develop deep control of his CLA.

- Learn the Natural Squat to find his balance point and create the potential to drop his centre of gravity through the hips and knees.

- Develop the neuromuscular timing and coordination of these two components to allow him to disperse his landing force.

## Forward Momentum Control

A good, dynamic Natural Squat is also necessary for forward momentum control to enable change of direction. The body counters forward motion effectively by dropping the centre of gravity. Bending at the hip and knee to drop the pelvis shares the often quite high forces involved throughout the lower limb.

### Clipboard Notes

A junior elite fencer presented with increasing knee pain. On demonstrating his technique, it was evident that he threw his forces entirely into his knee as he reached the point of impact in his attacking lunge. Once the front foot hit the ground, the knee continued to move forward over the ankle until it reached the limit of the ankle's range of motion and was passively blocked. A more experienced fencer will actively control his forward momentum by dropping into his hip, engaging his hip extensors in outer range. The forces are then shared dynamically between the hip and knee.

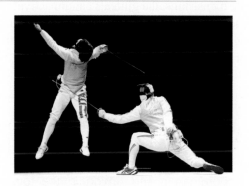
Fencer controlling forward momentum.

## The Support Strategy

The support strategy is the mechanism for managing unilateral (one-sided) weightbearing, whether it is for kicking a ball, running, high or long jumping or single leg landing. The quality of support will dictate how well the trunk is carried, and how well the athlete handles vertical force. Poor support strategy, which often shows up as collapse in the coronal plane of the pelvis, hip, knee or foot, is associated with increased stress through the pelvis and with groin, back and knee injury.

Any athlete involved in an activity requiring greater weightbearing through one side of the lower control zone, either in direct loading as mentioned with running, jump take-off or kicking, or in asymmetrical positions such as in curling or telemark skiing, requires testing and training of the support strategy. The Static Lunge shown in Chapter 5 is a classic test of support behaviour.

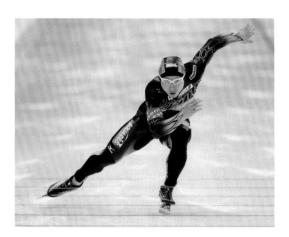

Shock absorption through a single leg requires the combination of vertical force management to ensure basic sagittal mechanics in the lower limb, support strategy to ensure that the leg being landed on has adequate control to keep forces in the sagittal plane, and the neuromuscular response to switch the right muscles on in time to prepare for impact.

Strong support strategy through the left leg is evident in the excellent alignment from foot to hip and across the pelvis. Once the support strategy is achieved, control must be further challenged by adding trunk rotation, moving one control zone on the other to ensure functional transference.

## Propulsion

Once you have achieved support, you can generate the next strategy – propulsion. Propulsion refers to the generation of forward, sideways and upwards motion. Effective forward propulsion requires a sound support strategy as the foundation for an up impulse against gravity and the ability to move the hip forward quickly over the foot. This relates to gluteal timing rather than gluteal strength. If this timing is poor, or if the body is trying to gain control through compression via the hamstrings, the gluteals cannot activate in time to engage in the movement. Many athletes seek help having performed gluteal strengthening exercises for many months with no results because the primary problem is timing, not weakness.

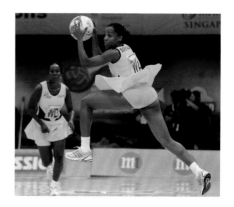

### Clinical Note

The Lunge Drive (Chapter 5) is a test for propulsion coordination and timing in the lower limb. The athlete should smoothly advance their body over the front support leg. If they don't successfully move the hip up and over the foot, the gluteals are not in a position to activate. When performed well, the final position is poised and relaxed (fig. 3.41a).

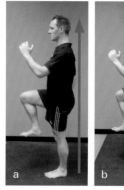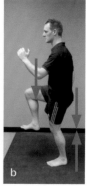

When a poor propulsive pattern is present, the body compresses and the stance leg remains flexed. The hamstring is firmly contracted and the pelvis is often tucked under in a posterior tilt. The balance point of the trunk is behind the hip, so the superficial abdominals are contracted and the toes are usually gripping to maintain control (fig. 3.41b). This pattern is common in athletes with recurrent hamstring injuries, where the hamstrings become dominant in controlling the stance leg and propelling the body over it.

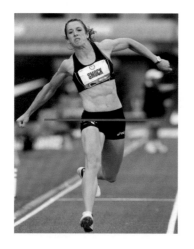

The CLA can critically affect the potential for the gluteal group to activate with appropriate timing and coordination in both support and propulsion. The pelvis provides a platform to carry the CLA, but if the CLA collapses from the vertical for any reason, it will place the lower limb and pelvis in a disadvantageous position for activation.

If, for example, an athlete (left) fails to rotate through the upper body, they may instead fall into the coronal plane. Once the shoulders have moved sideways beyond the hip, forces no longer transfer up the leg and diagonally across the entire trunk. They are blocked at the hip itself, increasing lower limb joint loading, demanding higher quadriceps and hamstring action, decreasing hip extension and impeding the ability of the gluteal group to fire. Everything above pelvis level becomes a passive weight to be carried, and pelvic muscle function becomes impaired no matter how strong the muscles are.

To restore the CLA and recover pelvic activation, the athlete must recover the movement impulse of *thoracic rotation.*

## Lateral Propulsion

The CLA concept is just as important for lateral propulsion, and its close relation, **lateral momentum control**. To achieve a good sideways or diagonal push, shoulder to pelvis alignment is critical. If the shoulders fall outside the line of the hip, the gluteal group is disadvantaged and force is generated predominantly by the quadriceps, hamstrings and TFL (and as such, more pressure is borne by ITB).

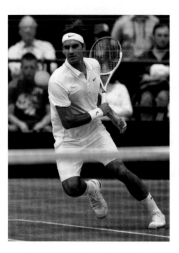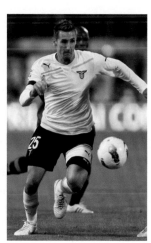

Note the CLA and effective relative position of shoulders to hips in these two athletes.

Again, the prerequisite for lateral momentum control is a good Natural Squat, as an athlete must be able to drop his centre of gravity quickly to convert forward or sideways momentum into downward motion in order to quickly change direction and generate propulsion. If he or she is not able to sit down to check their momentum, they will tend to plant the outside foot and the trunk will continue to move over it. The mind has changed direction but the body is still committed otherwise. This reduces the speed of change of direction.

Foot pressures also have a part to play in lateral momentum control and propulsion. The athlete will check their sideways motion with the outer aspect of the foot, but to break in the opposite direction, they must transfer that pressure across the foot towards the ball of the foot in order to be able to push off effectively. If they achieve this, they will create the double push, where the outside foot drives the body over the inside foot, which is then also in a position to push effectively. If the athlete stays on the outer border of his foot, he will instigate the block and pull strategy, where the outside foot checks the momentum but does not contribute any propulsive force. This leaves the inside leg to pull the body across. This strategy creates high load on the adductor group and can frequently be observed in athletes with groin pain.

## Balance

The ability of an athlete to place and control his or her centre of gravity over their stance limb requires a combination of factors. Apart from the primary balance systems of vision, proprioception (feedback from the body) and vestibular (inner ear) feedback, the athlete will need a support strategy that maintains the leg and pelvis as a secure but dynamic platform, have control of their CLA and the neuromuscular responses to make rapid, fine adjustments. Balance is therefore the result of a combination of good movement habits.

### Key Principle

- Rigidity impedes balance. Increased muscle tension is a common response when control is challenged, but it amplifies any off line forces acting on the body, creating balance problems out of small fluctuations which otherwise could be accommodated within the system.

- Soften and release tension to improve balance.

## Neuromuscular Response

The neuromuscular response will affect how well your body prepares for a movement, adapts to small fluctuations (either within the body or acting upon it from the outside), reacts to the unpredictable, and recovers from the unexpected. The concept covers a spectrum of possibilities, and we will focus on two of these, preparation for shock absorption and dealing with the unexpected.

### Preparation for Shock Absorption

For each step we take, the muscles of our lower limb must prepare for impact and weightbearing. This is a finely tuned operation – too little or too late from the muscles, and the joints collapse under pressure through lack of support. Too much activity around the joint deprives us of shock absorption.

Co-contraction, the cooperative coordinated contraction of muscle groups around a joint, is a primary mechanism for joint stability. However, there can be too much of a good thing – excessive co-contraction for too long a duration in a movement replaces the 'spring' potential of our joint with a fixed splint.

This is particularly prevalent in the knee, which creates a problem for the whole leg. The forces have to go somewhere, and if they are not absorbed in the knee, they are either forced downwards, causing a pronatory collapse at the foot and ankle, or they shunt up into the hip or sacroiliac joint. It is interesting to note that in athletes presenting with groin, hip, pelvic and back problems, many demonstrate this rigidity pattern in the knee.

## Personal Investigation: The Two-Step

Stand with your feet together and place your hands on your hips. This will help you to see whether you can keep your pelvis level. Now lightly step forward onto the front of the foot, and push back off it to the start position. The step should be light and quick, as if you had stepped on something hot just in front of you. Your other knee should also be springy.

You have two quality markers to look for. First, the step should be light, quick and springy. You should not become stuck with your weight on your front foot requiring definite push to make it back to the start position. The rhythm of the step should be even and continuous, with no discernible pause in the middle. This shows you that the muscles can work through both lengthening and shortening effectively.

Test one leg and then the other for comparative speed and rhythm.

The second marker is a level pelvis. If, as you step forward, the hip on that side pops up or out under your hand, the forces are not being absorbed and controlled in your leg. They are being shunted upwards. Although the obvious sign is a shift in pelvic position, the cause is a lack of absorption in the knee. Even if you practice pelvic control training, the knee behaviour needs to be normalised, otherwise the problem will persist because the forces have to go somewhere. If you block at the knee, the pelvis will be pushed out of place.

If this is your movement, shift your weight slightly forward on your feet and perform a few light, quick knee bends on the spot to remind your brain that the knee can move easily in the sagittal plane. Then repeat the forward bounce step as above, feeling for the same soft, quick bend in the knee.

It is not just running and jump landings where excessive co-contraction can occur. In lateral cutting manoeuvres, less-experienced athletes have been shown to co-contract more and flex the knee less than more experienced athletes, which is thought to be a protective strategy [120]. Functionally, their ability to drop their centre of gravity will be compromised, and this in turn will influence injury risk and performance.

Excessive co-contraction around the knee is also a feature associated with poor return to function after anterior cruciate ligament (ACL) reconstruction, and is thought to contribute to osteoarthritic changes in the knee by increasing joint compression [125].

## Clinical Note

Addressing coordination around the knee can start early after injury by using a simple exercise like Ball Bouncing (Chapter 6) to stimulate timing, overcome muscle inhibition and reduce excessive muscle 'fixing" around the knee. The ball introduces a modest control challenge, increasing the neuromuscular effect and integrating the trunk and pelvis with the injured leg at a very low load.

## Dealing with the Unexpected

The safety of the lower limb is also dependent upon trunk reactions. If the trunk is knocked into the coronal plane and cannot respond quickly enough to regain control, the loading angle on the lower body can amplify the forces. Lack of coronal plane control in the trunk has been associated with higher risk of knee injury [136].

### Clipboard Notes

A professional footballer had sustained a right hip injury, and had moved smoothly through the rehabilitation stages. He was managing Jump Landings and dynamic lateral control work well, and he had reached the stage where neuromuscular responses needed to be assessed and trained at a higher level.

Using Push Jumps (Chapter 5) to test his responses, it was found that pushing his trunk towards his uninjured (left) side triggered a quick response from his right trunk muscles, such that by the time he landed, his trunk was reoriented over his pelvis. However, pushing towards his previously injured (right) leg created a far greater coronal plane displacement of the trunk due to a delay in left trunk muscle reaction, such that he landed with his shoulders well beyond his pelvis. The angle of loading increased landing forces on this hip, increasing his potential for re-injury.

The rehabilitation priority was therefore to ensure that firstly there was sufficient strength in the athlete's lateral trunk muscles to reorientate his body, and then that they could react briskly to an external stimulus.

### Key Points

- The lower control zone has a number of key functions requiring an array of specific strategies.

- Regardless of how well a muscle can potentially activate, alignment of the body will dictate whether it can be used effectively. The right body part to the right place at the right time is what makes it possible for key muscles like the gluteals to fire.

- Unlocking the hips and reducing inappropriate over-activation of muscles is important for establishing normal movement control.

# ❸ The Upper Control Zone: The Shoulder Girdle

Whether you want power, fluency or precision from your arms, a stable shoulder girdle is essential to provide support and transfer of forces to and from the trunk. Compared with the pelvic girdle, the shoulder girdle is relatively delicate, but both depend on muscular attachments to provide a secure foundation for limb movements.

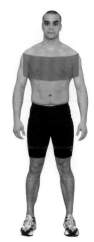

The scapula and the clavicle connect at the acromioclavicular (AC) joint, making a roof just above the ball and socket joint of the shoulder. Medially the clavicle articulates with the sternum (breastbone) at the sternoclavicular (SC) joint, joining the shoulder girdle to the axial skeleton at the front (fig. 3.45). Both joints are supported by strong ligaments.

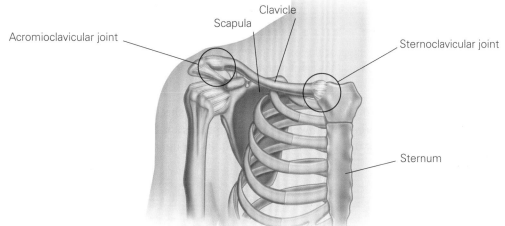

However, at the back of the shoulder girdle, the scapula does not attach to the ribs in the same way. The scapula needs to be very mobile in response to arm movements, so fixing it to the ribs with a network of ligaments would reduce the range of movement available to the arms. Instead, a coordinated muscular sling around the scapula allows it to support the arm but still be very mobile (fig. 3.46).

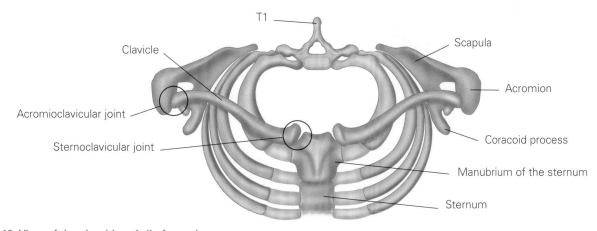

3.46 View of the shoulder girdle from above.
Note that the only direct bony attachment to the axial skeleton is at the sternoclavicular joint.

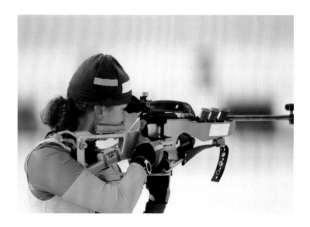

Some sports such as archery, dressage riding or shooting require a scapular position which is secure in a relatively static position (left). However, most sports need the scapula to be both *stable* and *mobile* simultaneously (fig. 3.48).

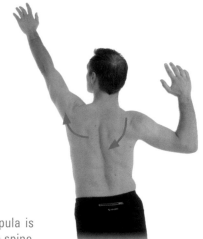

3.48 Dynamic scapular stability. To support the arm movements, the left scapula is rotating up and away from the spine, while the right scapula moves towards the spine.

Ideally, to produce or control optimum force, loading on the arm should be transferred to the axial skeleton over the largest possible surface area. The lower fibres of trapezius and serratus anterior are well designed for this function. These muscles work in partnership to secure the scapula to the rib cage while dispersing forces through their broad attachments.

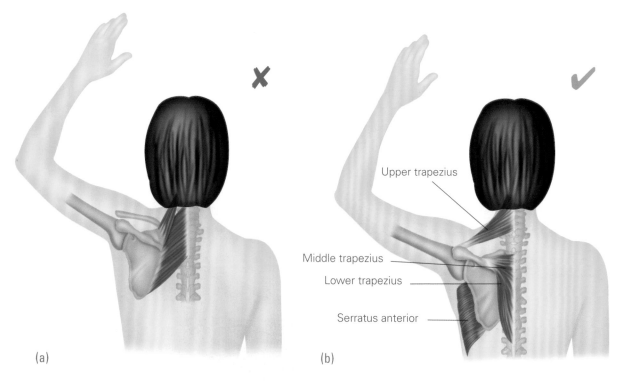

(a)

(b)

Upper trapezius

Middle trapezius

Lower trapezius

Serratus anterior

3.49 (a) Poor stabilising pattern: forces are transferred to the neck and upper back (small surface area); (b) ideal stabilising pattern: forces are distributed across a wide surface area.

## Personal Investigation

Can't feel your scapulae? This isn't unusual! Their position means that we can't see them, so it is harder to notice the effects of using different scapular muscles.

1. Reach under one arm and around to the scapula on that side. Feel the edges of the bone and keep your fingers on whichever part of the scapula you can easily reach. Ideally, have your fingers around the bottom point of the scapula.

2. Lift that arm to shoulder height. Press your arm forward without moving your trunk. Did you detect your scapula gliding forward around your rib cage? This is called protraction.

3. Without bending your elbow, pull your shoulder back as far as it will come. Can you feel your scapula gliding back around your rib cage towards your spine? This is called retraction.

4. Try shrugging your shoulder. Your scapula will feel like it is being pulled upwards. This is called elevation. You can press it downwards also, which is called depression.

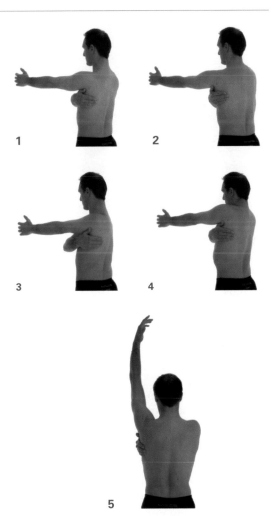

5. Put your feeling hand over as much of your scapula as you can reach. Lift your arm upwards in front of you. Can you feel your shoulder blade moving in response to your arm lifting? This is called upward rotation. Becoming more aware of your scapulae and their natural movements can make it easier to activate the correct muscles around them.

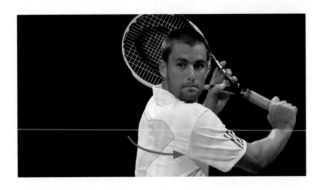

3.51 Scapula protracting to prepare for the backhand.

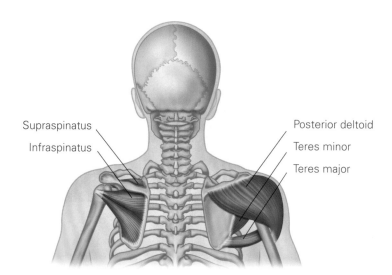

Supraspinatus

Infraspinatus

Posterior deltoid

Teres minor

Teres major

## The Rotator Cuff

The group of muscles collectively known as the **rotator cuff** controls the motion of the head of humerus, the "ball" in the ball and socket joint of the shoulder (glenohumeral joint). The "socket" part of the joint is the glenoid fossa of the scapula, so as the scapula moves so does the socket. The rotator cuff muscles act to keep the ball of the shoulder joint secured in the right position in the socket.

3.52 Subscapularis is located on the anterior surface of the scapula between the scapula and the ribs and attaches to the humerus.

The rotator cuff group comprises supraspinatus, infraspinatus, teres minor and subscapularis (fig. 3.52). Each of these muscles has a unique primary action, but they also act together as a stabilising unit. When used for primary action, subscapularis acts as an internal rotator, infraspinatus and teres minor as external rotators, and supraspinatus as an arm abductor (fig.3.53).

As stabilisers, these muscles exert a compressive force on the head of humerus to secure it in the socket during arm movements. In effect they suck the head of the humerus into the socket, providing a stable axis for arm movement. Without the rotator cuff's stabilising action, the more superficial movement muscles pull the head of humerus across the socket as they contract. The fixed point, or movement axis, is lost and the muscular pattern for force production and shoulder control altered. If the head of humerus is allowed to slide up or forward in the socket, it can press against bony and ligamentous structures in the shoulder, causing tissue trauma and painful pathologies such as tendonitis and instability.

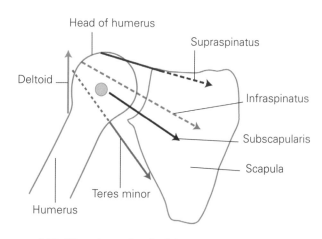

Head of humerus

Supraspinatus

Deltoid

Infraspinatus

Subscapularis

Scapula

Teres minor

Humerus

3.53 Directions of pull of the rotator cuff muscles.

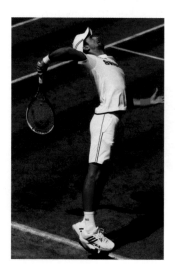

Rotator cuff training alone will not ensure shoulder health. Scapular stability is necessary to ensure that the socket is controlled and well positioned for whichever forces it must deal with. Trunk and pelvic stability is necessary to provide a supportive foundation for the scapula. If your trunk stability is poor and you have a weak CLA, it is likely that your scapulae will be dragged into a poor position. Pelvic control problems can also alter scapular positioning, either directly due to excessive dependence upon latissimus dorsi, or indirectly by failing to provide a supportive platform for the trunk.

To protect the rotator cuff, make sure that your pelvic stability, trunk stability and scapular stability are secure in order to support good shoulder mechanics prior to performing resistance work for the upper body. The rotator cuff is addressed along with scapular stability in Chapters 6–9.

3.54 External rotation of the shoulder around its axis.

# Force Management Problems in the Upper Control Zone
## Elevation Pattern

The lower trapezius-serratus anterior pattern is ideal for supporting upper limb forces, but compensatory patterns can cause problems around the shoulder girdle. Overuse of the upper trapezius and levator scapulae muscles directs forces to the cervical and upper thoracic spine. These spinal structures provide a relatively small surface attachment area and are not well suited to withstanding heavy loads. Lifting weights while using this pattern can cause stress and even injury to the neck, upper back and shoulders.

If upper trapezius is over-working, you will look as though your shoulders are pulled upwards, and you will feel tight and sore across the top of your shoulders.

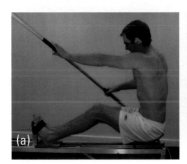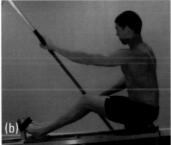

3.55 (a) Forces are supported by the neck in the weak elevated shoulder pattern, (b) forces are supported by the stronger chest wall with this secure scapular position.

> **Training Tip**
>
> Raising the shoulders brings forces above the upper control zone, directing them to the neck and disconnecting the entire upper body from the support below it. Maintain your upper body forces at mid-chest level.

The other outcome of sending forces to the neck and upper back is altered shoulder mechanics. The levator scapulae muscle, which attaches to the mid-cervical vertebrae, and rhomboid minor, which attaches to the upper thoracic vertebrae, pull the inner border of the scapula upwards. This tilts the scapula downwards. Normal biomechanics demand that as the arm is lifted, the scapula should rotate upwards, which moves the bony bridge above the shoulder away from the sensitive structures that run beneath. This avoids tendon compression that could eventually turn into tendonitis. Athletes with a downwardly rotated scapula therefore are at risk of developing an overuse injury of the shoulder. These athletes often appear to have very sloping shoulders.

## Depression Pattern

The next possible pattern is overuse of latissimus dorsi. From our discussion of the posterior oblique myofascial sling, we learned that latissimus dorsi activity can increase if the opposite GMax is weak. This can be observed when performing non-symmetrical activities such as standing on one leg or lunging. If the weightbearing side has an underactive GMax, the athlete will pull their opposite shoulder down slightly using latissimus dorsi.

Latissimus dorsi may also be used as a primary strategy to provide some fixation for the scapula even without the influence of the pelvis, especially in athletes who have been repeatedly told to pull their shoulders down. In this scenario, the scapula is pulled into depression and in some people, downwards rotation. This alters shoulder biomechanics in overhead activities and increases risk of injury.

**Key Point**

To maintain normal mechanics, it is more effective to cue young athletes to lengthen their neck or release their shoulders than to pull their shoulders down.

## Anterior Pattern

Overuse of the pectorals and anterior deltoid muscle to stabilise the shoulder girdle is exceptionally common in athletes who were made to perform press-ups before their stability system was sufficiently developed, and who perform heavy pectoral strengthening resistance exercises. These athletes' shoulders usually roll slightly inwards, giving the impression that there is a deeper groove than normal at the front where the arm joins the body.

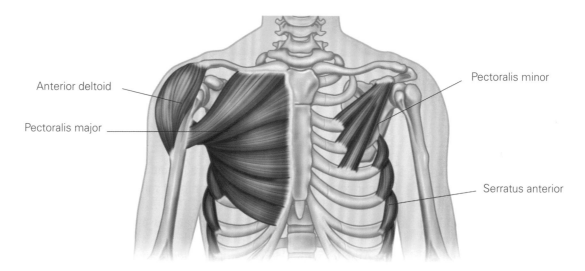

Anterior deltoid

Pectoralis major

Pectoralis minor

Serratus anterior

Chest and anterior shoulder muscles.

Pectoralis major is centrally secured to the ribs, sternum and clavicle and attaches to the humerus. It does not actually attach to the scapula and is therefore not an effective primary stabiliser of the shoulder girdle. Athletes with an anterior pattern try to bypass the scapulae by fixing their arms directly to the front of the chest wall, but as they are unable to secure the body of the scapula effectively against the ribs, the biomechanics of the ball and socket joint of the shoulder are altered.

Athletes with the anterior pattern are prone to the head of their humerus being drawn forward in the socket. This is usually prevented through delicately coordinated cooperative muscle action. If the scapula is positioned and supported well, the rotator cuff's compressive effect on the head of humerus should keep it secure in the socket. If the head of humerus is allowed to glide forward, the axis for movement is lost and the shoulder becomes vulnerable.

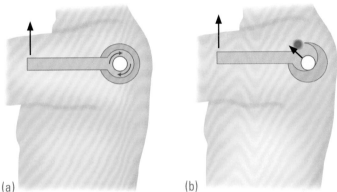

(a) The head of the humerus is maintained in a balanced position in the glenoid fossa; (b) stability is lost and the head of the humerus drifts forward and upward, stressing the soft tissues at the front of the shoulder.

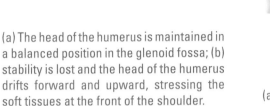

(a)　　　　　　　　　　(b)

Athletes are prone to this pattern if they have allowed their shoulder joint to repetitively slide forward during chest stretching or strengthening exercises. In exercises such as bench press, pec deck flyes and single-arm chest stretches on the wall, athletes can be observed pushing their shoulder joint forward as the arm moves backward instead of opening out the front of the shoulder and expanding the chest. This can lead to functional instability of the shoulder joint and potential tendon stress.

## Training Tip

To protect the shoulder joint, ensure that in activities where your arm is moving backwards into extension, the shoulder joint stays in position without drifting forwards. Focus on an expansion feeling where your arm joins your chest, opening and lengthening. Although this may feel as though you are not moving as far, you will be working more accurately in a position that will develop and support a stronger, more robust shoulder.

## Clipboard Notes

A world-class skier was experiencing shoulder problems in slalom. She showed a consistent anterior pattern in her upper control zone, and maintaining her arms in front of her provoked a shoulder ache. This athlete caught on to the front and back circle concept very quickly (see overleaf). She could flip between them readily, and could feel how the back circle created broad support for her arms, whereas the front circle virtually hung from her neck and stressed her anterior deltoids.

The beauty of this concept is that it does not ask for focus on specific muscles and does not pull the shoulders into a fixed position. The athlete does not have to worry about getting it right or wrong because it is a feeling that they can tap into at any time, and it can be used during general training.

**Personal Investigation: Front Circles and Back Circles (a Mind Game)**

The anterior patterner's brain is biased towards the front of the upper body and relatively blind to the back. It is possible to change this, however, if you are willing to work with awareness. You need to be relaxed to begin. Raise both arms in front of you, as if you were holding a large ball.

First, focus on the muscles on your front surface, from the palm of the hand, up through the biceps and around the chest. Feel where the support is – most people notice their neck once they tune in to themselves. Now change your awareness, tracking along the back of the hands, along the triceps and across the mid back to join up with the other side. Pause for a moment to feel this – it often feels as though your back has expanded just a little. Flip back and forth between the two circles to gain increasing awareness.

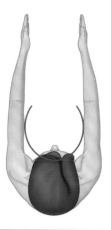 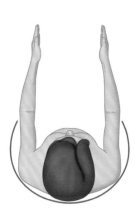

## Forward Scapular Tilt

This is a close relation of the anterior pattern. The relatively small pectoralis minor (see page 94) has a small attachment to the scapula and connects this point to the upper ribs. If you find the midpoint of one of your clavicles and press your fingers into the muscle tissue below that point, you will find your pectoralis minor – it is often quite tender! If pectoralis minor is your primary strategy for stabilising your scapula, it will tend to tip your scapula forward, raising the bottom of it slightly off the ribs at the back. The scapula is therefore not secured to the rib cage effectively, so forces must be transferred and supported elsewhere on the skeleton, with the most likely areas being the neck, upper back or chest.

## Retraction Pattern

This is usually an acquired strategy, where the athlete has been taught to keep his shoulders back, or back and down. The retraction pattern opens the front of the chest but compresses and narrows the back, maintaining the scapulae bilaterally in a relatively non-functional, biomechanically compromised position. Many people become fixed in this position of shoulder blades squeezing towards the spine, fearing that they will become round shouldered if they relax. Many trainers teach that if the shoulders are forward, then the solution is to pull them back. This does not just interfere with function of the shoulders. Pinning the shoulders back is also associated with diminished trunk rotation and less natural arm swing, which will affect running efficiency.

> **Training Tip**
>
> Whether the shoulders are too far forward or pinned back, the actual aim is to feel that the front and back of the chest is similar in length and in shape. To do this successfully, softly lengthen the spine through the top of the head and find the balance point where your weight feels as though it falls through the centre of your feet. This creates a postural foundation for the shoulders, and allows you to note whether you are shorter on the front or the back of your upper body, or whether the shape of your body is convex on one side and concave on the other. It usually only takes a small adjustment to nudge your shoulders into a workable position, and it should not provoke any sense of tension.

## A Whole-Body Approach

> **Personal Investigation**
>
> Sit in a slumped position looking straight ahead. Try to lift your arms as high as you can. Now lift yourself against gravity so that you are in a relaxed upright posture. Try lifting your arms again. Do you notice a difference in your range of movement? Your trunk position has influenced your arm movement.

Posture, trunk stability and scapular stability are directly related. A slumped spinal position and forward head posture alter shoulder biomechanics and make overhead arm movements difficult. Athletes with these deficits will react to a force demand on their arms or a body balance challenge by drawing their shoulders upwards or forward. These athletes look tense, their movement fluency is usually poor and their trunk appears disengaged. Simply telling them to keep their shoulders down will not help.

For explosive force production such as in a tennis serve, motion must move in a wave from the ground up, starting from the legs and pelvis, through the trunk to the shoulder girdle, and out into the arm and hand. If the athlete lacks control of their CLA or cannot rotate the pelvis or trunk adequately around it, they will overuse their shoulder muscles to compensate for the lack of force production. If the athlete has poor pelvic or trunk stability, they are likely to use a strategy in their upper control zone that sends forces to the wrong areas.

Some athletes have the correct pattern of activation but lack sufficient muscular endurance to sustain it for the duration necessary. As the stabilisers fatigue, other muscles are brought into play in order to maintain the position of the shoulders. Athletes required to hold relatively sustained postures in sports like shooting and archery are susceptible to this problem; however sports like kayak may provoke the same effect through sheer repetition of movement.

Similarly, the athlete's correct pattern may be available up to a certain level of load, but when this is exceeded, another muscular pattern emerges in order to cope. The increase in load may be actual weight to be lifted, or it may be the speed and complexity of movement involved. Progressing an athlete's training volume or intensity should therefore take into account their overall movement pattern quality throughout the drill or exercise rather than simply achieving a number of repetitions at a given load. If this is not the case, improvements will eventually plateau or the athlete will become injured.

Loading beyond capacity is likely to provoke coping strategies that eventually become movement dysfunctions. Loading must match the capacity to correctly perform the movement with an optimal pattern, especially in children or adolescents. This is particularly critical during adolescence. Following a growth spurt, it is not unusual for a young athlete to lose proprioceptive feedback from the spine and scapulae. If loading is increased at this time, it can result in impaired upper control zone force management and loss of integration with the central control zone.

The integrity and function of the upper control zone is highly dependent upon its integration with the rest of the body. Without a supportive pelvic platform to carry the trunk and create the CLA, and without the central control zone to share forces across the body, the upper control zone will be unable to maintain itself in a biomechanically advantageous position.

The examples that we have previously examined include:

- The importance of the CLA in reducing forces around the shoulder.

- The effect on the shoulder of inadequate pelvic support and of the posterior oblique myofascial sling.

- The importance of accessing myofascial support.

- The relevance of planes of movement.

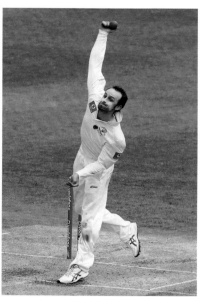

As shown here, the bowler's shoulder must be integrated with his central and lower control zones for optimal performance. Without a coordinated anterior chain, he cannot share the high forces of his action over a large surface area, and his shoulder would be vulnerable to repetitive joint stress.

Thoracic mobility is also essential for normal shoulder function. In this example, the footballer is failing to rotate his thorax to the right as he propels forward. If he did rotate his thorax, it would open the front of his right shoulder and create an effective myofascial connection diagonally across his trunk to his pelvis. Instead, he disconnects his right shoulder by rolling it into internal rotation and shunting it forward in the socket, which is stressful on the joint and ineffective for force transmission.

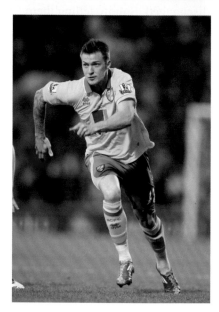

## Clipboard Notes

A 17-year-old tennis player joined the national junior tennis academy. Although she achieved reasonable results, she was technically poor on serve and ground strokes. She had unstable shoulders which she said felt like they "pop out of place," and an unstable rib that caused her pain and stopped her from playing and training effectively.

On-court analysis showed that the player produced all her power shots with her shoulders raised and pulled forward in a bracing position. She demonstrated poor engagement of her trunk musculature, and poor trunk and pelvis rotation. Her pelvic control was also inadequate.

There are several mechanisms to consider here. In the absence of a secure foundation for power generation in her pelvis and trunk, the player adopted the braced shoulder posture, which used strong anterior muscle tension to provide a degree of stability for her arms. This had unfortunate side effects. Playing with the shoulders raised disconnects the shoulders from the trunk, limiting the amount of power that can be generated and transferred from the lower and central control zones.

With the head of humerus positioned forward, it was not possible for the player to achieve the shoulder rotation required to hit an effective serve safely. For an effective serve, the shoulder needs to move rapidly from lateral to medial rotation around a consistent point. Without a secure axis of rotation, the head of humerus will shift in the socket. This player could not improve her service action without putting herself at greater injury risk.

### The following remedial programme was devised:

1. Improve central trunk and pelvic stability to give a sound foundation for movement that alleviates the need to brace her shoulders.

2. Begin scapular stability training in a position where her balance is not challenged in order to allow her to experience correct activation patterning.

3. Once scapular control is improving, begin awareness training for the axis of rotation in the shoulder joint. This should be done simultaneously with activation of rotator cuff muscles.

4. Gradually increase the balance and stability challenges, ensuring that the player does not lapse into shoulder bracing positions.

5. Strengthen the entire system while simultaneously working on rotational action in the pelvis and trunk on court.

**Key Points**

- Performance and health of the arms, shoulder girdle and upper trunk are dependent upon an athlete's posture, control and movement coordination.

- Forces from the upper limbs should be dispersed across large surface areas.

- The health of the rotator cuff is dependent upon scapular control, which should be established before undertaking resistance training for the arms.

**Chapter Summary**

- Muscles can be grouped according to their characteristics, but these groups overlap and our understanding of this will continue to evolve as more research becomes available.

- The behaviour of our muscles and their relationships within patterns helps us to understand athletic movement. If the movement does not seem fluent, or if injuries occur, it is helpful to identify the patterns that might be the root of the problem.

- Poor patterns are usually the result of timing and coordination problems between muscle groups. Muscles that are habitually underactive need to be activated so that the pattern becomes efficient.

- Understanding key force management strategies helps us to interpret technical problems and certain types of injury presentations.

- Understanding the anatomy of stability gives us a foundation to start assessing movement to see how it is applied to body control. We will investigate this in Chapter 5.

# 4 | Key Concepts for Efficient Movement

Posture
Breathing
Low-Stress Abdominals
The Listening Foot
The Relaxed Face
Effortless Control
Compete in the Moment

Big changes emerge from simple activities that unlock old habits and create a relaxed, receptive start point. The JEMS fundamentals in this chapter introduce you to your neurological body, the wiring that animates and influences all those muscles and joints. Before leaping into drills and exercises, take the time to settle into and connect with your body. Fluency and efficiency start here.

# Posture

Posture is fundamental to efficient movement but is frequently misunderstood. We often talk about good or bad posture as if there were only these two polarities to choose from, but this is not the case. Posture is a dynamic event, and we all fluctuate through a spectrum of relative body positions, depending upon our activities.

Ideally, posture is a dynamic experience, whether you are in motion or in stillness. Once upon a time, we spoke of dynamic posture and static posture, but this in itself is deceptive. Even when standing still and breathing, the body is active and moving in subtle ways to maintain your balance and control with minimal effort. When allowed to make these subtle automatic adjustments, the body absorbs your natural, postural fluctuations so that you feel balanced and still. The body is never truly static except for very brief moments, and actively trying to prevent motion through muscle activation tends to create rigidity and loss of physical performance.

Instead of static posture, it is more accurate to think of active stillness. This stable platform is created when an athlete feels connected through the feet into the ground, places their balance point centrally over their feet, and can breathe without restriction.

Ideally, in an effective posture, nothing is locked or fixed, even when you are just standing quietly. You simply and buoyantly support yourself against gravity, and allow your body structures to move and interact in their least stressful, most effective relationships. An effective posture should make movement easier, helping you to establish a central axis for balanced motion.

The traditional view of posture is one of pure vertical body alignment. We are told: "Stand up straight, head up, shoulders back, stomach in" in order to achieve this alignment, but it is costly in terms of effort to bring all these body parts into line and sustain them in this perfect position. Increasing the effort increases the muscle tension, and it is hard to move freely when everything is holding tightly. It is also difficult

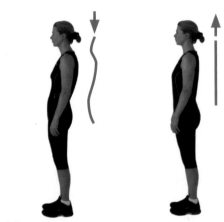

(a) Compression causes buckling,
(b) elongation restores alignment.

to translate this position into motion – you know where this position is when you are standing still, but how does it relate to sporting movement when your shoulders and spine must change their positional relationships?

The effect of effort can easily be seen in young athletes who are told to either sit up or stand up straight. They try to straighten up by increasing back muscle tension. They then can't move freely or they fatigue quickly, so they collapse into their original posture. They become caught in a cycle of straightening and collapsing and fail to achieve the central axis that would permit a more relaxed and efficient movement. Sensation has a key role to play for these young athletes.

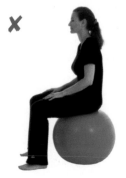
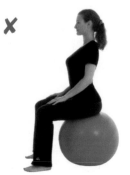
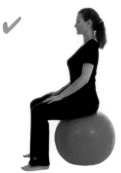

## Sensation, Tone and Posture

Posture is intimately connected to sensation, and this is a key through which we can access the nervous system. We all have a certain amount of muscle activity at rest, and this is referred to as tone or tonus. This can vary in response to what is happening to us physically, psychologically and emotionally, and can have a dramatic effect on posture. Some of us have too much and hold ourselves in tension. Others have too little and struggle against gravity.

Children and adolescents are great examples. Many present as low tone, switched off and even floppy. Their movement is non-dynamic and inaccurate in the early parts of a training session, and they cannot maintain an upright posture for any length of time, despite frequent reminders. This presentation can be quickly overcome with tone raising activities, and these involve increasing sensory input into the body. Bouncing a ball as hard and fast as they can; rhythmically slapping up and down their arms and legs with their hands; firmly shaking their limbs so that the vibration moves throughout the whole body; and practicing sharp, quick footwork, especially in patterns that require crossing the midline of the body, are all examples of sensory engagement. Warm-ups are therefore critical: planned well and executed with accuracy, a good warm-up will improve performance in a session beyond recognition.

The overly tense athlete will benefit from a similar approach, even though it seems contradictory. The key is the sensory input – if the body can sense itself, it can recalibrate its tension, whether it is too high or too low. The vigorous input creates a relaxation response once the activity is completed, leaving the body relaxed and prepared.

---

**Training Tip**

Having used these techniques with many athletes over the years, I have found a positive effect when tone calibration tasks are used for pre-activation purposes in the weights gym. Anecdotally, tone calibration tasks such as seated or standing Ball Bouncing have shown an increase in power output on weightlifting tasks such as power clean and squat in both male and female athletes.

---

## The Four Locks

Collapsing with low tone is not conducive to athletic performance, but nor is the opposite, which is creating too much spinal tension. Both strategies cause shortening in the body, and as we are learning, compression is the enemy of performance. Athletes can actively block force transmission in their bodies through an extension pattern that focuses on four main areas. In each case, the postural dysfunction is associated with an attempt to stabilise and control motion. The upper lock occurs at the top of the neck, and appears as the back of the neck, shortening into what was once known as a poke chin posture. This lock blocks neurological postural communication through the body and can directly switch off the deep abdominal stabilisers. It also affects spinal posture all the way to the pelvis, and as such can influence the performance of pelvic muscles such as GMax.

The second lock is the scapular lock, which is created when the athlete attempts to keep his "shoulders back" too rigidly as he tries to avoid a round shouldered posture. The third lock is the rib lock, which tilts the rib cage upwards at the front, and creates an area of fixed tension between approximately T9-11. This is usually a response to trying to "stand up straight". Both of these locks interfere with counter body rotation, disconnect the upper and lower body, and therefore block the flow of force through the body. This diminishes the sharing of forces over large surface areas and decreases efficiency. The compressive action at the back of the rib cage also interferes with the breathing action, making it difficult for the athlete to expand into the back and access the lower, larger parts of the lungs.

The fourth is the lower lock, which occurs at the junction of the sacrum and the lumbar spine. This gives the appearance of an anterior tilting pelvis, and creates a situation where the back extensors take the primary role in stabilising the lumbar spine and pelvis against the forces of the legs. This lock inhibits the lower abdominals and gluteals.

An example of this is runners who pin their shoulders back (scapular lock), creating spinal extension (lower lock) which in turn pushes their hips backwards. The movement impulse should be forward, yet they look as though they are running through their own resistance. These athletes should be encouraged to relax and lengthen their spines as they run, using the balloon cue described below. This restores the CLA and the capacity for normal rotation, and sets up more efficient myofascial relationships.

The postural and exercise performance cues throughout this book focus on actively opening and lengthening the spine to address the four locks and promote more effective postural control.

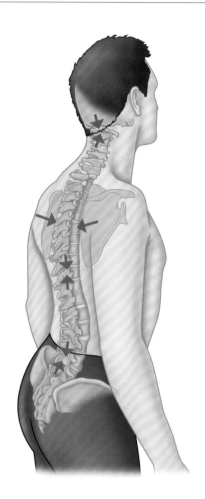

## Finding a Posture You Can Live With

The good news is that the skeletal alignment model is appealingly simplistic but not entirely accurate. Posture isn't just about your skeleton: your nervous system powerfully influences your posture, making it possible to work more effectively with less effort. As gravity presses down upon our bodies, some parts can buckle forward and some buckle backwards. Trying to pull all these parts back into line is addressing the symptoms but not the cause of the problem. Perhaps instead we could get to the root of things by simply learning to withstand compression. How do we do this? Resisting gravity can be quick and easy using neurological reflexes and sensory feedback to stimulate your posture. Visualisations and imagery are useful here. Improving your posture is not about hard work, but about awareness of a new sensation.

Stand in a relaxed, almost slumped posture. Imagine for a moment that a very large helium balloon on a string is attached to the back of the top of your head. Make it real for yourself by giving it a colour. Helium rises, so the role of the balloon is to gently lift the weight of your head up off your body. This releases the spine from the compression of gravity. Allow your body to decompress and lengthen without straining. Breathe freely now that the weight of your head has been lifted.

Now switch your balloon off. Feel how you collapse under the influence of gravity. Make a mental note of your shoulder position. Switch your balloon on again and you will find that your chest has opened and your shoulders have spread apart. This has happened even though you weren't thinking about pulling your shoulders back. Switch your balloon off again and put your hand on your lower belly. Switch on the balloon and you will find that your stomach moves inwards and possibly upwards. You have activated your trunk stabilisers without needing to think about it.

You have achieved all of this by cleverly stimulating a reflex which was triggered by your head position. Most of us carry our heads slightly rotated backwards. Ballooning encourages you to gently rotate the head slightly forward, decompressing the back of the neck and encouraging the deep postural muscles to switch on.

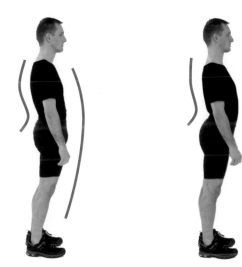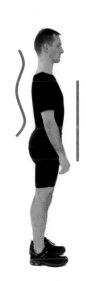

4.4  (a) Buckling against gravity, (b) over-strain, (c) ballooning for relaxed elongation.

Now we can replace the word posture with the concept of *self-carriage*. Some people can't get past the idea of posture being anything but an upward strain, but self-carriage is a more buoyant approach. Feel what it is like to carry yourself lightly.

Athletes in such diverse sports as swimming, triathlon, karate, kayak, weightlifting, biathlon, football, athletics, tennis, golf and gymnastics are all applying the balloon principle, and they are finding that it unlocks their movement and provides a balanced, relaxed and dynamic foundation for their movement. It doesn't matter what position you are in: once you learn the feeling of low-effort alignment triggered by your head position, you can apply it in any situation.

## Clipboard Notes: Movement Dysfunction

A female long jumper presented to the clinic with a long history of severe shin pain. Although she had received substantial treatment including surgery, she was unable to run without increasing her pain.

This athlete's natural posture produced an inefficient running and walking style that led to overuse of the muscles on the front of her lower leg. In an effort to run tall, she threw her shoulders back and raised her chin, which forced her hips backwards, arched her back, and made it impossible for her to use her hip muscles effectively. This forced her to overuse the small muscles of her lower leg as she tried to pull herself over her foot when transferring her weight, rather than pushing herself over her foot with the strong gluteal muscles of her hip.

By using the balloon cue, the athlete was able to lengthen the back of her neck, relax her shoulders and bring her hips under her trunk. This position felt strange at first, as she was accustomed to thinking that her slightly backward-bent posture was in fact upright. Keeping the balloon cue in mind, she was asked to simply maintain the posture and roll onto her forefeet to initiate the movement. There was an immediate change in her movement pattern. Her stride length and forward propulsion increased, and she could feel the muscles on the back of her leg, from her calf to her hip, pushing her forward on each stride.

The athlete's coach had identified a technical problem with her running style, but had been unable to change it. That style had eventually led to injury. Simple postural cueing enabled the athlete to access the muscles she needed to develop more efficient, less stressful movement.

*Having trouble ballooning?* Occasionally it happens. You may be lifting the top half of your body but disconnecting it from your bottom half. The curve in your spine appears to deepen, your ribs tip upwards at the front, and your pelvis tips in the opposite direction. This effectively shortens your body at the back and lengthens it at the front. If you suspect you might be doing this, place your hands on your rib cage, fingers at the front and thumb at the back.

When you perform the balloon postural cue, check that your fingers are not pointing upwards and your thumb downwards. If they are, relax the front of your rib cage back down so that your hand is level. Tilt it again so that the fingers point upwards. Can you feel that your whole rib cage is rotating up at the front and down at the back? Relax the front back down until your hands are level again. Picture your rib cage sitting balanced and level on your spine.

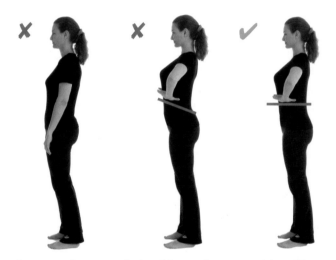

*Try this alternative visualisation:* imagine your spine as a long, sealed rubber tube, something like a bicycle inner tube. The tube runs from your tailbone all the way to your head. Now imagine filling that tube progressively with air from the bottom of the tube to the top. What happens? Most people feel their rib cage and pelvis come back into line as they inflate the inner tube, and as this occurs, the back of their neck releases and the spine lengthens all the way to their tailbone. If this image works better for you than ballooning, use this one as you move.

## Posture is Not Just About Your Body

Although muscle patterns and the way you react to gravity can affect posture, they are not the only factors to consider. Did you realise how much you are communicating with your posture? Imagine for a moment what these statements might look like in a person's posture: "I'm tired" (so don't ask too much of me); "I'm not that confident right now" (so I'll make myself a little smaller so as not to attract attention); or "Some day if I try hard I might be a winner" (but I haven't had any results yet and I don't want anyone to think I'm cocky).

Your thoughts, attitudes and mood can deeply influence your posture. Posture is one of the ways you can tell the world who you are. Decide what you want to say and wear it.

### Key Concept

Better posture should not be a strain. Allow your body to lighten up in order to decrease pressure on your joints and move freely. An ideal natural posture should be comfortable, repeatable and sustainable. Efficient posture is the foundation for movement: your effort should be directed towards your sporting activity, not just holding yourself up against gravity!

Use light, effortless self-carriage as the starting point for each exercise.

## Breathing

Breathing is intimately related to both posture and stability. As discussed in Chapter 2, the diaphragm, TrA, the pelvic floor and multifidus all work together to provide primary stability for the trunk. Poor posture may change the breathing pattern by compressing the rib cage, and influence trunk stability by altering the activity of the diaphragm and TrA. Inefficient trunk control strategies may change the breathing pattern due to recruitment of global muscles that inhibit rib motion, and this abnormal muscle activity can distort posture. A poor breathing pattern can maintain these patterns and make them difficult to change. In order to improve posture, breathing or stability, all three must be addressed.

Although we all breathe, we don't necessarily do it in the same way, and some breathing patterns are more effective than others. A surprising number of athletes have suboptimal breathing patterns, and when tested, these athletes often demonstrate associated stability or balance problems, hyperventilation symptoms or performance differences between static and dynamic situations. Without an effective breathing pattern, stability training does not produce the best results.

When breathing normally, the lower ribs should expand in an outwards and upwards direction. However, if athletes have poor trunk stability, they may try to support themselves by using their external abdominal obliques as stabilisers. If this occurs, it is difficult for them to expand the lower ribs upward and outward with the obliques pulling the ribs down and in. The athlete has to find another way to breathe, and the most likely strategy is to breathe in the upper chest instead. Physiological efficiency is compromised as the upper lobes of the lungs have a relatively small surface area for gas exchange compared with the lower lobes.

An athlete with this breathing pattern looks like their upper chest wall is moving up and down instead of their lower ribs moving in and out. They look tense across the shoulders and tilt their head slightly back, which makes it difficult to efficiently activate the deep stabilisers of the abdomen. They may be repeatedly told by their coach to pull their shoulders down, or simply to relax, but unless their breathing pattern is retrained they can't respond to these instructions. This pattern is seen in, but is not exclusive to, asthmatic athletes.

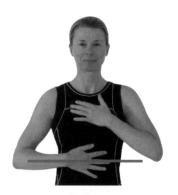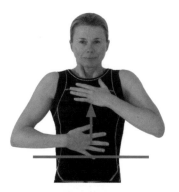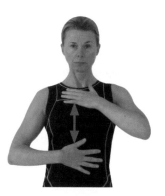

Do you know what your normal breathing pattern is? Fortunately it is not difficult to work out your own breathing pattern and learn how to breathe more effectively. Place one hand on your upper chest and the other over your lower ribs. Breathe normally and note which hand seems to move more. Now take a slightly deeper breath. If your hands move apart or towards your head, you are using a piston breathing pattern. This means that your chest wall is moving up and down as you breathe instead of expanding outwards. It is likely that you are not inflating the largest part of your lungs efficiently.

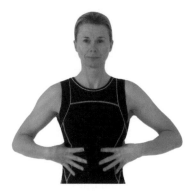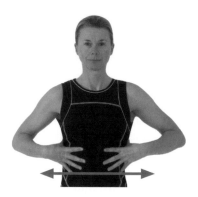

Now place your hands around your waist, and gradually work them upwards until they cover your lower ribs. Place your fingers to the front and your thumbs to the back. The space between your fingers and your thumb will be wrapped around the side of your rib cage. Take a gentle breath in. Your ribs should move out into the space between your fingers and thumb. If they didn't, it is likely that you felt your chest move upwards, or forward into your fingers. Breathe quietly and notice whether your ribs move underneath your hands. You should see your fingers move slightly apart as you breathe in. Gradually increase the size of your inwards breath. You should start to feel your ribs move outwards and slightly upwards as you breathe in, and feel them move back down and in as you breathe out.

Now take a full breath in: make sure that the ribs move into that space between your fingers and thumb. Return to normal breathing. Now focus on your out-breath. The air should move freely out of your lungs without you needing to make any effort. The abdominals should only be used to breathe out under forced conditions, such as coughing, sneezing and extreme effort. Over-using them for normal breathing will affect their normal action. If you find that you are squeezing the air out with your abdominals, move one hand down over your belly button and focus on keeping these muscles relaxed throughout the breathing cycle.

This basic breathing exercise is useful to perform prior to starting your stability programme. It helps with your posture and makes it easier to activate the correct stabiliser muscles.

## Breathing and Intra-Abdominal Pressure

The diaphragm, pelvic floor, TrA, internal obliques and multifidus create a container that controls pressure within the abdominal cavity. Intra-abdominal pressure (IAP) has a stabilising effect on the spine [49], and the greater squeezing force of the superficial abdominals further raises IAP to reinforce the spine in response to sudden load. Increasing the pressure in the abdominal cavity by breathing in or holding our breath is a natural strategy for increasing spinal stability when producing forceful movements [37]. This should only be temporary however. Holding your breath can put the abdominal organs and muscles under immense pressure.

Athletes with poor local stabiliser function can often be observed performing relatively low-load activities using breath holding and excessive superficial abdominal muscle activity to stabilise. Apart from the musculoskeletal risks associated with a faulty deep local stabiliser system, prolonged or repeated spikes in IAP have been linked to hernias and prolapses [22, 20, 29].

---

**Personal Investigation**

Not sure about breathing in or breath holding? If you're sitting down, stand up. Did you breathe in or out? Still not sure? Try lifting something with one arm. Did you breathe in, out, or hold your breath? Which one felt more comfortable? It might surprise you to discover that you breathe in as you naturally access one of your body's normal stabilising strategies.

Breathing is a natural part of movement. The habit of breath holding, however, can interrupt this natural response. Better awareness of your breathing pattern can improve your potential for stability.

---

**Key Concept**

Breathe normally at all times during your exercises.

## Low-Stress Abdominals

There has been a great deal of confusion about how the abdominals should be trained to work in order to increase stability around the central control zone. Some athletes have been taught to simply pull their stomach in, but this can lead to incorrect muscle patterning, a decrease in trunk mobility and problems with breathing. Some have been taught to brace their abdominals, and others have been taught a hollowing manoeuvre, all in the name of trunk stability.

In Chapter 2, you learned that transversus abdominis, a local stabiliser, is supposed to work at low levels over long periods in response to movement, and that it should normally activate automatically to do this. When you performed the balloon postural cue (page 106), you allowed your body to decompress. As you released your spine and allowed it to lengthen, you had the sensation of your lower abdomen automatically drawing inwards and upwards gently. This did not require conscious muscular effort and concentration, so it will have had little effect on your breathing other than perhaps to make it a little easier. You should still feel that you can move freely and dynamically. This is the sensation that you are aiming for when training to move fluently at low effort.

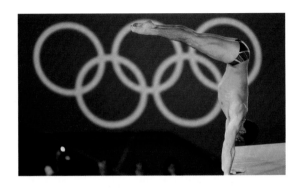

Deep abdominal support, shown here as a hollowing action with a lengthened spine, enables the diver to maintain a secure trunk and support isolated hip extension from a flexed position.

This is an entirely different feeling from that which you would experience withstanding a heavy blow from an opponent, as you might in a combat or contact sport. The more superficial (global) abdominals must react to brace the spine for impact. An impact or unexpected load can cause a sudden forced bending or twisting movement of the spine. If your ribs are knocked sideways, for example, the spine is subjected to a rapid side-bending stress, compressing the spinal structures on one side and over-stretching them on the other. Powerful global muscles, like the external obliques and quadratus lumborum, help to maintain the alignment of your ribs relative to your pelvis. Higher-load core strengthening programmes therefore have a role to play in sports where the ability to brace your body is important.

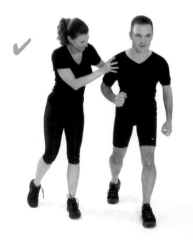
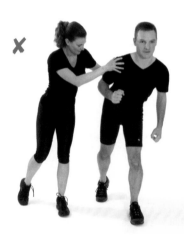

Bracing helps to keep the trunk positioned over the pelvis despite strong coronal plane pressure.

Bracing generates a high level of global tension as a protective measure. It acts like a momentary suit of armour in the face of great force, but as mentioned in Chapter 1, the suit of armour strategy will restrict your dynamic movement if this is your only source of stability. As we have noted previously, athletes in contact sports need to recognise the difference between training to brace and training for dynamic stability. Training to brace enables short bursts of high effort against strong resistance. Training to be dynamically stable fosters fluid, unrestricted movement with strength and control.

If your sport requires stillness, bracing yourself may feel as though it makes you stronger, but if overdone, can actually decrease your stability by amplifying the small natural fluctuations in balance that occur in our bodies constantly, especially with breathing. As mentioned in the section on posture (page 102), aiming for active stillness rather than a fixed, static posture allows your body to absorb these fluctuations. Achieving a deeper level of stability releases excessive muscle tension and allows you to feel more grounded. Most sports require smooth movement and freedom of breathing. Constant bracing of your trunk with high abdominal tension restricts both of these. If you perform stability exercises with high levels of tension, the benefits are difficult to transfer back to your sport. When performing the exercises in this book, aim to build confident, controlled, fluid movement.

To be functionally stable, we must use combinations of abdominal muscle activity. With transversus abdominis providing a foundation, the other abdominal muscles act as layers of increasing support in response to the loading on your body. Remember though that with a greater proportion of superficial abdominal muscle activity to stabilise, there will be a corresponding decrease in mobility. A balance is necessary.

This balance could be demonstrated in a well-coordinated golf swing or tennis ground stroke. In both of these situations, the local or deep stabilisers should provide a firm trunk axis, with the more superficial muscles taking on a powerful movement role as well as controlling the trunk through the movement.

In both sports, the pelvis and shoulders must rotate with slightly different timing to optimise efficiency and power. The pelvis actually starts to rotate forward to initiate the swing-through before the shoulders have fully rotated backwards [10], which temporarily lengthens the trunk muscles. This sudden stretch stores elastic energy like a rubber band, increasing muscular efficiency when the upper body begins its swing through. If an athlete is using abdominal bracing as his primary stabilising strategy, he will lock his ribs and pelvis together and therefore find it difficult to separate the upper and lower body as is necessary for efficient technique.

The exercises in the next chapters will give you some cues to focus on to make sure that you are using an appropriate abdominal strategy. The main thing to remember is that if you are holding your breath or working hard to maintain your position, you are not using your most efficient pattern.

## Clipboard Notes

A professional footballer presented with a history of chronic groin problems. He was a very powerful-looking player, yet on simple low-load testing he struggled for control, demonstrating lip biting, bracing and breath holding in order to perform the basic test movements. Many footballers and rugby players who present with persistent back and groin problems can demonstrate this behaviour. They may have excellent core strength and can withstand sudden bursts of force, but they lack low-load or low-threshold stability.

These athletes will often say that they know that they are fit, but yet they are always more out of breath than their teammates. In most of these cases, adding simple Phase 1 and 2 activation exercises (see Chapters 6 and 7) on a daily basis prior to training, significantly improved symptoms and prevented recurrence to a surprising extent.

These athletes are subject to body contacts of varying severity throughout a game, and it is possible that these sometimes painful knocks are sufficient to alter their muscle activity patterns. By supplementing the existing higher-load programme with low-load preparatory switch-on activities, hamstring, groin and back symptoms and injury rates decreased throughout the footballer's whole team.

## Key Concept

Aim for fluid strength and elastic movement rather than rigid resistance.

To develop deep local stabiliser effectiveness, breathe normally and use the lowest amount of muscle activity necessary to control the exercise perfectly. This can be difficult at first, because athletes are accustomed to experiencing muscle work rather than movement quality when performing trunk exercises. Remember that the deep local stabiliser muscles should give long duration support but allow for fluent dynamic action.

It is widely thought that the trunk and pelvic stabilisers should be trained statically first, usually using voluntary contractions, followed by increasing levels of motion control, finally arriving at neuromuscular reactions. However, our deep stabilisers respond automatically to the impulse to move, the feedforward action. Hence, even in Phase 1 (Chapter 6), we approach the training of the abdominals in a way that relates to the natural behaviour of the muscle, with a movement stimulus to provoke a stabiliser response, but at a sufficiently low load that the body does not need to compensate with global overactivity. You are aiming to develop efficiency. If you use high effort for low-level exercises, what are you going to use in a high-level situation?

# The Listening Foot

Balance, pelvic stability and posture are all heavily influenced by sensory information from the foot. The sole of your foot is sensitive for a good reason: it is constantly sending information into your central nervous system so that you can instantly and unconsciously adjust your body's alignment [113]. It also promotes a strong and stable pelvis in running, jumping or any other weightbearing exercise, by triggering a connection called the *positive support response*, and this forms the foundation for closed kinetic chain exercise.

When the sole of the foot is stimulated by weightbearing, it activates the extensors of the knee (quadriceps) and hip (gluteals) to withstand the load and prevent the joints from collapsing. Effective stimulation of the positive support response reflex requires the joints of the lower leg to adapt to the ground surface so that the sole of the foot (the plantar surface) can gather comprehensive information from across the whole surface. The brain compares this sensory input in order to decide where we should position our centre of gravity, so the sole is critical for dynamic balance.

In Chapter 1 we introduced the concept of functional rigidity. A functionally rigid foot and ankle complex will react to a balance or stability challenge by stiffening the muscles below the knee. This will sometimes show up as a shortening or narrowing of the foot, gripping the floor with the toes, wobbling from one side of the foot to the other, or having part of the foot lift off the floor. If any of these reactions appears, the foot can no longer "listen" to the floor. The available sensory information from the foot is impaired, so its role in balance and stability is diminished.

Excessive muscle activity around the foot and ankle usually indicates underactive gluteal muscles, which will influence propulsive power. Because of its relationship with the gluteal group, the rigid foot is also associated with groin, pelvic and lower back problems. Functional rigidity patterns in the feet and lower leg show up frequently in athletes, and are also associated with overuse injuries, such as shin splints and Achilles tendonitis.

Rigidity may develop in response to poor stability elsewhere in the body, or sensory issues in the foot itself, e.g. in skiers who excessively tighten their boots, or footballers who down-size their boots to improve their feel. It may be the result of a past ankle sprain or knee surgery, where rotational mobility of the bones of the lower leg, the fibula and tibia, has been lost. In losing this rotational capacity, the normal locking and unlocking mechanism at the knee is diminished in gait, and this in turn can create overactivity in other muscles such as the hamstrings, to compensate.

The listening foot is one of the most important components of functional motor patterning. You will not achieve good transfer of gluteal activation and strength in your sport if the information coming up from your foot is poor. This connection via the positive support reflex helps to ground you, as is necessary in golf or judo, but it also fires up the muscular chain in your legs, which allows for the short foot contact times necessary for running and jumping.

---

**Personal Investigation**

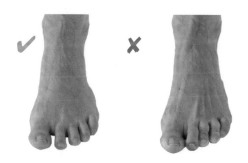

If you are not sure whether you have the functional rigidity pattern, take a look at your stance foot when standing on one leg. Are the tendons on the tops of your feet and front of your ankles markedly visible? Are your toes curling under or lifting off the floor? Is your ankle making small adjustments while your foot maintains its broad floor contact as it should be, or is your whole foot rocking from side to side? If you close your eyes, does your foot narrow and tighten? If so, you may want to use the technique for developing a listening foot, outlined overleaf. Many athletes find that they have poor awareness and sensitivity in their feet and ankles, but are surprised to find that their balance and gluteal activation improves quickly when they improve their foot mobility and control.

---

## Technique to Develop the Listening Foot

Sit upright on a chair with both feet on the floor and no socks or shoes. Feel the surface of the floor under your feet, and with one foot at a time, explore shifting the pressure from one part of your sole to another.

Now place your hands around the top of your lower leg, just below the knee. This is purely to help you to sense the motion. Your knee will remain completely still. Using as little muscle effort as possible, slowly move the pressure towards the outside of your foot while keeping the toes relaxed on the ground. You should find that your lower leg rotates with this movement. Move the pressure back across your foot the other way, and you should detect the rotation of your lower leg in the other direction.

Make this movement as smooth and slow as possible, aiming to eliminate any unnecessary tension until you can freely move the pressure from the outer to the inner portion of the sole of the foot. Repeat as often as you like throughout the day.

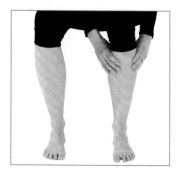 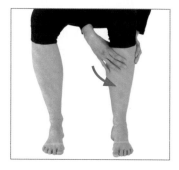 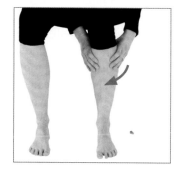

> ### Key Concept
>
> Aim for a supple, adaptable foot in all weightbearing exercises. Remember to check your foot to ensure that it is not rigid during the movements.

## The Listening Foot and Knee Health

Restoring normal rotational mobility of the lower leg has direct benefits for the knee. A small but critical muscle called popliteus diagonally crosses the back of the knee and is an important stabiliser and source of feedback for the knee in motion [100]. Popliteus is involved in rotation between the femur and tibia (upper to lower leg) which is an important component of walking and running. It also stabilises the knee most directly when its ligaments are least able to do so, the range between 30 and 50 degrees of flexion. This is particularly critical, as it is the range in which sudden change of direction or cutting manoeuvres predominantly take place [80].

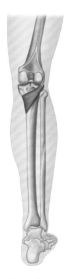

If you have lost rotational mobility in your lower leg, as can happen following anterior cruciate ligament surgery or a severely sprained ankle, it can affect the function of popliteus and alter the balance of muscle action around the knee. The listening foot exercise can help to restore this mobility, and control can then be stimulated with weightbearing exercises which may include:

1. balance tasks, especially those that involve the free limb reaching in diagonals in all directions over a smoothly bending stance knee (Chapter 6).

2. balance with a softly pulsing knee action (Chapter 6) to ensure that you are not using excessive hamstring/quadriceps co-contraction as a compensatory mechanism.

3. exercises in the 30–50 degree range of knee flexion, beginning with relatively static movements that provoke rotational control such as the Medicine Ball Square Rotation and Single Leg Balance with Medicine Ball Movements (Chapter 7), moving on to more dynamic challenges such as the Mini Trampoline Leaps (Chapter 9).

All of these should be practiced without foot rigidity.

## Internal Foot Balance

Apart from its implications for the function of the whole leg, one of the casualties of the functionally rigid foot is a seldom mentioned group of muscles called the lumbricales. These small muscles attach to the flexor tendons of your second, third, fourth and fifth toes on the underside of your foot. Weakness in these muscles changes the muscle patterns in the foot, leading to common problems such as hammer toes and claw toes. The lumbricales, shown here, strengthen and support your toes to push off in gait, but if they are weak, the body finds alternatives, such as your toe flexors and even your calves, as they attempt to compensate during push off.

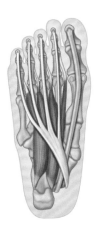

## Personal Investigation

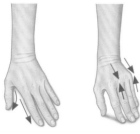

Place one hand palm-down on your thigh. Keeping your fingers straight, shorten your hand by dragging the pads of your fingers along your thigh towards your palm. This lifts the knuckles and creates a "tent" shape with your hand. Notice that you do not need to curl your fingers and that your thumb is not involved. This mirrors the lumbricale action that you are about to explore with your foot.

Sit on the front of a chair with your feet flat on the floor. Take a look at the shape of your feet. The lumbricale-deficient foot tends to look concave (hollow) across the forefoot. This may be accompanied by toes that have curled under or seem to have lifted slightly from the floor.

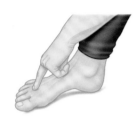

To begin, lengthen and spread your toes as much as you are able to, using your hands if necessary. Feel the joints where your toes meet your foot. These are the joints that will be lifting.

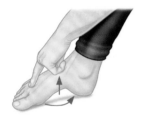

Gently shorten your foot and draw up the joints under your finger by dragging your toes in the direction of your heel. Your toes remain straight and long throughout the movement, even though you may feel the temptation to curl them. The calf and Achilles area should stay relaxed.

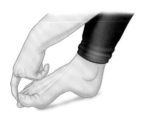

The lumbricales do not attach to your big toe, so you should be able to pick it up easily while maintaining the contraction with your other toes.

You may find this very difficult at first, and it can take practice before the body understands the motion and can relax its muscles enough to perform it. However, restoring your foot function will decrease harmful joint stress in your toes and help to rebalance the foot.

## The Relaxed Face

Clenching the teeth, biting the bottom lip, sticking the tongue out of the side of the mouth, and folding the lips over the edges of the teeth, are all behaviours that we use when we need a bit more control. We often think of them as indicators of concentration, but in fact they are telling us about our stability. These fixing behaviours appear when we are not using our balance and stability mechanisms effectively. If you are doing this as you perform a training exercise, you may manage that exercise a little better at the time but the benefit transference to your sport will be poor.

Immobilising the jaw affects the relationship between your head, neck and shoulders, so a short-term benefit of compensating for a weakness can come at a longer-term cost.

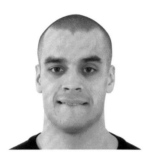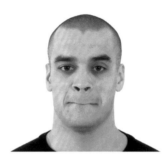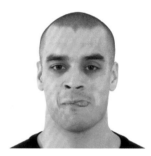

Initially, you may find that an exercise that was easy when you braced with your face (above) is almost impossible when you keep it relaxed. Be positive: now you know what your real level is and can progressively improve. To prevent facial fixing, you can whistle, count or repeat a word or phrase to yourself.

### Clipboard Notes

An international-level sprinter presented with a long history of hamstring problems. She was asked to demonstrate some simple movements in her evaluation, including a lunge, which was a part of her normal strength programme.

The athlete performed the movements well, but used firm lip bracing throughout. When asked to verbalise a simple phrase while performing the movement again, the athlete could barely keep her balance. Without facial fixing, she could barely stand on one leg, let alone perform some of the higher-level drills.

Throughout virtually all of her non-track training, the athlete used facial fixing but on the track, aimed to keep her face relaxed. The pattern that she trained off-track was not the one she needed when competing. It had just not been noticed until the injuries were impeding her performance. This was one of the critical corrections needed to improve the athlete's neuromuscular pattern. By eliminating her compensatory behaviour in order to build truly sound foundations, she went on to run personal bests without injury.

## Eye Fixing

Staring at a fixed point will help your balance as you perform standing exercises, but it will not improve your sporting performance if your sport requires that you have to move your head and eyes. Try to move your head and your eyes from time to time during standing movements to make sure that your body control is developing independently.

> **Key Concept**
>
> Aim for minimal tension in the face at all times.

## Effortless Control

Sometimes tension behaviours can be overcome with a change of mental emphasis. It is customary for athletes to perform exercises with maximal effort in training. They often display this effort visibly, even when performing exercises that are not heavily loaded. Many athletes look like they are trying hard as they train. They are then asked to appear relaxed when competing. This is contradictory.

For all of the exercises in this programme, the aim is to demonstrate effortless control. This does not mean that there is less commitment to the exercise. There should be total commitment to a perfect performance, but by aiming for an effortless-looking movement, unnecessary muscle activity can be avoided, leaving only the most efficient pattern.

**Clipboard Notes**

An elite sprinter was performing Pulley Pushes as outlined in Chapter 8. He was performing to the best of his ability and really trying hard, but he was finding the resistance quite a challenge. He felt that the weight was perhaps too great to enable a good performance.

He was asked a few simple questions. When he races, should a sprinter look as though he's trying really hard, or should he look smooth and fluent? Who wins, the athlete who makes it look hard or the one who makes it look easy? These were easy questions for the athlete to answer.

This led naturally to the next question: "Why is it that in all your training, you make it look like you are using high effort, but you want to compete looking relaxed?" This is a learned behaviour and nothing to do with the actual demand of the exercise. It also trains a different motor pattern to the competition pattern, so it is a faulty training strategy.

This athlete had developed the look of effort when training to communicate to his coach and peers that he was giving 100 per cent. Many athletes have a similar behaviour. He was asked to try the Pulley Push again, but this time to demonstrate a picture of effortless control and focused power. The athlete stepped up, performed the motion, and nearly fell over with the unexpected increase in speed and ease with which he moved. He was shocked: the weight was exactly the same but his mind set had changed completely and with it had come a better performance.

The same technique was used with a power lifter. The power lifter was using effort behaviours to communicate his strength to others in the gym. It looked and sounded impressive, and he believed that it was necessary in order to lift a heavy weight. A quiet observation was made that perhaps he might look more intimidating if he could lift a very heavy weight without apparent effort, rather than making it look like a strain. Adopting this attitude improved his technique and overcame a performance plateau, allowing him to lift greater weights. The athlete's effort behaviours had been holding him back.

## Key Concept

Focus fully but make it look easy.

## Compete in the Moment

Sometimes we forget to just move. Technique is incredibly important, but sometimes we have so much to think about that the movement starts to fragment into a sum of its pieces. We start to work against ourselves.

Train the skill components in drills and exercises. Let them embed the right patterns in your nervous system. Understand what they are all about. Be aware of these patterns as you move in training. Then integrate your brain and body by *remembering the feeling* of the peak moments that you produce.

When it's time to compete, the brain and the body have to come together. This is not the time for your brain to be analysing every movement. It is the time to be in the moment. When the drills are over and it's time to really move, *feel it*.

The concepts in this chapter are foundations for the entire programme. Keep them in mind as you train. Successful transference of your training to your sporting movement depends upon these simple principles.

# 5 | Functional Asessment

There are so many elements that could be included in a chapter on functional assessment. To gather the most specific information in the quickest way possible, my array of tests will differ depending upon the sport, and even the athlete's role in that sport. I would not evaluate a swimmer, a golfer and a footballer in exactly the same way, as they have very different requirements. However, there are some basic tasks that everyone should be able to do. The choices I have made here are based on identifying basic movement strategies. They ask the question: "How do you respond to a simple movement task?" Once you have completed these, I have added a number of additional possibilities to demonstrate how you might tailor your testing to meet the demands of your sport.

*How prepared is your body for the demands of training and competing? How well does it match the musculoskeletal requirements of your sport? How well do you manage forces?* By assessing simple movements it is possible to create a profile of your basic control. By identifying the mobility and stability demands of your sport, increasingly specific tests can be added to guide you towards the type of exercise you should be incorporating into your programme.

The components of a capsule functional assessment are:

• sensory communication and central longitudinal axis control.

• functional mobility specific to the training and competitive demands of the sport.

• function of the lower control zone and pelvic stability.

• function of the central control zone and trunk stability.

• function of the upper control zone and scapular stability.

The sequence of tests covers the basic foundations that athletes in any sport should be able to perform well. These are low-load movements designed to expose fundamental motor control deficits. An athlete should be able to perform these simple movements without difficulty. Surprisingly, many elite athletes struggle with this level of testing. Most athletes are skilled at compensating and can hide movement dysfunctions easily when performing fast, loaded or complex movements. By using simple tests, it is easier to detect control problems.

Testing for movement quality and control is difficult to quantify absolutely objectively. Rating the degree of dysfunction from minor control problems to major instability is subjective and based on experience with this type of testing. For this reason, the degree of dysfunction has been eliminated from the scoring procedure. Each test has a list of possible errors; you only need to decide whether the error is present. Total up the number of errors to score the movement; the aim is to achieve a score of zero. The higher the score, the more control dysfunction has been identified. The result should give you an impression of overall functional control.

If you have limited time, you can simplify the testing further. If the movement is performed with none of the errors, it passes. If any errors appear, it fails. Think of the tests as a series of checks that will give you an insight into your movement control.

Once you can perform these foundation movements effectively, additional movements can be added to assess control at higher load and skill levels. The functional checks outlined opposite can be used to supplement the structural and physiological testing provided by sports medicine and sports science personnel as a part of athlete profiling. As a coach or athlete, these checks will highlight areas that need to be worked on as part of training.

**Should any of the tests cause pain, seek the advice of a qualified medical professional.**

## Scoring

For all of the tests except balance, perform the movement three times and score the third one. If the pattern is inconsistent, watch a further three movements and score the most frequently occurring problems. You are aiming for a score of zero. A result of greater than zero indicates that problems should be addressed. A score of two or more indicates a high-priority issue. The total score for the selected tests can be kept and the scores can be compared when the athlete is reassessed at a later date. In this way they can be monitored for changes in their physical profile.

## Automatic Points

### Foot Fixing

As discussed in Chapter 4, an indicator of possible stability problems is the use of excessive tension around the foot and ankle. When weightbearing normally, the foot should relax into the floor with small adjustments occurring in the ankle to account for balance fluctuations. You should not see the foot itself shortening, narrowing or lifting any part of its sole from the floor. These signs indicate that the foot itself is becoming rigid in response to fluctuations in balance. This is a poor balance strategy which is often associated with decreased pelvic stability and hip control on the same side.

Note what the foot looks like prior to the test movement and compare it to its behaviour during the movement. If any of the foot rigidity signs appear and are sustained throughout the test, an automatic one point is added.

### Facial Fixing

As mentioned in Chapter 4, lip biting, clenching of the teeth, pressing the lips together very firmly, or poking the tongue out, are all facial fixing behaviours that can enhance central stability. Even if you think it is only happening because you are concentrating, it is more likely that it is helping you to maintain control. These tiny movements can subtly influence your trunk stability and make test movements look very good when in fact they are not completely sound. On clinical testing of a simple test movement like a Static Lunge, some athletes have changed from a low score, indicating reasonable control, to a maximum score, indicating very poor control, simply by eliminating their facial fixing.

The test movements are very simple and should be performed without effort. If any of the facial fixing behaviours appear during a test, it will mask potential problems, so the test must be repeated without the fixing behaviour. Repeat a simple word or phrase during the test movement to eliminate facial fixing. This keeps the face mobile and relaxed without adding complexity to the task. Whistling can have the same effect. This is preferable to the more commonly used technique of placing the tongue on the roof of the mouth behind the top teeth, as some athletes will press their tongue firmly enough up into their palate that they are able to increase their trunk tone for increased stability. If the facial fixing cannot be eliminated, an automatic point is added to the test score.

If you eliminate the facial fixing, be aware that you may shift your need to fix instead of stabilise to somewhere else in the body. You may increase foot fixing, or even stiffen your elbows or hands to increase limb tension in an attempt to stabilise. More subtly, you can even fix with your eyes: people using this strategy adopt a staring quality to their gaze. If you are observing your own movements in a mirror, you are unlikely to be fixing your gaze; however if you are observing someone else, ask them to look at you as they perform the movement as this stops them from adopting the glassy-eyed stare of visual fixing.

All of these strategies can mask an athlete's true level of control on testing. If you do not account for them, you may be missing possible control problems that may occur when normal breathing and dynamic movement are required in more complex situations. Lack of attention to detail during testing can lead to failure to identify problem areas, and this in turn can misdirect conditioning and injury prevention programmes.

### What to Do Next

If your scores are coming in higher than one on basic assessment movements, you will need to address the problems. For each exercise, a short list of relevant initial exercises is provided to get you started on your way to improving.

# Capsule Functional Assessment

This is a small collection of key tests that provides a baseline impression of your current movement readiness. It provides a jump-off point for designing your programme. The capsule tests are widely applicable, so they can be used for just about anyone.

## Section 1. Simple Sensory Communication Test

The following Simple Sensory Communication test (SSCT) looks at some fundamental foundations for movement control that influence lower limb support development. Performance in this test examines:

- the sensory communication between your foot and your central nervous system.

- body orientation and control of your central longitudinal axis over each leg.

- the ability of your body to make fine adjustments without inappropriate muscle tension, so that you can easily move your limbs independently without affecting your trunk position or balance.

### ○ Test 1: SSCT (Eyes Open)

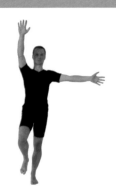

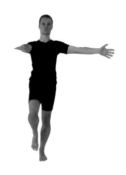

Stand on one leg with both arms above your head. Maintain a soft knee.

Move one arm down to your side and back up. Move the other arm down and back up.

Move both arms out in front of you. Take one arm out to the side and back to the front. Repeat with the other arm.

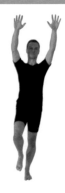

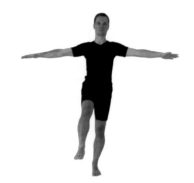

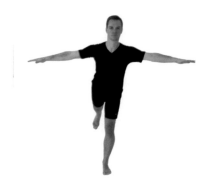

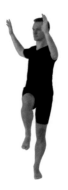

Lift your arms to a horizontal position and bend your elbows. Keeping your pelvis facing forward, turn your upper body to the left and to the right.

Move your free leg out in front of you as far as you can.

Bending your knee a little more, take your leg out as far behind you as you can.

Move your free leg out to the side as far as you can. Take it across your body to the front. Take it across your body to the back.

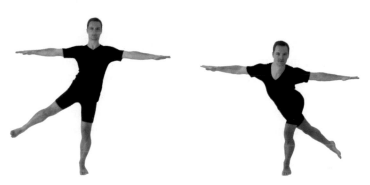

**Performance points to note:**

- Does your trunk tend to tip to one side more consistently than the other? This is a loss of the CLA into the coronal plane.

- Has your foot become rigid in response to this challenge, or is it relaxed and adapting well to your movement to help you to balance?

- Poor control strategies emerge as fixing behaviours, and common observations include adductor, hip flexor, foot, latissimus dorsi and upper trapezius tension. In each case, the adjacent body segments become locked together preventing smooth motion.

| SCORING | For both of the balance tests, score only for the worst error that you see. For example, if you wobble but then touch the floor for support, you will score 3 points | |
|---|---|---|
| | Relaxed, accurate performance | 0 |
| | Wobbles but does not touch the floor | 1 |
| | Violent wobbling or shifting of stance foot to regain balance | 2 |
| | Needs to touch the floor at any time | 3 |
| | Facial fixing | add 1 point |
| | Foot fixing | add 1 point |
| | **Total:** | |

**What should I do to improve my performance?**

A training athlete should not test poorly on eyes open balance testing. If your balance is poor at this stage of testing, focus on pelvic stability work and establishing a listening foot.

**Key exercises are:**

- Basic Balance: Eyes Open and Eyes Closed (Chapter 6)

- Progressions for balance training (Chapter 7)

- Listening Foot (Chapter 4)

- String of Pearls Bridge, Clam, Standing Knee Press (Chapter 6) and progressions for pelvic stability

## ○ Test 2: SSCT (Eyes Closed)

The body has three main balance systems: vision, somatosensory and vestibular. The *somatosensory system* provides feedback from the skin, joints, tendons and muscles to tell your nervous system where you are in space. The *vestibular system* is the delicate balance organ of the inner ear, and it responds to changes in your head position and movements of the head. These three systems work together to maintain your balance. If you close your eyes, you eliminate one of the three systems, and this exposes how well the other systems are working.

As we discussed in Chapter 3, some athletes are over-dependent upon their vision to stay balanced, which makes them vulnerable to injury if their eyes are moving or engaged in another task. Their body orientation may change quickly as would happen on take-off for a pole-vaulter. They may be quickly scanning their environment as they run, or catching a ball on the move as in basketball or netball. They may be a skier who encounters poor conditions like flat light but needs to be making split second adjustments to the surface under their feet. Vision is not enough if you are running over uneven ground: you need your somatosensory system to be very responsive in order to make quick, fine adjustments for balance and the safety of your ankles and knees. You may have to move in poor or patchy light as a dancer may have to on stage, so your eyes cannot give you consistent feedback. You need the other balance systems working well to cope with these situations.

Testing with your eyes closed can tell us a little about how well your balance system really works and how much you depend upon your eyes. Testing poorly on this can indicate an over-dependence on vision for balance, and inadequate somatosensory feedback from the body. The reflex that links hip and knee muscle activity to sensory feedback from the sole of the foot is involved in this, so problems with feedback can also compromise pelvic and leg stability.

Repeat the same sequence as Test 1.

| SCORING | | |
|---|---|---|
| | Relaxed, accurate performance | 0 |
| | Wobbles but does not touch the floor | 1 |
| | Violent wobbling or shifting of stance foot to regain balance | 2 |
| | Needs to touch the floor at any time | 3 |
| | Facial fixing | add 1 point |
| | Foot fixing | add 1 point |
| | **Total:** | |

**What should I do to improve my performance?**
- Basic Balance: Eyes Open and Eyes Closed (Chapter 6)
- Progressions for balance training (Chapter 7)
- Listening Foot (Chapter 4)
- String of Pearls Bridge, Clam, Standing Knee Press (Chapter 6) and progressions for pelvic stability
- Static Lunge: Eyes Closed (Chapter 7)

## Section 2. Functional Mobility

Functional mobility differs from flexibility in that it represents relationships between body parts rather than muscle length alone. Investigating functional mobility highlights the effect of one body part's movement on another in the movement chain so that the relationship is easily seen. This relates both to the concept of relative flexibility and also to body awareness.

The ability to move one body part independently from another is called *dissociation*. Dissociation problems can be caused by poor stabilising patterns, which do not allow you to be both fully mobile and stable at the same time. If an athlete can only maintain stability by limiting limb or trunk motion, they are in fact functionally rigid rather than dynamically stable. They may appear to have true physical restrictions in mobility, but these limitations may in fact be due to excessive activity in global muscles responding to inadequate postural or motor control. They may be fixing instead of being stable. The movements below are simple, but each one represents an important movement element. It is helpful to video the movement if you are new to evaluating movement in this way. You are looking for the ability to move only one body part, unless otherwise stated, and symmetry of the movement from right to left.

### O Test 1: Double Arm Raise — Shoulder/Trunk Relationship

The relationship between shoulder and trunk movement can be influenced by poor shoulder mobility and poor trunk control. In this test you are assessing:

- trunk stability in the sagittal plane.

- active shoulder mobility.

- the effect of shoulder movement on trunk posture and control.

The movement is performed in a standing position, and the best place to view is from the side. If you are rating someone else, instruct them to raise his or her arms straight above their head. Do not give any further instructions regarding the quality of the movement: you want to see what their natural response will be.

**Performance points to note:**
The ideal response would be to see the arms move through a 180-degree arc, with the pelvis maintaining its position. The CLA is maintained in the sagittal plane. There are several possible movement dysfunctions, which may interrupt an ideal shoulder/trunk relationship:

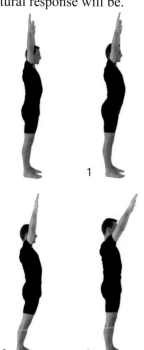

1. Forward tilt of the pelvis. This will pull the lumbar spine out of neutral into extension, causing the CLA to collapse in the sagittal plane. This may be due to inadequate shoulder mobility, underactive transversus abdominis (TrA), or poor awareness of lumbar spine position.

2. The pelvis slides forward, shifting the bodyweight towards the front of the feet and once again pulling the lumbar spine out of neutral. The CLA has collapsed in the sagittal plane. The same factors as above may contribute with the possible addition of a stiff thoracic spine limiting shoulder motion.

3. The shoulder mobility is limited to less than 180 degrees. This is not necessarily a problem for all sports, but any sport that requires a controlled trunk position with overhead arm activity or incorporates overhead arm activity in cross training will need to address this.

SCORING

| | |
|---|---|
| Pelvis level | 0 |
| Pelvis rotated forward (spinal curve deepens) | 3 |
| Pelvis shifted forward | 3 |
| Shoulders less than 180 degrees | 3 |
| **Total:** | |

**Further testing**

If you find that the performance is poor in standing, Double Arm Floor Press eliminates the pelvic component and allows you to focus on the relationship between trunk and shoulder.

**What should I do to improve my performance?**

- Floor Press (Chapter 6)

- Greyhound (Chapter 6)

- Wall Press (Chapter 6)

- Latissimus Dorsi Stretches (Chapter 10)

---

### Clinical Note

In addition to these motor control exercises, soft tissue release of the muscles that restrict upward shoulder movement is advised where muscle shortening limits range of movement. The new shoulder mobility must be integrated with the trunk for functional carry over. Greyhound in Chapter 6 is a good start point.

---

## ○ Test 2: Seated Hamstring Test — Hamstring/Trunk Relationship

Hamstring tightness is often blamed for lower/back pain, and in many sports is thought to impact on performance. However, proprioceptive awareness of lumbar position and the ability to control it also play a part. This test was originally developed for sprint kayak, football and martial arts, but has become a useful marker for any sport as it demonstrates available hamstring length against a neutral spinal position as well as proprioceptive problems in the lumbar spine. Performance in this test examines:

- active hamstring length.

- trunk proprioception and control (how well the trunk supports itself against a lengthening hamstring).

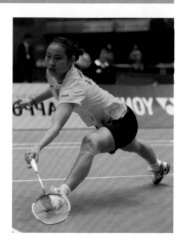

Sit on a chair with your foot on the front of a Swiss Ball. Sit up onto your sitting bones so that your spine is in neutral. Maintain this spinal position and push the ball out away from you until you feel the limit imposed by your hamstrings.

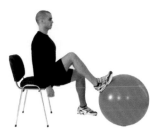 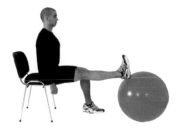

**Performance points to note:**

An ideal performance will show an athlete who can maintain a neutral spine with their leg straight and hip at 90 degrees. The problems associated with this movement will be:

1. Your pelvis slips into backward rotation before the hamstrings reach a tension point. This indicates poor proprioception and control around the spine.

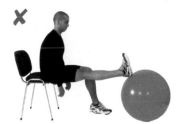

2. You cannot straighten your knee. This indicates hamstring length restriction.

3. You slip into backward pelvic rotation once the hamstrings are under tension. This indicates greater relative flexibility in the spine than in the hamstrings.

4. You tip your pelvis sideways to relieve the pressure on your hamstrings.

| SCORING | | |
|---|---|---|
| Neutral spine is maintained | 0 | |
| Spinal position is lost at any time | 3 | |
| Knee fully straightens | 0 | |
| Knee cannot straighten | 2 | |
| **Total:** | | |

**What should I do to improve my performance?**

• Straight-up Hamstring Mobility (Chapter 6)

• Standing Leg Swing (Chapter 6)

• Tail-up (Chapter 9)

• any trunk stability exercise in an unsupported neutral spine position, e.g. Wall Press and Ball Bouncing (Chapter 6) or, at a more advanced level, OTT (Chapter 7)

## ○ Test 3: Total Body Rotation

This movement looks at the total available rotation from the foot to the top of the spine. Few sports require only one body part to rotate. Usually rotation occurs as a result of many parts contributing to the total motion. Coordinated multi-joint motion is also necessary to maintain balance and postural control as the head moves [107]. In the more comprehensive Functional Mobility Testing section (page 152), tests to examine each component are available. Performance in this test examines:

• total joint rotation availability from foot to head.

• correct foot pressure changes in response to rotation.

Stand with feet hip-width apart. Turn and look behind you, noting a spot that you can comfortably see. Do not strain yourself. The test seeks to determine what movement is naturally available to you. Turn back around the other way, noting a spot that you can comfortably see.

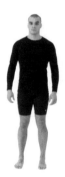 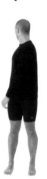 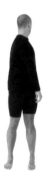

Once you have noted how much motion is available, turn your attention to your feet. Note the pressure changes in your feet as you turn. It should follow the same pattern: as you turn to the left, the left foot pressure moves towards the outer part of the foot, and the right foot pressure moves to the inner part of the foot. In other words, the pressure moves in the direction of the turn.

**Performance points to note:**

1. Note whether the feet alter their pressure in the correct pattern.

2. Note whether rotation is markedly restricted in one direction.

**Scoring:** Imagine standing in the middle of a circle and that circle is cut in half from front to back. Each of these halves will be divided into three even slices.

You will take your position measurement from where your nose is pointing.

| SCORING | | |
|---|---|---|
| | Head position is limited to the first 1/3 | 3 |
| | Head position reaches the second 1/3 | 2 |
| | Incorrect foot pressure response | 3 |

## Section 3. The Lower and Central Control Zones — Pelvic and Trunk Stability Relationship

### ○ Test 1: Static Lunge (Eyes Open)

The Static Lunge is the least complex of the lunge group of exercises and is therefore suitable as a baseline assessment. It is alternatively known as the *Split Squat*, but considering it as a Static Lunge establishes it as the starting point for a clear path of progression.

The Static Lunge is used instead of the commonly used Single Leg Squat as a baseline test because it reduces the weightbearing load requirement of the test leg. This means that the neuromuscular pattern and coordination is examined more clearly without strength issues being an obscuring factor.

If an athlete fails at this level, they will need a supported level of exercise in order to establish the coordination, timing and patterning of the movement. They can then strengthen into the movement. If they pass at this level, they can move on to more highly loaded assessments.

The Static Lunge gives insight into:
• pelvic stability: the support strategy.

• eccentric GMax activation through range.

• loaded functional hip mobility through range.

• control of the leg between the hip, knee and foot.

• central axis control for the trunk.

• basic balance.

Stand with one foot in front of the other, hip-width apart. Raise your back heel. Put your arms straight out to the side. Keeping a vertical trunk, drop your pelvis straight towards the floor until your knee approaches 90 degrees of flexion. Your body weight should not be moving forward. Your back knee should move straight to the floor.

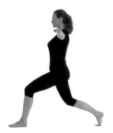 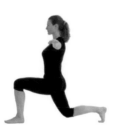 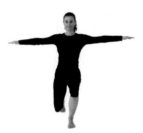

**Clinical Note**

The most critical problems with coordination of the required muscle action in this test occur in the first half of the movement. This means that if the person to be tested does not have sufficient strength to perform the full movement, as they may be when recovering from injury, their support strategy can still be assessed through a smaller range of motion.

Strength comes into play the further into range you move. If the early part of the movement is good, but control is lost when the lunge is at its deepest point (the mid to outer range) eccentric strength of GMax will be a training priority.

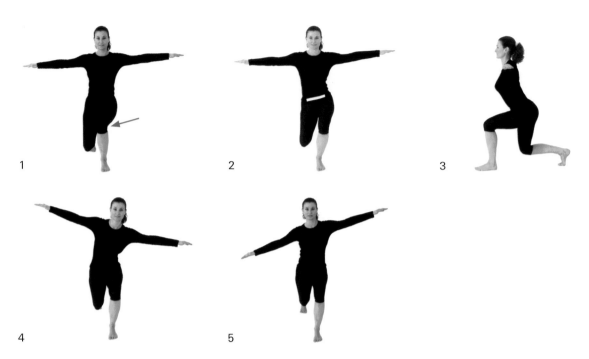

**What would a poor performance look like?**

1. Knee moves inwards. If this is the case, it is unlikely that GMax and GMed are functioning correctly.

2. Pelvis tips sideways. This demonstrates loss of control in the coronal plane for the pelvis, and indicates a GMed dysfunction.

3. Hips move backwards. This may appear as the lumbar spine deepening its curve when observed from the side, and indicates that GMax is either not functioning well eccentrically (as it lengthens), or functions poorly in outer range (when it is longest). Instead of the hip moving downwards, it is moved backwards where it is easier to access the back extensors and hamstrings to assist.

4. Trunk tips sideways. This demonstrates a loss of central axis control.

5. One arm drops lower than the other. This may indicate a dependence on latissimus dorsi on that side.

| SCORING | | |
|---------|---|---|
| Knee moves inwards | 3 | |
| Pelvis tips sideways | 3 | |
| Hips move backwards (lumbar curve deepens) | 3 | |
| Trunk tips sideways | 3 | |
| One arm drops lower than the other | 3 | |
| Lip biting or facial fixing | 1 | |
| Foot fixing | 1 | |
| **Total:** | | |

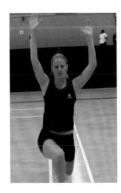

This athlete is performing a Static Lunge poorly. The pelvis has tipped downwards on the left and the knee has moved inwards. Note that the left hand is lower than the right with the elbow bent. She is trying to use her left latissimus dorsi to compensate for poor right gluteal activation.

## ○ Test 2: Static Lunge (Eyes Closed)

The Static Lunge (Eyes Open) tests whether the pelvic stabiliser muscles are capable of controlling the movement, and looks at the relationship between sensory feedback and pelvic control. The procedure here is exactly as Test 1, only with the eyes closed.

| SCORING | | |
|---|---|---|
| Knee moves inwards | 3 | |
| Pelvis tips sideways | 3 | |
| Hips move backwards (lumbar curve deepens) | 3 | |
| Trunk tips sideways | 3 | |
| One arm drops lower than the other | 3 | |
| Lip biting or facial fixing | 1 | |
| Foot fixing | 1 | |
| **Total:** | | |

### Clinical Note

If an athlete presents with latissimus dorsi tightness that does not resolve with soft tissue treatment, it is worth using the Static Lunge test to assess whether the arm drops or trunk tips, indicating latissimus activity as a stabiliser. The athlete may need pelvic control work to resolve the issue.

**What should I do to improve my performance?**

- String of Pearls Bridge, Hip Pops, Hip Swivels (Chapter 6)
- Clam, Standing Knee Press (Chapter 6)
- Supported Lunge (Chapter 7)
- Lunge progressions (Chapter 7)

## ○ Test 3: Dynamic Lunge

Testing both Static and Dynamic Lunges is often questioned. Why not just test the higher level? The issue is one of specificity. The Static Lunge tests the support strategy in its best-case scenario: the movement is not complex and the body is not translating over the ground. It simply identifies whether the muscle coordination, control and strength in the necessary range is available to provide support. The Dynamic Lunge brings a whole new element into play; that of preparation. Where the Static Lunge identifies that the support strategy is accessible and the muscles are able to activate appropriately, the Dynamic Lunge tests whether they can do so in time to prepare for weightbearing. It is the neuromuscular extension of the more basic test.

This clarifies the action plan. If the Static Lunge is sound but the Dynamic Lunge is poor, then neuromuscular (feedforward) drills such as the two-step from Chapter 3 are the priority. They teach the leg to prepare and shock absorb, and to coordinate the knee with the hip. If the Static Lunge is poor, the pattern is not available in the first place. Early activation and strength through range are necessary. Exercises like the Supported Lunge will be an appropriate start point.

By understanding the different features of the two movements, your testing will generate the most appropriate action plan. In addition to the behaviour of the hip and knee, the Dynamic Lunge examines the effectiveness of the athlete's total body management. The trunk should be carried in balance, requiring low-threshold control, proprioception and a sense of verticality. In the stepping leg, the athlete must absorb forces in the hip as it bends into the lunge, allowing the full foot to contact the floor. If the hip timing is off, or the athlete cannot use their hip extensors eccentrically into sufficient hip flexion range at the higher speed required by the Dynamic Lunge, forward motion will not be contained. The athlete will end up on the front of their foot, the heel will lift and their calf will be working hard. The forward force increases the load on the knee, and decreases the ability to perform a return motion without using the trunk to drive backwards.

Performance in this test therefore examines:

- higher-level trunk control and proprioception as the trunk is carried by the pelvis over the ground.

- neuromuscular preparation for support.

- the ability of the athlete to push effectively from the leg instead of throwing the shoulders back to generate momentum.

Start standing straight with feet together and arms straight above your head. Step forward into a lunge while maintaining an upright trunk, then push back to the start position. When moving back to the start position, check that the motion is initiated from the foot, not by driving the shoulders back to generate momentum.

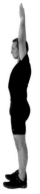
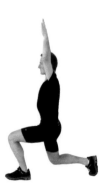

| | | |
|---|---|---|
| **SCORING** | Knee moves inwards | 3 |
| | Pelvis tips sideways | 3 |
| | Hips move backwards (lumbar curve deepens) | 3 |
| | Trunk tips sideways | 3 |
| | Trunk collapses forward | 3 |
| | Front heel lifts from floor | 3 |
| | Moving shoulders back initiates return to start position | 3 |
| | Lip biting or facial fixing | 1 |
| | Foot fixing | 1 |
| | **Total:** | |

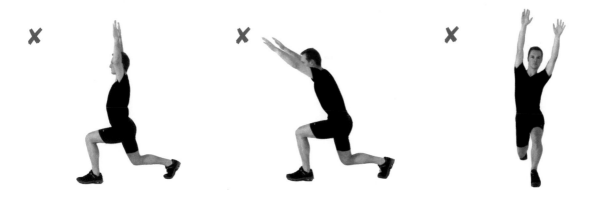

This test can also be performed with the eyes closed, for the same reasons as mentioned for the Static Lunge.

### What should I do to improve my performance?

• The Two-Step (Chapter 3) for neuromuscular preparation

• Wall Press (Chapter 6) for trunk proprioception

• Overhead lunge holding horizontal stick stretched above the head, focusing on pressing up on the collapsing side (an adaptation of Chapter 7's Lunge exercise progressions)

## ○ Test 4: Lunge Drive

The Lunge Drive is a test of the forward propulsion strategy as needed in running and bounding. It examines the coordination and timing of the hip over the foot.

Start in a split stance, with both hips and knees bent. The back heel is lifted from the floor. Right leg is forward and left arm is forward. Move the body forward onto the forward stance leg, lifting the left knee and reversing the arms.

The trunk should be carried smoothly forward and upward over the foot, and the end position for the stance leg should be long and straight through the hip and knee. The balance point is directly over the foot and there is no excessive muscle activity in any one area. When performed well, the final position is poised and relaxed. When a poor propulsive pattern is present, the body compresses and the hip and knee remain flexed, the hamstring is firmly contracted, and the pelvis is often tucked under in a posterior tilt. The balance point of the trunk is behind the hip so the superficial abdominals are contracted and the toes are usually gripping to maintain control.

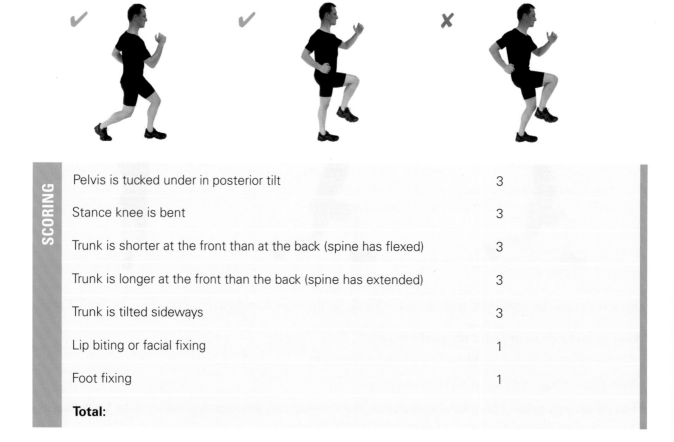

| SCORING | | |
|---|---|---|
| Pelvis is tucked under in posterior tilt | 3 |
| Stance knee is bent | 3 |
| Trunk is shorter at the front than at the back (spine has flexed) | 3 |
| Trunk is longer at the front than the back (spine has extended) | 3 |
| Trunk is tilted sideways | 3 |
| Lip biting or facial fixing | 1 |
| Foot fixing | 1 |
| **Total:** | |

### What should I do to improve my performance?

There are several factors involved in this test:

- The support strategy: if your Static Lunge test is poor, your support leg will not accept weight effectively as the hip carries the body up over the foot. Address this first

- To improve hip timing from flexion to extension, use Ski Jumper (Chapter 7)

- You may need to improve the hip bending action on the lifting side. See Seated Knee Lift clarifying test

## ○ Test 5: Natural Squat

The subject of squatting seems to provoke much debate which largely revolves around the loaded barbell squat. However, in Chapter 3, I introduced the Natural Squat as a key movement for agility and shock absorption that demonstrates that the athlete can drop and recover their centre of gravity smoothly and easily. My emphasis is therefore on the balance point for the body weight and the ease of joint motion.

Apart from snatching, it is rare to need your arms fully stretched upwards while you are in deep squat. The priority movement I need to assess in most of my athletes is whether they can compress the three-joint spring of the ankle, knee and hip in balance: that is the purpose of the Natural Squat test. (As an aside: if an athlete needs to achieve a squat position with his arms overhead as he would with Olympic lifting, then test appropriately and differentiate out the mobility components of shoulder and spinal restriction.)

As previously noted in Chapter 2, mobility needs to be available before it can be functional. Sometimes a movement dysfunction can appear significant, but it is simply the body accommodating a single joint restriction. Symmetry and motion availability in the ankle, knee and hip are necessary for a full, evenly weightbearing Natural Squat.

Take up a position with your feet just a little more than hip-width apart, and arms folded in front of you at shoulder height. Feet face forward with no more than a five-degree turn out. It is a great deal easier to perform this movement with feet facing further outwards, but again, this is not about how much load you can push in a static position. Imagine you are a skier who has to land a jump – it won't work if your skis are pointing away from each other.

Keeping the elbows up, sit down into your feet. Aim towards a horizontal thigh. Hips, knees and ankles should remain aligned. Your feet should neither roll inwards nor outwards. The movement impulse should clearly be *downwards* in a concertina-like folding of hip, knee and ankle. There should not be greater forward displacement of the trunk than downward displacement of the pelvis.

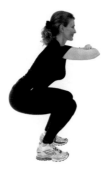 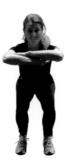

Think of the pelvis as an elevator carrying the trunk down and then back up. The shape of the trunk changes very little. However, if the pelvis halts its downward progression, the spine in many cases continues the motion by folding into flexion (forward curl) or compressing into extension (excessive lumbar curve). The pelvis should also lower centrally between the two legs. A pelvis that deviates to one side indicates uneven weightbearing or a joint restriction in hip, knee or ankle. The mobility in these joints should be checked in this case. Ultimately you are aiming to feel balanced and capable of moving in any direction.

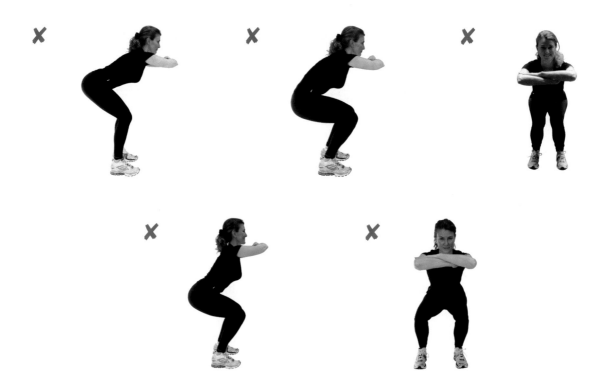

| SCORING | | |
|---|---|---|
| Thigh does not reach a horizontal position | 3 | |
| Knees and ankles collapse inwards or outwards | 3 | |
| Angle of trunk tilts too far forward | 3 | |
| Change in trunk shape, either into flexion or extension | 3 | |
| The pelvis does not sit centrally between the legs | 3 | |
| Balance point is in heels | 3 | |
| Facial fixing | 1 | |
| **Total:** | | |

### What should I do to improve my performance?

There are several factors involved in this test:

- Balance Point practise (Chapter 3)
- Wall Squat (Chapter 6)

## ○ Test 6: Standing Knee Lift

Performance in this test examines:

- the ability to easily position the CLA over each stance leg indicating predominantly coronal plane control of thorax on pelvis.

- lateral pelvic stability.

- the foot-hip connection for support.

- the hip flexion pattern.

Stand with feet together and arms out to the side at shoulder height. Lift one knee to hip height. Replace the foot and swap sides. It is most useful to alternate sides on each repetition. This exposes issues and makes them easier to see.

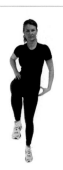

### Technical Note

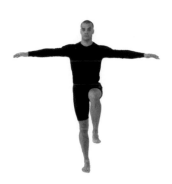

It has been noted that elite athletes slightly elevate their pelvis on the lifting (flexing) side in sprinting [8]. This allows the athlete to advance the pelvis on that side smoothly by minimising soft tissue resistance, and enhances push-off on the stance side. Although this is spoken of as a locking of the stance side for push-off, I consider it to be just as much an unlocking motion to allow the pelvis to advance. This positive pelvic elevation should not be confused with a hip hitch.

Normal, positive pelvic elevation on the lifting side does not pull the trunk into side-bending. On your stance leg, the greater trochanter (the bone that you can feel on the side of your hip) remains aligned with the ridge of your pelvic bone (the iliac crest). Hip hitching on the other hand tends to pull the greater trochanter significantly under the pelvis on the stance side and shortens your trunk on the lifting side as the pelvis is dragged upwards. Vertical alignment is lost.

Practically, just aim to press out strongly with your stance leg into the floor while maintaining an upward impulse through your spine as you lift your other leg. This is more likely to bring about a sound pattern than trying to find the ideal amount of pelvic lift.

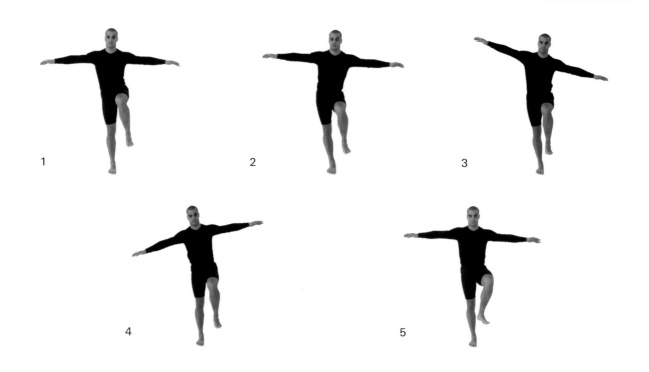

**Performance points to note:**

1. Hip hitching. This is a fault in the hip flexion pattern. Instead of lifting your leg cleanly in the sagittal plane while maintaining your CLA, you hitch the pelvis upwards, shortening your side and creating spinal side-bending.

2. Stance hip moves out to the side. The pelvis should remain straight and level throughout this movement; however, if GMed is weak, it will not keep a firm control over the femur-to-pelvis relationship. This either appears as the pelvis dropping on the lifting side or permitting the hips to drift sideways. An athlete showing this response may find that driving sideways off this leg, landing on it or jumping off it is slower or less powerful than the other side.

3. One arm moves lower. This indicates possible use of latissimus dorsi to compensate for decreased trunk or pelvic stability.

4. Trunk tips sideways. This loss of the central axis is usually a compensatory response to loss of pelvic position but can also indicate that the body is not well balanced over the stance side.

5. Leg does not lift straight. Weakness in iliopsoas may cause you to recruit other muscles to flex the hip.

6. Lifting the leg causes the spine to extend.

7. Lifting the leg causes the spine to flex.

**SCORING**

| | |
|---|---|
| Hip hitches up on the lifting side/trunk shortens on that side | 3 |
| Stance hip moves out to the side | 3 |
| One arm moves lower | 2 |
| Trunk tips sideways | 3 |
| Leg does not lift straight | 2 |
| Spine extends | 3 |
| Spine flexes | 3 |
| Facial fixing | 1 |
| Foot fixing | 1 |
| **Total:** | |

---

**Clinical Note**

If the athlete presents with persistent quadratus lumborum tightness, it is worth testing to see if they use hip hitching in association with hip flexion. This may be a contributing factor.

---

**What should I do to improve my performance?**

A stance leg problem is a support issue:

- Clam, Standing Knee Press (Chapter 6)

- String of Pearls Bridge, Hip Pops, Hip Swivels (Chapter 6)

- Supported Lunge (Chapter 7)

- Lunge progressions (Chapter 7) particularly with your arms stretched upwards to improve the CLA and minimise the effect of latissimus dorsi overuse

Although this test is often thought of in terms of the stance leg, it can flag either stance leg problems (support), or lifting leg problems (control of the trunk against hip flexion). To differentiate between an issue in the stance leg or the moving leg, first assess the support behaviour by testing Static Lunge. If the lunge is sound, it is less likely that the problem is primarily support in the stance leg.

To further examine the hip flexion pattern, use the Seated Knee Lift test overleaf. Sitting diminishes the weightbearing component, so the test can focus more on the effect of leg loading on the trunk. If this provokes a higher score, then your priority is development of the hip flexion control. If instead the movement pattern is improved, then your priority will be on support and pelvic control.

---

○ **Clarifying Test: Seated Knee Lift — Trunk Control Against Hip Flexion**

Many athletes experience the sensation of tightness in their hip flexors. Usually we tend to think of stretching a tight muscle, but what if stretching doesn't seem to help?

If your trunk stability is poor, you may use your hip flexors to enhance control. Constant activity of the hip flexors in a stabilising role can cause the perception of tightness in the hip, but unless you improve your central control, the hip flexors will continue to work in this way, making stretching ineffective. It also means that the hip flexors may not contract effectively through the full range. Your hip flexion action may actually be quite weak, especially if your trunk is not sufficiently stable to support a strong hip flexion action (i.e. does not provide an adequate fixed point for muscles to pull from). Even international-level competitors have had to start with this most basic of exercises to establish a normal relationship between the trunk and hip flexors.

This test also enables you to see whether you can achieve a straight hip flexion action. There are a number of muscles that contribute to hip flexion, and each can pull in a slightly different direction. If you find as a cyclist that one knee is always closer to the cross bar, or as a runner that one foot always seems to place itself too far under your body, this may apply to you.

Sit on the front of a chair with both feet on the floor hip-width apart. Make sure you are sitting directly on your sitting bones. Lift both arms out to the side until they are level with your shoulders; this will help you to monitor your trunk position. Relax your breathing. Keeping your weight evenly pressing through both of your sitting bones, lift one knee and hold it in this position for 5 seconds. Your arms should not have moved, and you should see no visible abdominal activity occurring. Check that you can still breathe by expanding your lower ribs. Your knee should be in line with your hip. Your lower leg should hang straight to the floor without turning.

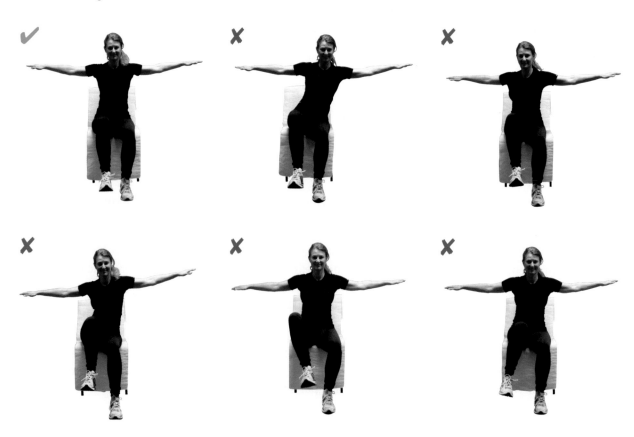

**Performance points to note:**

- Your ribs draw downwards and inwards. This suggests that you are overusing your oblique abdominals.

- Your trunk shifts sideways. Coronal plane collapse is due to poor stability.

- Your trunk shortens on the lifting side. Coronal plane collapse due to poor stability.

- You collapse your trunk forward. This is a sagittal plane collapse.

- Your belly button turns towards the lifting leg. This is a transverse plane collapse.

| SCORING | | |
|---|---|---|
| Ribs draw downwards/trunk tips forward | 3 |
| Trunk tips sideways away from lifting leg | 3 |
| Belly button turns towards the lifting leg | 3 |
| Trunk shortens on lifting side | 3 |
| Leg does not lift straight | 3 |
| Facial fixing | 1 |
| Foot fixing | 1 |
| **Total:** | |

**What should I do to improve my performance?**

- Greyhound (Chapter 6) to learn to flex the hip cleanly against a controlled trunk

- Seated Knee Lift (Chapter 6) to increase load on the hip/trunk relationship

- Pelvic Side Tilts (Chapter 5) to lengthen through the side of the trunk

If the score is low, you may progress to the next test.

## ○ Test 7: Seated Knee Lift on a Ball

The Seated Knee Lift on a Ball is quite a sensitive test which examines trunk control and vertical alignment of the trunk on the pelvis. It will highlight any asymmetry in weightbearing between the left and right sides of the pelvis as well as control of the CLA.

Performance in this test examines:

• trunk control.

• vertical alignment of the trunk on the pelvis and control of the CLA in all planes.

• symmetry of weightbearing through left and right sides of the pelvis.

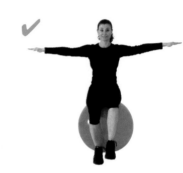

Sit on a Swiss Ball with your hips and knees at approximately 90 degrees and your feet together flat on the floor. Position your arms so that they are parallel to the floor. Maintaining an upright trunk, lift one knee so that your foot comes off the floor.

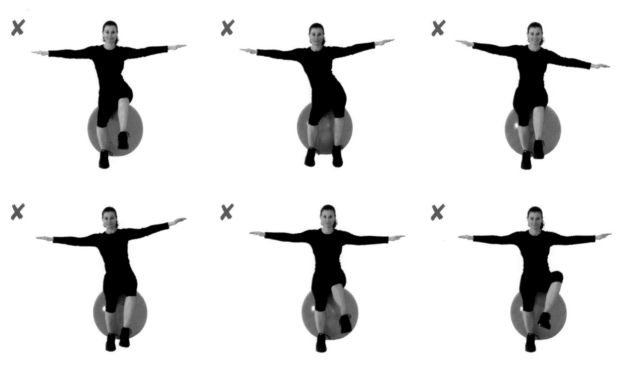

| | |
|---|---|
| Hip hitches up on the lifting side/trunk shortens on that side | 3 |
| Pelvis moves out to side | 3 |
| One arm drops lower than the other | 3 |
| Trunk tips sideways | 3 |
| Leg does not lift straight | 3 |
| Belly button turns towards the lifting leg | 3 |
| Facial fixing | 1 |
| Foot fixing | 1 |
| **Total:** | |

**What should I do to improve my performance?**

• Seated Knee Lift (Chapter 6)

• String of Pearls Bridge, Hip Pops, Hip Swivels (Chapter 6)

• Clam, Standing Knee Press (Chapter 6)

• Ball Bouncing (Chapter 6)

## Section 4: The Upper Control Zone — Scapular Stability

### ○ Test 1: Diamond — Scapula/Shoulder Relationship

This simple test looks at active shoulder external rotation mobility with respect to scapular control. Tennis players, volleyball players, swimmers and handball players should all be able to perform the movement well.

Performance in this test examines:

• scapular control against the rotating arm.

• external rotation mobility and control of the shoulders.

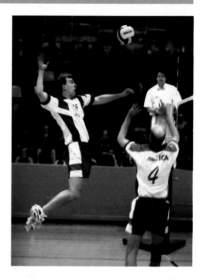

Lie on your stomach with your forehead resting on the floor. Place your arms in a diamond shape on the floor so that your fingertips touch. Draw your scapulae away from your ears just enough to lengthen your neck. Lift the forearms and hands off the floor and hold them there for a count of 5.

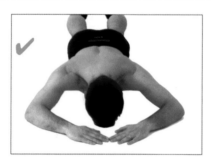
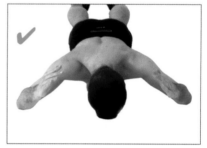

**Performance points to note:**

1. Scapulae moving towards the ears instead of maintaining a consistent position. This indicates a shoulder dissociation problem or a scapular stability problem.

2. The arms raise less than 10 cm from the floor. This indicates insufficient shoulder mobility which may be due to stiffness or poor patterning of the movement.

3. One or both shoulders sink towards the floor as the arm lifts.

4. Hands turn palms upwards instead of wrists and forearms lifting.

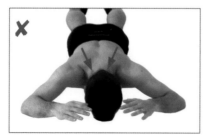
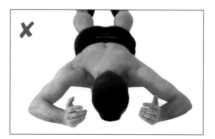

| SCORING | | |
|---|---|---|
| Hands turn palms upwards instead of wrists and forearms lifting | 3 | |
| Shoulders move towards ears | 3 | |
| Hands lift less than 10 cm | 3 | |
| Shoulder sinks towards floor | 3 | |
| **Total:** | | |

---

**Clinical Tip**

This test can help a clinician to identify a cause for persistent upper trapezius tightness.

---

## What should I do to improve my performance?

- Diamond (Chapter 6)
- Superman (Chapter 6)
- Wall Press (Chapter 6)
- Shoulder Stretch (Chapter 10)

## ○ Test 2: Wall Press — Scapula/Trunk Control Relationship

The Wall Press is a low-load movement that looks at coordination of the shoulder girdle with the trunk and pelvis. It does not require strength but does require coordination so it sheds light on low-threshold control and proprioception through the spine.

Performance in this test examines:

• scapular control.

• sagittal trunk control.

• coordination of upper body to lower body.

Stand with your palms flat against a wall at shoulder height in front of you. Your arms should be straight. Stand tall, then bend your elbows to perform the press-up movement, keeping your body alignment consistent. Press out again.

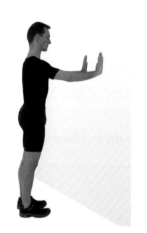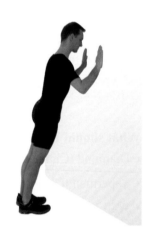

**What would a poor performance look like?**

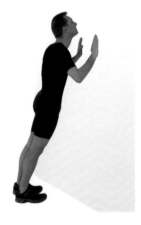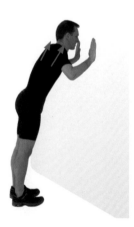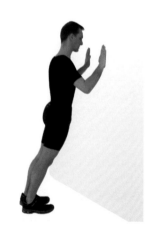

1                   2                   3

1. The chin tilts upward. This rotates your head backward on your neck, putting it into extension and switching off your local trunk stabilisers.

2. The shoulders hitch up towards the ears, or wing off your rib cage. This indicates poor scapular stability.

3. The pelvis drifts forward relative to the trunk. This means that the trunk stabilisers have switched off.

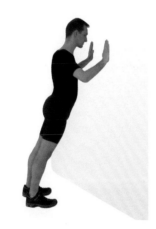
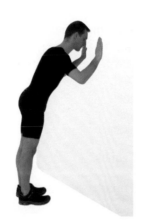

4

5

4. The stomach protrudes. You are not using TrA to control your trunk.

5. Upper body bends forward and leaves your hips behind. You have found a way to avoid using your abdominals and load your upper body.

| SCORING | | |
|---------|---|---|
| Chin tilts upward | 3 | |
| Shoulders move up, or scapulae wing off the rib cage | 3 | |
| Pelvis drifts forward | 3 | |
| Stomach protrudes | 3 | |
| Upper body bends forward | 3 | |
| **Total:** | | |

---

**Clinical Tip**

This test can help a clinician to identify a cause for persistent upper trapezius tightness.

---

**What should I do to improve my performance?**

- Wall Press (Chapter 6)
- Greyhound (Chapter 6)
- Ball Bouncing (Chapter 6)

## Section 5: Basic Global Control

This exercise requires coordination of all three control zones.

Performance in this test examines:

- scapular control.

- pelvic control.

- trunk control.

- the coordination of all three control zones.

### ○ Superman

Start on your hands and knees. Hands should be positioned under your shoulders, knees under hips. Press out with one heel and stretch out with the opposite fingertips so that you have a straight line from fingers to heel. Your chest and pelvis should be parallel to the floor.

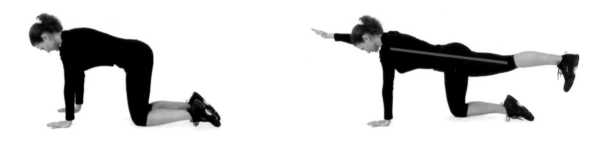

**What would a poor performance look like?**

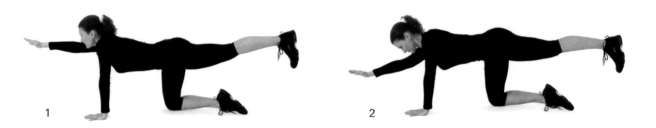

1

2

1. Head drops or rotates up and back. This is a poor head control response to loading of the shoulder girdle and trunk.

2. Chest drops on the unsupported side. This indicates an upper control zone weakness which could implicate both scapula and rotator cuff stability on the supporting side.

3. Scapula on the supporting side lifts off the ribs. This indicates poor activation of stabiliser muscles.

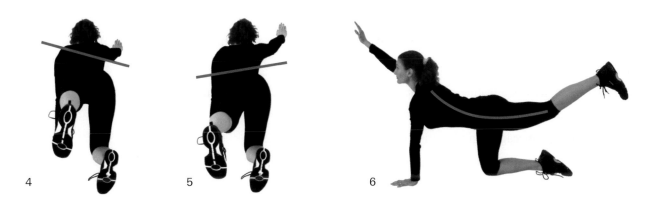

4. Pelvis rotates upwards on the unsupported side. This is usually an indicator of poor inner-range GMax activation, reduced hip mobility or a dysfunctional hip extension movement pattern.

5. Pelvis rotates downwards on the unsupported side. This indicates weakness in GMed on the supporting side.

6. The spine moves from neutral into a deeper curve. This indicates a proprioceptive deficit in the trunk as the spine moves out of its neutral position into extension in response to a hip extension stimulus. The TrA will switch off in this circumstance.

| SCORING | | |
|---|---|---|
| Head position is lost | 2 |
| Shoulders move up, or scapula wings off rib cage | 3 |
| Chest drops on unsupported side | 3 |
| Pelvis rotates upwards or downwards on unsupported side | 3 |
| Stomach protrudes/spinal curve deepens | 3 |
| Facial fixing | 1 |
| **Total:** | |

**What should I do to improve my performance?**

- String of Pearls Bridge, Hip Pops, Hip Swivels (Chapter 6)
- Clam, Standing Knee Press (Chapter 6)
- Superman (Chapter 6)
- Supported Lunge (Chapter 7)
- Wall Press (Chapter 6)

Once you have completed the Capsule Functional Assessment, you should have an impression of your overall foundations for movement. You may have performed well in some sections but not in others. You may have highlighted a difference between one side and the other. Note your findings and see if they relate to injuries or technique issues that you may have. The programmes outlined in Chapters 6–9 provide exercises to address problem areas that you may have identified.

# Expanding the Assessment Parameters

Having used the set of basic tests to establish your overall motor control profile, you can then extend the testing according to your capabilities and the demands of your sport.

In order to progress the testing procedure, additional elements can be added. These may include:

• more comprehensive sports relevant mobility testing

• dynamic force management: jumping and landing

• momentum control: forward and lateral

• control in multiple planes

• control of external forces: predicted and unpredicted

• increased dynamic demand

• increased cognitive demand (body control is maintained when the mind is distracted)

• increased speed

• increased load

• increased skill

The testing difficulty level is limitless and can become increasingly sports relevant. It is important to expose limitations and assess coping strategies, so depending upon your capabilities or those of the athletes you work with, you can progress as far as is necessary using the methods listed above.

For example, after testing the Static and Dynamic Lunge with a tennis player, you may add rotation to the movement. If the player performs this well under controlled circumstances, they might be asked to perform a deep Dynamic Lunge to catch a low-thrown ball. This would look at automatic postural control responses, pelvic and trunk stability, functional strength through the available range, balance and recovery. By increasing the dynamic demand as well as adding a cognitive task, additional systems are examined for their effect on the soundness of the basic movement. Despite the added coordination requirement, the trunk, pelvis and leg should still be controlled and efficient during the lunge.

Similarly, a basketball player may have good trunk control in slow, focused movements but has to cope with a variety of dynamic demands when playing. You may therefore test his Jump Landings by pushing him from the side as he jumps to see whether his trunk control is sufficient to counteract an external force. You want to see how far he lands from his take-off point, how far his central axis is pushed off line under resistance conditions, and how he positions his legs on landing. The basic tests are applicable to all sports. The list opposite provides options to gain further insight, assuming that you have already tested the basic movements. If you are not sure which additional tests will be relevant to your sport, use the list opposite as a guideline. The list is by no means comprehensive: there are many additional tests that can reflect the demands of your sport.

| Features of the sport | Examples | Jumping Landings | Cross and Stop/Leap and Return | RotationalControl | Lunge progressions | Seated Lumbopelvic Mobility | Leg Swings | Press-ups | Double Arm Floor Press | Supine Hip Flexion | Locomotor Thoracic Rotation | Chicken Wings | Step-ups | Seated Forward Trunk Tilt | Vertical Hip Release | Active Rotation of Pelvis on Trunk |
|---|---|---|---|---|---|---|---|---|---|---|---|---|---|---|---|---|
| Multidirectional/move off either leg equally/ jumping | Football, tennis, handball, skiing | • | • | • | • | | • | | | | | | | • | • | |
| Symmetry of body alignment | Equestrian, sprint and distance running, jump sports | | | | | • | • | | | | | | | • | | |
| Control of pelvic motion in a seated position | Equestrian, rowing, kayak | | | | | • | | | | | | | | | | |
| Hip bending mobility and control | Rowing, cycling | | | | | | | | | • | | | | | | |
| Even pressure and power through both legs | Cycling, running sports | | | | • | | | | | | | | • | | | |
| Arm motion | Volleyball, tennis, golf, waterpolo, swimming | | | | | | | • | • | | • | • | | | | |
| Control of spinal angle/ coordination of trunk angle with hip bending | Show jumping, skiing, golf, kayak, rowing, throwing sports | | | | | | | | | | | | | • | • | |
| Kicking sports | | | | | | | | | | | | | | | | • |

As for the Capsule Functional Assessments, scoring can be as simple as a pass/fail rating. However, if you wish to score numerically, a system has been provided.

# Functional Mobility Testing and Mobility Training

The mobility tests listed in the Capsule Functional Assessment can be augmented with additional movements relevant to your sport. Checking mobility is as important as checking any other factor influencing stability. Insufficient mobility or a distorted pattern for achieving mobility is often associated with poor stability. If you don't have sufficient mobility in the right planes, something somewhere else will compensate instead.

Many of the following tests can be used as exercises as well as for assessment. They comprise movement elements that train awareness and control as well as mobility. If you or an athlete you are working with struggle to perform a movement, it is advisable to practise it in order to improve. There are as many tests for mobility as there are for sporting movements, and it is impossible to account for all of them in one resource. The exercises listed below can be used to augment the more familiar procedure of muscle length testing for sports where very specific flexibility is required.

## ○ Test 1: Ball Follow

This is a useful test to gain an impression of total body movement.

Two people hold a Swiss Ball up between them using one hand. They should start with their hands directly opposite each other with fingertips pointing upwards. One person leads the movement in any direction, trying to push the other into large changes in position. The first point to look for is good transference of body weight during a movement. Some athletes are surprisingly static, preferring to reach awkwardly to the side instead of shifting their weight for a smoother performance.

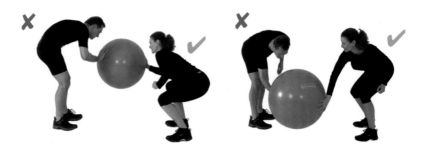

The athletes should be able to keep their trunk relatively upright by bending their hips, knees and ankles. If they do not bend sufficiently in the legs, it will look as though they are leaning forward, collapsing their trunk and losing contact with the ball. Upper zone control is also tested with this movement. The athletes should be able to keep their shoulders quite relaxed, they should not draw their shoulders upwards, and their scapulae should not lift off their rib cage.

| SCORING | | |
|---|---|---|
| Movement is not smooth and fluent | 2 | |
| Shoulders are tense or hunched | 2 | |
| Hips don't bend | 3 | |
| Weight is not shifting from side to side with the movement | 3 | |
| **Total:** | | |

## ○ Test 2: Vertical Hip Release

This is a small movement that tests hip/trunk timing and movement proportion. As we noted in Chapter 3, it is not a squat: the objective is to keep the trunk in a relaxed neutral position while bending the hips and knees. It is a quick test for athletes in any weightbearing sport to examine active hip-to-trunk coordination in the sagittal plane.

The movement is simple. Stand with feet hip-width apart. Keeping the body upright, bend at the hips and knees so that your centre of gravity moves straight downwards.

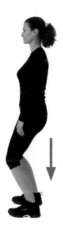

**What would a poor performance look like?**
There are several possible movement dysfunctions that can interrupt the hip/trunk relationship.

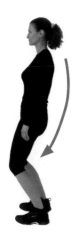 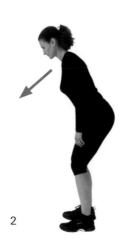 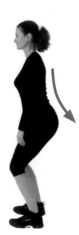

1          2          3

1. The hips do not bend in proportion to the knee. The hip has relatively little bend and the trunk may look like it is tipping slightly backwards. Poor eccentric GMax performance is associated with this pattern.

2. The pelvis immediately moves backwards. This enables an athlete to avoid controlling their hip with eccentric GMax contraction.

3. The athlete excessively curves their lumbar spine. This is often associated with faulty squat training.

4. The knees fall inwards and the arches of the feet flatten.

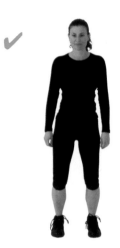
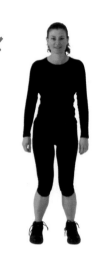

| SCORING | | |
|---|---|---|
| Trunk tips forwards | 3 | |
| Trunk appears to tip backwards | 3 | |
| Lumbar spine curve deepens | 3 | |
| Knees fall inwards | 3 | |
| **Total:** | | |

---

### Clinical Tip

If an athlete has persistent hip flexor tightness, check the Vertical Hip Release to see if they are willing to let go of their anterior thigh muscles to achieve a balanced position. Work with their Balance Point as described in Chapter 3.

---

**What should I do to improve my performance?**

- Improve hip awareness with Hip Pops (Chapter 6)

- Improve hip-to-trunk alignment as well as knee control with Supported Lunges (Chapter 7)

- Achieve awareness of separation between a controlled trunk and a flexing/extending hip with Greyhound (Chapter 6)

## ○ Test 3: Double Arm Floor Press — Shoulder/Scapula/Trunk Relationship

This test enables you to look at the relationship between the shoulder, the scapula and the trunk. The test was initially introduced for swimmers but has become standard for any athlete requiring good shoulder mobility.

Start by lying on your back with your knees bent and feet on the floor. Keeping straight elbows, move your arms over your head, keeping the movement in line with your shoulder joint. Your hands should finish in a palms-up position. Your spine should lengthen along the floor, with your arms moving smoothly over head.

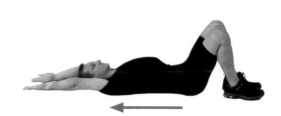

**What would a poor performance look like?**

Several possible movement dysfunctions commonly appear with this movement:

1. The lumbar spine lifts off the floor. If the shoulder or thoracic spine have lost mobility or latissimus dorsi is tight, the athlete will allow their lumbar spine to deepen its curve in order for the hand to reach the ground.

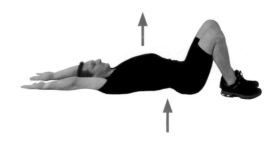

2. The elbow bends, or the arm moves outside the line of the shoulder. Both of these indicate insufficient mobility at the shoulder.

3. The scapula becomes clearly visible more than 3 cm beyond the line of the chest wall. This indicates that the scapula is compensating for reduced shoulder mobility and possibly stiffness of the thoracic spine.

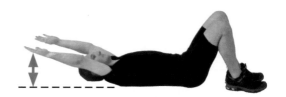

4. The arm does not reach the floor when the elbow is straight and the arm is in line with the trunk.

---

### Clinical Tip

An athlete in an overhead sport, e.g. a throwing sport or gymnastics, may present with low back pain and appear to have quite an extended spine. Use this or the Double Arm Raise test to see if the lower back is compensating for insufficient mobility in the shoulder. It may shift your treatment focus from the back as the site of pain to the shoulder as the main driver for the dysfunction.

| SCORING | | |
|---|---|---|
| The lumbar spine lifts off the floor | 3 |
| The scapula becomes visible outside the line of the chest wall | 3 |
| The arm does not reach the floor | 3 |
| **Total:** | |

**What should I do to improve my performance?** If the primary problem is shoulder mobility:

- Latissimus Dorsi Stretch (Chapter 10)
- Greyhound (Chapter 6)

---

**Clinical Tip**

If your finding correlates with test results that show overuse of latissimus dorsi in the Lunge and the Standing Knee Lift, you will also need to address pelvic stability.

---

## ○ Test 4: Supine Hip Flexion

This test of available hip mobility was introduced to the collection when evaluating rowers, cyclists and skiers, as well as those performing deep squats. It is used to determine whether backward pelvic rotation in response to hip flexion is due to primary stiffness in the hip or to a hip-pelvis coordination and control problem.

Lie on your back with one leg straight and the other hip bent to 90 degrees. Place your hands on your raised knee. Keeping the straight leg pressed to the floor, move your other knee slowly towards your chest. You should manage an additional 30 degrees before you feel your pelvis start to move.

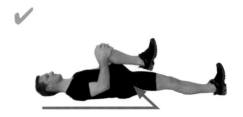

Hip stiffness will cause the pelvis to rotate backwards rather than the hip freely flexing. You will see the other leg lifting slightly off the floor when this occurs as hip flexor tension pulls the femur up when the pelvis rotates.

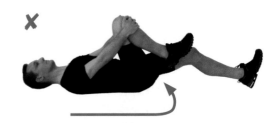

If this test appears normal, but the athlete tilts the pelvis backwards in response to active hip flexion, the Seated Knee Lift and Standing Knee Lift tests should be examined to investigate the athlete's movement patterning and hip flexor strength.

The figure shows an athlete with poor left hip mobility. When her right hip is flexed as her right knee moves up, her pelvis remains level and her spine is not stressed. When her left knee moves up, the pelvis tips sideways to compensate for the left hip stiffness. The spine is forced to rotate.

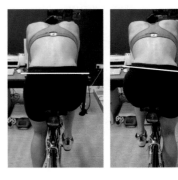

**Scoring** is a pass/fail. To pass, the additional 30 degrees of hip bending will not cause any pelvic tilting. If you are numerically scoring, a fail will incur 3 points.

**What should I do to improve my performance?**
• Hip Ranger (Chapter 9)

## ○ Test 5: Seated Lumbopelvic Mobility

It is easy to see why these tests are relevant to seated sports such as rowing, paddling and equestrian events; however, they also give additional insight into the symmetry of weightbearing in any athlete.

The tests can be practiced as exercises if a problem is found.

### ○ Test 5.1: Pelvic Forward and Backward Tilts

Athletes who use their back extensors and hip flexors to stabilise the pelvis on the trunk have difficulty with this movement, partly due to the physical restriction of tight muscles, and partly due to poor awareness. Because of this, they may have difficulty achieving and maintaining a neutral spinal position.

Sit on a Swiss Ball with feet flat on the floor. With minimal ball movement, collapse your spine so that you feel yourself roll off the back of your sitting bones, causing the lower spine to form an outward curve. If your sitting bones were arrows, they would be pointing forward. Then lift your body upwards and roll up and over your sitting bones, causing the spine to form an inward curve. Your sitting bones will be pointing backwards. Finally settle your weight straight through your sitting bones which will give a neutral position. Your sitting bones will be pointing straight downwards.

It is possible to perform this test on an ordinary chair, but it is easier to detect problems using a ball.

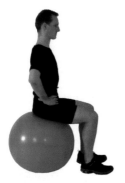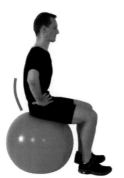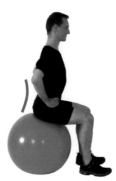

**Scoring** is a simple pass/fail. If you are numerically scoring, a fail will incur 3 points. To pass, the spine and pelvis should move into a lengthened outward curve as pictured above, and then into a shortened inward curve. The head should stay in a constant position. In a failed test, the spine shape changes very little, but the ball moves significantly forward and backward. The head can be seen to move backwards and then forwards.

○ Test 5.2: Pelvic Side Tilts

Athletes who stabilise by shortening one side of the trunk with latissimus dorsi and quadratus lumborum will have difficulty with this movement. You will have noted this when you tested the Static Lunge and the Standing Knee Lift.

Pelvic side-tilting can expose weightbearing asymmetries and central axis control problems. It is often uneven in athletes with groin problems or chronic back and hamstring pain. It should also be checked when evaluating chronic shoulder problems, as an inability to perform a lateral pelvic tilt changes the trunk's ability to lengthen, and this in turn can affect shoulder mechanics.

Sit on a Swiss Ball with both feet on the floor. Press one side of your pelvis down into the ball so that the pelvis tilts sideways. The hip and shoulder on that side will seem to move away from each other as your side lengthens and your spine curves gently. Your head should stay in the same position. Usually one side moves better than the other. The head will seem to move sideways on the side of poor lumbopelvic movement. The trunk tips sideways instead of releasing on the lengthening side.

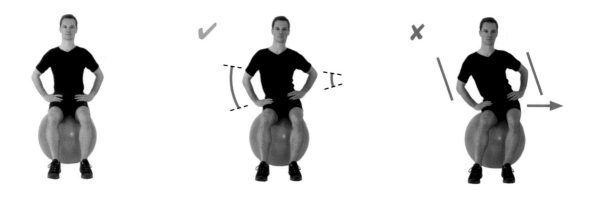

**Scoring** is again a simple pass/fail. If you are numerically scoring, a fail will incur 3 points. To pass, the movement is symmetrical, with the head staying in the centre as the pelvis tilts.

### What should I do to improve my performance?

If you cannot press your pelvis down on one side, lift your arm up on that side and rest your hand on your shoulder blade. Your elbow will be pointing upwards. Stretch your elbow up as you press your pelvis down on that side.

## ○ Test 5.3: Knee Creepers — Rotation of the Pelvis

As your foot moves forward in walking or running, the pelvis advances on that side while the opposite shoulder moves forward to create a spiral or rotation in the spine. This rotation and counter rotation is a fundamental component of efficient locomotion. Athletes are usually unaware that they rotate far more on one side than the other. The ability to smoothly rotate the pelvis is also necessary to kick a football, strike a golf ball, hit a strong tennis forehand and advance one hip in a dressage saddle. Lack of rotation causes an increase in coronal plane movement and this is rarely desirable from a technical perspective in any sport.

Sit on a chair or Swiss Ball with your arms crossed over your chest. You will keep your chest facing forward throughout the movement.

Make sure that you start with your knees level. Slide one knee forward and the other one back and note how far you move. Start again with knees level. Repeat the movement with the other side.

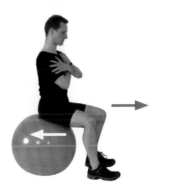
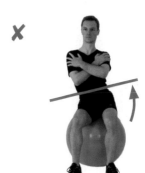
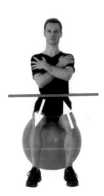

**What would a poor performance look like?**

Problems that you might see include:

- A difference in the amount of rotation between the two sides.

- An inability to keep the chest facing forward.

- A tendency to hitch the hip upwards instead of sliding it backwards.

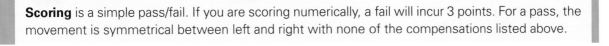

**Scoring** is a simple pass/fail. If you are scoring numerically, a fail will incur 3 points. For a pass, the movement is symmetrical between left and right with none of the compensations listed above.

## ○ Test 6: Seated Forward Trunk Tilt

Sports such as golf and kayaking require a forward tilt of the trunk and pelvis on the hips. A simple forward tilt maintaining a neutral spine minimises pressure on the structures of the back and creates a good axis for rotation. However, few athletes can manage the movement with a neutral spine.

This test is best done with a partner who can observe you while you perform it.

Sit on a chair or ball with both feet on the floor and knees at 90 degrees. Place your hands behind your head and sit directly onto your sitting bones so that your spine is upright. Tilt your whole trunk forward, bending only at the hips. Count to 10 and return to the start position.

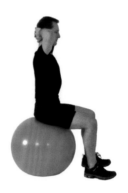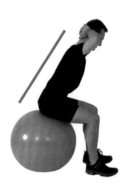

### What would a poor performance look like?

The shape of the spine should not change at any time during the movement. If there are problems with this movement, you will see one of two things:

1. The spine collapses and the trunk bends. The spine looks like an outward curve.

2. The lumbar spine deepens its natural inward curve, causing the spinal muscles running down either side of it to over-work.

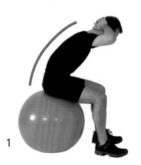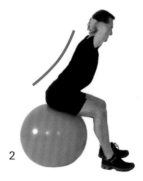

1                      2

### What should I do to improve my performance?

• You need to develop awareness and control of your CLA, and learn to bend in your hips instead of your spine.

• Ball Bounceing (Chapter 6)

• Greyhound and progressions (Chapter 6)

• Seated Knee Lift (Chapter 6)

• Wall Squat (Chapter 6)

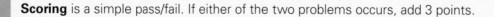

**Scoring** is a simple pass/fail. If either of the two problems occurs, add 3 points.

## ○ Test 7: Seated Thoracic Mobility

Stiffness in the mid-back is a common complaint. It may be caused by postural problems, holding sustained positions such as driving or sitting at a computer, or may indicate overuse of secondary stabilisers to compensate for poor primary stability.

To investigate thoracic mobility, sit on a chair or ball with feet hip-width apart and your weight straight through your sitting bones. Cross your arms over your chest so that the backs of your hands are placed on the sides of your face. Keeping your weight evenly distributed through both sides of your pelvis, turn your trunk and head as one unit.

Your starting posture will make a difference to this movement. If you sit upright too rigidly, supporting your weight in front of your sitting bones, the joints of your spine are more compressed and the muscles are under tension. This will decrease your available movement. The balloon position is sufficient as a starting posture.

### What would a poor performance look like?

1. Visible asymmetry in available motion.

2. Shifting the hips away from the direction of rotation.

3. Moving the arms to give the impression of more rotational movement.

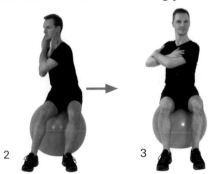

The measurement marker is the point at which the arms cross over the chest.

| SCORING | | |
|---------|---|---|
| Cross point less than 30 degrees from the front | 3 | |
| Cross point between 30 and 60 degrees | 2 | |
| Cross point between 60 and 90 degrees | 0 | |
| Shifting of hips sideways | 2 | |
| **Total:** | | |

### What should I do to improve my performance?

• Thoracic mobility can be restricted due to joint and muscle stiffness and to overuse of the oblique abdominal muscles to stabilise. To rebalance your trunk stability strategy, you need to learn how to activate TrA without over-recruiting the obliques

• Greyhound, Ball Bouncing, Superman and Wall Press (Chapter 6) can be progressed into OTT and progressions (Chapter 7)

• Exercises to address rotational mobility include: Thigh Slides and Total Body Rotation (Chapter 6); Revolving Lunge and Hip and Spine Twist (Chapter 7); Corkscrew (Chapter 9)

## ○ Test 8: Locomotor Thoracic Rotation

This version of thoracic rotation testing is the one most relevant to gait.

Sit at the front of a ball or chair with both feet flat on the ground. Place your hands on your thighs. Keeping your head still, turn your shoulders by sliding one hand forward and the other back along your thighs. You should be able to maintain a vertical CLA with your head facing forward and shoulders relaxed. Your hands should easily reach your knees. Note any difference between left and right rotation.

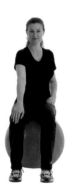 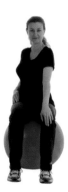 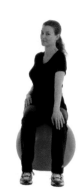

Some people use a compensatory strategy of keeping their thorax still and simply moving their arms. To ensure that this is not happening, watch the sternum to see that it is turning from side to side.

| SCORING | | |
|---|---|---|
| Head turns with shoulders | 3 |
| CLA tips or bends sideways | 3 |
| Shoulder raises as arm slides backwards | 2 |
| Asymmetry between left and right rotation | 3 |
| **Total:** | |

### What should I do to improve my performance?
Practice this simple movement regularly in order to improve your thoracic rotation.

## ○ Test 9: Active Rotation of Pelvis on Trunk

Kicking sports require the ability to sustain a firm trunk position over the supporting leg while rapid lower-body rotation occurs. Testing of footballers has shown that this is not always present. Poor stability and restrictions in internal hip rotation of the supporting leg can cause a collapse into spinal side-bending or extension. Groin and back problems can be associated with a poor performance of this movement.

Stand upright with arms out to the side and lift one knee until it is approximately level with your hip. Move the knee across your body, keeping the chest facing forward. Your knee should move easily past your supporting leg.

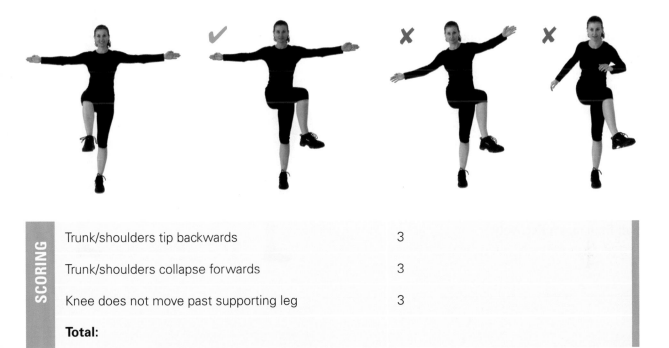

| SCORING | | |
|---|---|---|
| Trunk/shoulders tip backwards | 3 | |
| Trunk/shoulders collapse forwards | 3 | |
| Knee does not move past supporting leg | 3 | |
| **Total:** | | |

### What should I do to improve my performance?

This test requires good rotational mobility of the pelvis on the stance leg and the pelvis on the trunk, but also demands a secure, vertical trunk.

- To train rotation around the CLA, develop OTT and progress to OTT Scissors and Floor Bridge (Chapter 7), progressing to Twisted Floor Bridge (Chapter 8)

- To train body alignment over the stance leg, use Basic Balance (Chapter 6)

- To improve mobility of pelvis on trunk, use Corkscrew (Chapter 9) and Pelvic Rotation Over a Fixed Foot (Chapter 6)

## ○ Test 10: Standing Leg Swing

This movement checks for a fluid sagittal leg movement pattern on the foundation of a secure central axis and controlled pelvis. All runners should be checked for this balance and symmetry.

Stand on one leg and swing the other leg fully back and forth, allowing your arms to move normally. Your trunk should stay vertical and your leg should swing in a straight line. Your pelvis should remain in a constant position so your spine should move very little.

### What would a poor performance look like?

Your powerful leg muscles need a stable attachment to pull from to achieve their most efficient performance. The muscles involved in this test are attached to the pelvis. If you observe your lumbar spine deepening its curve when you move your leg back and flattening its curve as you move the leg forward, you are not maintaining the pelvis in a stable position for your legs to pull from most effectively.

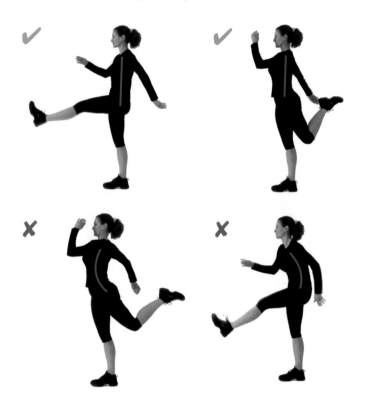

| | | |
|---|---|---|
| **SCORING** | Trunk tilts sideways | 3 |
| | Pelvis rocks forward or backwards | 3 |
| | Balance is poor on one side | 3 |
| | Any fixing behaviour | 1 (add a point for each behaviour observed) |
| | Jerky, non-fluent movement | 1 |
| | **Total:** | |

### What should I do to improve my performance?

- Greyhound, Superman and Wall Press to secure your CLA, and Basic Balance (Chapter 6)

- Hip Pops to learn how to straighten your hips without bending your spine (Chapter 6)

- Quadricep and Hip Flexor Stretches to improve muscle length (Chapter 10)

## ○ Test 11: Windscreen Wipers — Active Shoulder Internal Rotation

Rotation at the ball and socket shoulder joint is essential for overhead sports [29]. Diamond shown earlier, investigates active external rotation and its relationship to scapular control. This test examines control and range of internal rotation.

Lie on your back with your elbow bent to 90 degrees, your upper arm level with your shoulder, and the back of your forearm and hand as close to the floor as possible without pushing. Relax everything before you start. If you feel that your shoulder lifted closer to your ear when you positioned your arm, release it

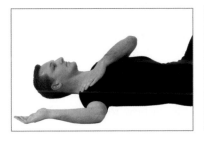 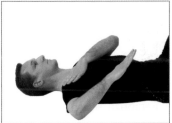

back down so that it is level with your other side. Place your other hand over the front of your shoulder. This hand will monitor the movement of the head of the humerus (the ball) in the socket of your shoulder joint.

> **Note:** if your pectorals are tight, you may not be able to rest your elbow on the floor without your shoulder joint pushing up or forward. You must begin with your shoulder in an optimal position, so until you gain more muscle length, place a small folded towel under your elbow to lift it slightly and take the pectorals off stretch.

Keeping your elbow secure on the floor, lift your forearm so that your arm rotates and your hand now points to the ceiling. Imagine this position as the zero position, with the floor being the 90-degree mark in each direction. This completes phase 1 of the test. Keep moving in the same direction until you cannot continue without shifting your shoulder position. This completes phase 2 of the test.

**Performance points to note:**

1. You should be able to perform this movement without feeling your shoulder pushing upwards or rolling forward into your hand. If you detect the head of the humerus pushing into your hand, it means that it is losing its position in the socket by sliding forward. If this happens repeatedly as it can when throwing a ball, swimming, spiking a volleyball or serving in tennis, it stresses the structures at the front of the shoulder. Painful shoulder instability can occur as a result. This motion dysfunction will occur in phase 1 of the test, before muscle tension becomes involved.

2. The shoulder mobility required for different sports varies widely. However, you should be able to reach 70 degrees with your forearm, which means that you can touch the floor with your fingers if you bend your wrist (a handy tip from the movement expert, Shirley Sahrmann [116]).

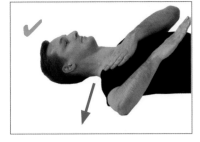 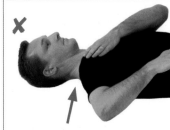

3. If you lack shoulder mobility, you might compensate by rolling your scapula forward. This will feel as though you are closing the space at the side of your neck.

Phase 1: A pass or 0 score means that the ball of the shoulder stays in a consistent position throughout the first phase of the movement.

Any movement of the ball constitutes a fail, or 3 points.

Phase 2: To gain a pass or 0 score, you reach 70 degrees (finger touch) without the shoulder shifting forward or upward.

A fail, or 3 points, demonstrates insufficient mobility.

**What should I do to improve my performance?**

- Establish scapular stability and learn how to separate ball-in-socket movement from scapular movement with Diamond (Chapter 6)

- Mobilise the shoulder with Chicken Wings (Chapter 9)

- Practice Windscreen Wipers as described above

# Jumps

We often assume that athletes can jump and land effectively; however, even in sports where this is a necessary component, movement dysfunctions are common. Sports such as volleyball and basketball are obvious candidates for testing jumps and landings, but it would equally apply to footballers, handball players and skiers.

## ○ Test 1: Jump Take-offs

A common error is overuse of the upper body and spine on take-off. To look at this, first perform a natural jump and feel how high you have moved off the ground.

Next, put your hands on your head and try the jump again. There should not be a dramatic difference in height although it might feel higher in effort.

You should not feel your shoulders drive back either – this would indicate that you are not maintaining a neutral spinal position in the air. Your trunk should look as though it is driving upwards, not backwards.

Your knees should not draw together on take-off. Your hips, knees and ankles should remain parallel as you dip slightly before take-off and launch yourself upwards.

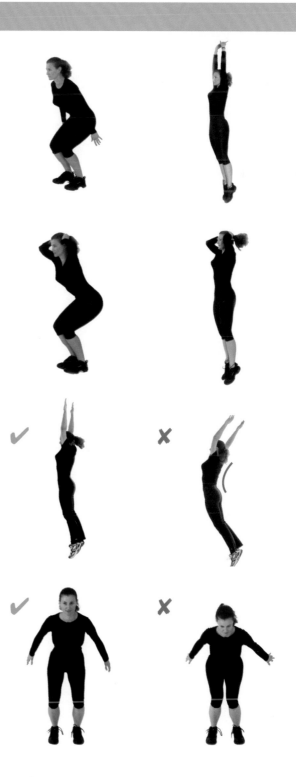

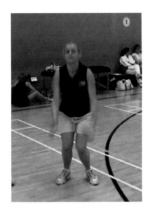

An athlete demonstrating poor knee control on take-off.

| SCORING | | |
|---|---|---|
| Marked drop in jump height with hands on head | 3 | |
| Shoulders driving backwards | 3 | |
| Knees drawing together | 3 | |
| **Total:** | | |

On the pass/fail system, presence of any of the above will rate the test as a fail.

## O Test 2: Single Leg Jump Take-offs

Greater hip and knee control is necessary to generate a good jump off one leg. The pelvis must remain level and the knee aligned with the ankle and hip. Marked loss of power is often associated with poor pelvic control.

| SCORING | | |
|---|---|---|
| Loss of pelvic alignment on preparation for take-off | 3 | |
| Knee moves inwards or outwards | 3 | |
| **Total:** | | |

On the pass/fail system, presence of either of the above will rate the test as a fail.

# Landings

Landings are a common source of injury for athletes. Poor landing technique has been positively linked with anterior cruciate ligament (ACL) injuries [55] and high loading on other knee structures [24]. Female athletes in particular have demonstrated insufficient sagittal joint control, higher ground force reactions and poor lower limb alignment [13, 80, 41]. However, poor landing strategies can be observed in male athletes also.

A good landing should absorb force through the hips, knees and ankles; the muscles on opposite sides of the joints work in partnership to allow the extensor group to first quickly lengthen and then shorten again to absorb and control joint bending. This does not necessarily come naturally to some athletes. Instead of springs in their joints, the supporting muscles fail to change length in a coordinated fashion and the athlete lands with their joints locked, causing a jarring sensation and reducing their ability to move easily from the landing position.

Landing with a relatively straight knee absorbs less energy and can therefore be associated with higher ground reaction forces and greater knee stress [19]. In the knee, movement strategies that reduce the transfer of force up the kinetic chain through coordinated hip and knee bending are thought to reduce the risk of non-contact ACL injuries [110]. Trunk compensations for blocked landing include excessive forward trunk tipping to absorb force [101].

---

**Movement Quality Tip**

Develop an eye for shock absorption. If the athlete blocks their joints, there is no sense of spring – the joints may bend on landing but stay fixed in a narrow range. This is over-contraction and it makes it very difficult for the athlete to move dynamically immediately after landing. The joints should bend but look as though they have some vertical play. Test your eye: ask the athlete to land and move off quickly on a diagonal. Is their response brisk and immediate or sluggish and effortful?

---

Another landing problem is the issue of landing heavily. The heavy lander does not maintain a functional level of tension in the muscles during the landing, switching off on impact. These athletes usually exhibit too much motion in the joints, giving an appearance of joint folding. In this case, elastic energy storage in the muscle-tendon unit is diminished and a quick take-off in any direction is virtually impossible.

## ○ Test 3: Jump Landings

Landing should occur with the legs in normal alignment. If landing on both feet, legs should be parallel, and if landing on one foot (see below), the alignment rules that we investigated in the lunge apply. To do this, you need good sagittal control in your hips and knees so that the force of landing is absorbed vertically. Without this control, the force seeps out of the sagittal plane and the knees move towards each other on impact. This is an extremely common landing pattern in female athletes and in children.

| SCORING | | |
|---|---|---|
| Hips, knees or ankles blocking/non-shock absorbent | 3 | |
| Loss of balance on landing | 3 | |
| Loud/heavy landing | 3 | |
| Trunk tips forward | 3 | |
| Knees move together | 3 | |
| **Total:** | | |

## ○ Test 4: Single Leg Landings

To progress this investigation of landings, take off into a jump off two feet but land on one foot. You are looking for the same issues as you did in the Lunge in terms of pelvic and lower limb control, but the speed of muscle activation has increased.

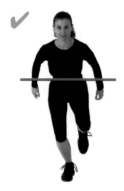 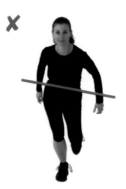 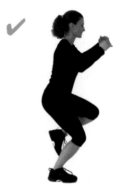 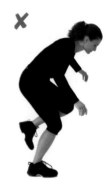

| SCORING | | |
|---|---|---|
| Knee moves inwards | 3 |
| Pelvis tips sideways | 3 |
| Hips move backwards (lumbar curve deepens) | 3 |
| Trunk tips sideways | 3 |
| Trunk collapses forward | 3 |
| Wobbling | 1 |
| Lip biting or facial fixing | 1 |
| Foot fixing | 1 |
| **Total:** | |

Depending upon the dynamic demands of the sport, this theme can be extended. For example, landing with the eyes closed to observe the athlete's anticipatory preparation for landing, or jumping sideways and landing on the outside leg with balance.

**What should I do to improve my performance?**

Phase 1 exercises to build activation and awareness include:

• Clam (Chapter 6)

• Standing Knee Press (Chapter 6)

• String of Pearls Bridge (Chapter 6)

• Vertical Hip Release (Chapter 5)

• Natural Squat (Chapter 3) progressing to pulses at different depths of the Natural Squat

• Lateral Pulses (Chapter 3)

Phase 2 exercises for integration include:

• Supported Lunge (Chapter 7)

• Supported Single Leg Squat (Chapter 7)

• Static Lunge and progressions (Chapter 7)

• Space Invaders (Chapter 7)

• Sway (Chapter 7)

# Higher Level Trunk Control Testing for Jumps and Landings

Trunk control and activation of preparatory or feedforward neuromuscular responses when landing from a jump are critical for athletes who can be contacted while in the air. This anticipatory action is extremely fast to restore and maintain joint stability [74] and minimise risk of injury. Footballers, netball and basketball players fall into this category.

## ○ Test 5: Push Jumps

1. Evaluate a jump with a light sideways push to the pelvis and ribs while in the air. You want to see that the trunk remains straight and the landing is not far from the take-off spot.

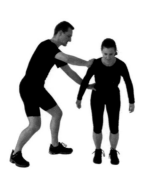 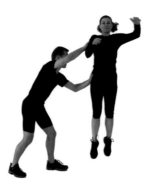 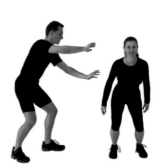

2. Add light resistance only to the ribs. This puts a higher demand on the trunk to stabilise itself in the coronal plane.

3. Compromising vision's contribution to landing control can change the motor pattern [117]. Engage the eyes by throwing and catching a ball during the movement to see if this influences landing control.

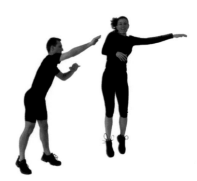

4. Repeat the movement but land on one leg. *For safety, this should always be the opposite leg to the side being pushed.*

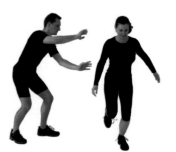

| SCORING | | |
|---|---|---|
| Trunk is off-centre on landing | 2 | |
| Landing is rigid or heavy if compared to a basic jump | 2 | |
| Knee alignment is lost | 3 | |
| **Total:** | | |

**How do I improve jumps and landings?**

You need to be willing to bend your hips and knees freely to generate and absorb force. To do this, you need an active GMax and GMed to control the hip joint and knee alignment.

• Phase 1 activation and awareness exercises include: String of Pearls Bridge, Hip Pops and Wall Squat (Chapter 6).

• Phase 2 integration exercises include: Natural Squat with Pulses (Chapter 3), and lunge progressions (Chapter 7).

These exercises can be progressed into jumping and landing tasks, starting very simply with no distraction and aiming for quiet landings with springs in ankles, knees and hips. Basic jumps can be further challenged by:

1. Adding a visual distraction such as catching and throwing during jumping.

2. Jumping and turning the body in the air to land with feet at 90 degrees to the start position. This can be progressed to a 180-degree turn (see Rotational Control).

3. Jumping in different directions.

4. Adding a mild push while in the air, aiming to land securely.

# Higher Level Pelvic Control Testing
## Support Strategies

### ○ Test 1: Lunges

Lunge testing can be progressed almost indefinitely to meet the demands of your sport. This is a sequence used for an international-level badminton squad. Interestingly, the badminton players performed poorly at first and thought that it was an unreasonable level of testing. The former Olympic Gold medallist who coached in the national programme performed it perfectly.

Start in the lunge position as previously outlined.

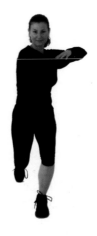

1. Add rotation to the lunge. With arms crossed in front of you, keep your head facing forward and turn your shoulders in the direction of the front leg. All movement markers are the same as for the Static Lunge. Turning the shoulders should not cause the knee to collapse inwards. In order to be truly systematic, you would test a Static Lunge with added rotation before a Dynamic Lunge.

2. Perform the same movement, but allow the head to turn with the shoulders. The knee should still be facing straight ahead.

3. Perform the rotation movement in conjunction with the Dynamic Lunge. Start with arms crossed in front of you. As you step forward, turn your shoulders, keeping your head facing straight ahead.

4. Perform the same movement, allowing the head to turn.

5. Perform multidirectional lunges with sound form and no trunk rotation. Include side-steps, angled steps, forward and backward steps.

6. Perform multidirectional lunges returning to stand on one foot.

## ○ Test 2: Step-ups

The Step-up combines support with propulsion, and examines force management between the foot and the hip. For those who need to produce force from alternate or single leg, and those who need to propel forward or upward, this test is a useful one.

Stand with one foot fully on a standard step and check that your pelvis is level before performing the movement. Raise your body onto the step by pressing through your foot. Maintain your balance on the supporting leg. Slowly reverse the movement and return to the start position. You are only watching the working leg.

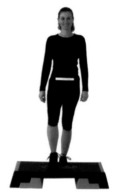
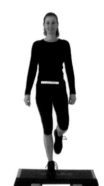

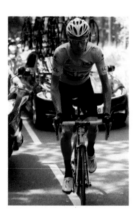

Right leg demonstrates sound force containment between foot and pelvis as the pedal is pressed down.

### What would a poor performance look like?

1. The pelvis not remaining level throughout the entire movement.

2. The hip moving out to the side.

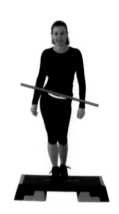

3. The knee falling out of alignment with the hip and ankle.

If you see the pelvis tip down on one side, the hip move outwards, or the knee move inwards, the muscular force you are producing is being lost sideways and is not being used effectively to propel you. The force you produce should be contained between your foot and your hip, like a cushion of air pressure between two plates. If this pressure is maintained, you can absorb shock effectively and the force you produce can be controlled and focused in the most effective direction.

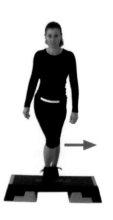

**SCORING**

Pass if none of the markers listed above are observed. Fail if any of them are observed. If you are numerically scoring, 3 points for each marker can be given.

## How should I improve my performance?

Phase 1 exercises for activation and awareness include: Clam, Standing Knee Press and String of Pearls Bridge (Chapter 6)

Phase 2 exercises for integration include: Supported Lunge, Supported Single Leg Squat, Static Lunge and progressions, Space Invaders, Sway (Chapter 7)

---

### Clipboard Notes: Functional Application of Testing

A road cyclist finds that his right knee habitually drags towards the crossbar of his bike as he rides. His leg action is deviating from the straight sagittal plane to the coronal plane. It is altering the angle of pressure through his pedal and putting the muscles of his hip at a disadvantage. This makes driving off a left-hand curve less powerful, and also puts more stress on his lower back.

To determine the appropriate course of action, we would need to test three main movements. First we need to know whether the knee moves inwards due to a problem flexing the hip on the trunk. We would use the Supine Hip Flexion test to make sure that the athlete has sufficient available hip mobility to perform the task. Then we would use the Seated Knee Lift test to see whether the cyclist is able to lift his thigh in a straight line. Having investigated the hip flexion phase, we then need to see whether the cyclist can exert pressure through the pedal with a level pelvis and straight leg action, so we would choose the Step-ups test to investigate this relationship. All three tests investigate movement capability and control in the sagittal plane.

## Momentum Control

The Standing Knee Lift is a static method for testing stability of the pelvis when weightbearing on one leg, but the lateral hip-trunk control relationship can be tested more dynamically. Any sport that requires lateral hip control is a candidate for this type of testing, so it is as relevant to downhill skiing as it is to multidirectional sports.

### ○ Test 1: Side Squat and Return — Lateral Control

Where initially we thought that it seemed necessary to observe athletes working very dynamically to pick up lateral momentum control strategies, it has become apparent over many years that an athlete's natural response to lateral movement can be identified using the most basic of tests.

Begin with feet together and arms crossed across the chest. Step to the side and sink straight down into a Natural Squat before returning smoothly to the start position.

**Performance points to note:**

1. The trunk should be carried straight to the side and downwards. If the shoulders tip towards the outside leg, it indicates that you are not cleanly bending the hip and not accessing outer-range hip extensors (GMax) adequately. For a clean test, the trunk will sink vertically.

2. If the outside heel does not contact the floor, it is also an indicator that the hip is not fully bending.

3. The movement should be one continuous motion. In athletes who tend to over-control and lack fluency, the movement looks as though it is made up of four distinct phases: sideways, down, up and back. This indicates that they lack the fine coordination to control the body as it moves across their base of support, and the timing to press back out from the floor.

The major factor in all three cases is a lack of hip bending.

| SCORING | | |
|---|---|---|
| Trunk tilts from sideways at any point | 3 | |
| Heel does not contact floor | 3 | |
| Motion lacks fluency | 2 | |
| **Total:** | | |

**What should I do to improve my performance?**

Focus on achieving a smooth, even Natural Squat (Chapter 3) and progress to Ski Shifts (Chapter 7)

## ○ Test 2: Cross and Stop — Lateral Control

From a standing position, take a sideways leap off your left leg onto your right leg, bring your left leg across the front of the right leg and use it to push into another large sideways leap to balance on your right (outer) leg.

**What would a poor performance look like?**

1. If timing and coordination are a problem, you won't be able to organise your trunk in space to land balanced and upright on the outside leg.

2. Your pelvis will not be level on landing if GMed and the other hip abductor muscles are weak or their response is poorly timed. Your pelvis will be higher on the landing leg side and lower on the non-weightbearing side.

3. If GMed and the other hip abductor muscles lose control of the pelvis-femur relationship, your knee will move inwards.

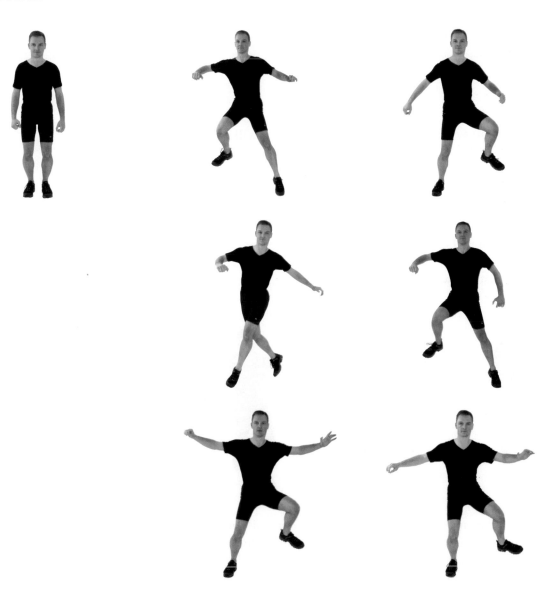

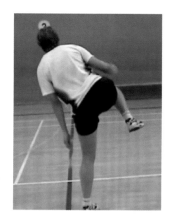

An athlete failing to control her trunk momentum.

| SCORING | | |
|---------|---|---|
| Trunk tips sideways | 3 | |
| Pelvis tilts sideways | 3 | |
| Knee moves inwards | 3 | |
| **Total:** | | |

On the pass/fail system, presence of any of the above will rate the test as a fail.

## O Test 3: Leap and Return — Lateral Control

This time, you will land on your outside leg and immediately push off it in the opposite direction. Don't be concerned about the leg that you finish on. It is the leg that controls momentum and pushes you back to the start point that you will be scoring.

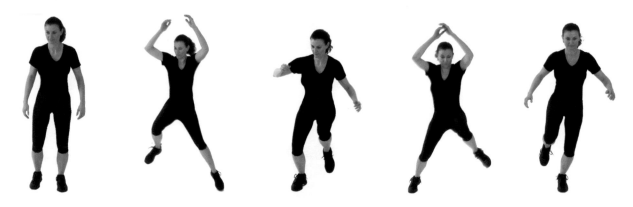

The main problems are the same as for the Cross and Stop test, and are usually easier to see. If there is a tendency for the hip to collapse and the pelvis to tilt sideways due to a GMed weakness, you will usually see the trunk move past the hip on landing instead of arranging itself in the air in preparation for landing. With this pattern, you will use trunk momentum to try and assist you with jumping back when you should be using GMed strongly. This is not a powerful strategy and puts stress on the inner knee.

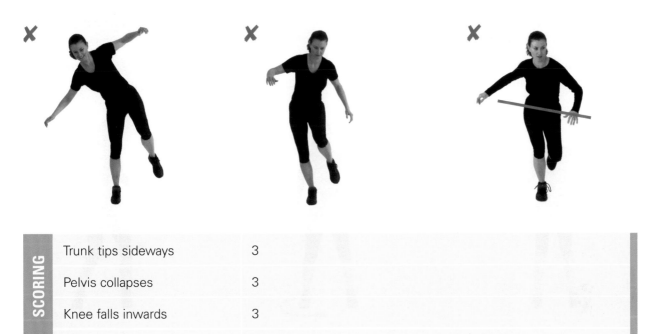

| | | |
|---|---|---|
| **SCORING** | Trunk tips sideways | 3 |
| | Pelvis collapses | 3 |
| | Knee falls inwards | 3 |
| | **Total:** | |

On the pass/fail system, presence of any of the above will rate the test as a fail.

These tests also relate to cutting manoeuvres, where inadequate planning and postural adjustment have been found to increase rotational and sideways stress on the knee structures [6]. More complex dynamic tasks introducing unanticipated changes of direction can be designed to investigate these patterns at a higher level.

**What should I do to improve my performance?**

Phase 1 exercises for activation and awareness include: Clam, Standing Knee Press (Chapter 6) and rotational Natural Squat pulses (Chapter 3)

Phase 2 exercises for integration include: The Two-Step (Chapter 3), Supported Lunge, Space Invaders and Sway (Chapter 7)

## ○ Test 4: Rotational Control

Over-rotation on landing from a turning jump can greatly increase the risk of knee injury. If your sport is multidirectional and involves jumping, this simple test highlights a major control problem.

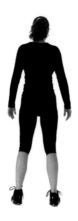
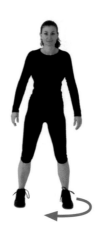
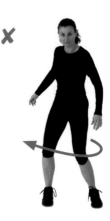

Stand with feet hip-width apart. Soften your knees and hips, then jump to land facing in the opposite direction. Ask someone to watch your knees: they should not continue to rotate or fall inwards. This is a basic pass or fail movement. If you land with good knee alignment, you pass the test.

For court sports such as handball, netball or basketball, add a higher level of testing by working with a partner and have them challenge your anticipatory responses by getting you to catch a ball thrown to you just as you are landing.

## ○ Test 5: Forward Control

This is a difficult movement to score objectively but it is interesting to see differences in strategy between athletes. Problems are usually obvious. Slow changes of direction and a toppling forward of the trunk indicate momentum control problems.

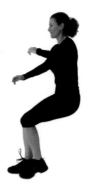
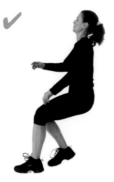
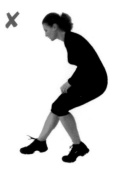

Ask someone to observe your movement. You will run as fast as you can in a forward direction, and react to a clap or noise to brake and reverse your direction to run backwards for a few steps. Your hips and knees should bend to drop your centre of gravity.

**Performance points to note:**

1. Height of pelvis from the ground.

2. Number of steps needed to brake.

3. Head/pelvis relationship: has the trunk tipped forward?

Your centre of gravity is located at around the level of your pelvis. To control momentum, drop your pelvis quickly to initiate the change. A higher pelvis and forward head posture is less effective for braking (see bottom right hand picture, page 180). Agile athletes may additionally angle their trunk slightly backwards to initiate and prepare for the brake, and they shift their weight off their toes back onto their midfoot to make effective counter movement possible. The combination of factors makes it possible for these athletes to use fewer steps to achieve a brake.

Athletes who manage forward momentum poorly, collapse their trunks forward and increase their step rate, rather than using the braking mechanism of dropping their centre of gravity. The movement of the head with respect to the pelvis can be clearly seen. Athletes using this strategy tend to drop their heads forward but do not effectively drop their pelvis. This makes it difficult to produce an effective counter movement and requires a greater number of steps to achieve a brake.

**What should I do to improve my performance?**

When you need to check forward momentum, focus on dropping your hips.

## ○ Test 6: Brake and Turn

To combine braking and turning, sprint forward, brake on command and turn 180 degrees to run in the opposite direction. Look for the same ease of movement on left and right turns. Some athletes will avoid one side by pushing off with the same foot regardless of which way they are turning.

---

**Clipboard Notes**

During routine screening, a professional footballer was found to have decreased control of his right leg and pelvis and greater foot rigidity on that side. His right Static and Dynamic Lunges were not well controlled, nor was his Standing Knee Lift. On the Brake and Turn test, he turned and pushed off well to the right but performed poorly to the left. On further questioning, the player admitted that he would do anything to avoid pushing off his right leg when he turned. He would literally run around the ball so that he could move off his left leg. His right leg was not painful but he did not have confidence in it.

The Single Leg Wall Press, cueing the player to lift himself up and place his trunk over his right leg, some lunge training with corrections and external resistance with hand pressure, and a small amount of Listening Foot exercise increased the pelvic stability responses in the right side. The player became aware of his gluteal group, and as he repeated the movements, the leg started to respond. When tested again on Brake and Turn, he had improved. The player was relieved: this problem had bothered him but he had not known what to do about it. Assessing simple movements made it possible to identify a performance problem and correct an asymmetry.

## Scapula/Trunk Relationship Control

The Wall Press is the basic movement for foundation testing but it is a very low-load exercise. If an athlete can perform it well, it is necessary to increase the load to control a larger proportion of body weight.

### ○ Ball Press-up

With thighs on a Swiss Ball, position yourself so that you look straight at the floor with your head, neck, and spine in a straight line. Perform a press-up by bending your elbows and make sure that you do not push the ball backwards. You are looking for the same issues as in the Wall Press (Chapter 6).

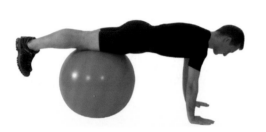 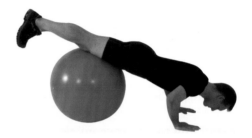

| SCORING | | |
|---------|---|---|
| Head rotates backwards/drops down | 1 | |
| Shoulders move up towards ears/scapula wings off rib cage | 3 | |
| Lumbar spine curve deepens | 3 | |
| Stomach protrudes | 3 | |
| **Total:** | | |

## ○ Full Press-up

Surprisingly few athletes can be tested to the level of a full press-up. Most show scapular control problems at much lower loads. However, a well-coordinated athlete with ideal functional motor patterns should be able to perform a full press-up correctly.

Start in a plank position with arms and trunk straight and hands positioned under shoulders. Lower yourself to the floor and press back up to this position. All the same observation points apply, with the addition of hip flexion. The hips should remain straight, but athletes who do not have adequate trunk control can commonly be observed using a combination of hip flexor and back extensor activity to control the trunk/pelvis relationship.

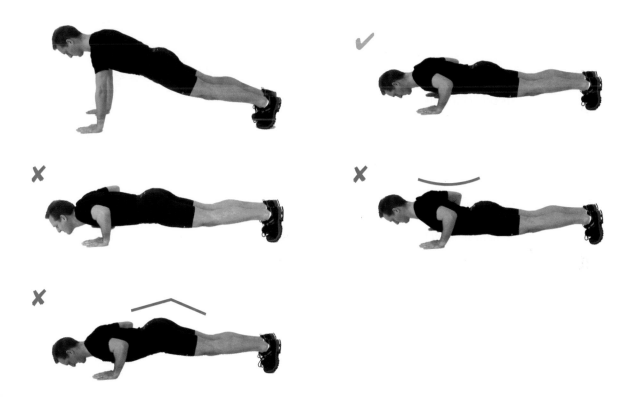

| SCORING | | |
|---|---|---|
| Head rotates backwards/drops down | 2 | |
| Shoulders move up towards ears/scapula wings off rib cage | 3 | |
| Lumbar spine curve deepens | 3 | |
| Stomach protrudes | 3 | |
| Hips flex/bottom sticks up | 3 | |
| **Total:** | | |

## Functional Assessment in the Elite Environment

A great deal of money is invested in athlete screening, or profiling as it is now more commonly known, but the return from this investment is variable depending upon the integration of the multidisciplinary team and the administrative structure of the sport. In order to justify the cost of profiling, a clear action pathway should be established. First it is important to establish the expectations of a profiling procedure. Why do we do it?

Most commonly, profiling is seen as an injury-prevention measure, and as such is usually performed by sports medicine personnel. It is normally expected that if no issues are identified, the athlete should be able to cope with normal training and competition demands without breaking down, and able to make technical improvements where necessary. Including functional tests in the profiling procedure can also give us an insight into an athlete's movement efficiency and any technical difficulties that may be persistent. To achieve this, the professionals involved in profiling must have sufficient knowledge of the sport's mechanics and a good relationship with the coach.

The barriers to gaining insight into functional reasons for injury or technical barriers are:

1 Insufficiently sports relevant tests.

2 Insufficient technical knowledge in the tester.

3 Insufficient communication between coach and tester.

4 Insufficient time allowed for testing.

From a technical movement perspective, there are many possible tests to examine whether an athlete can create and control forces to a level that meets the demands of their sport. The questions you may want to ask when selecting tests will include:

• What are the main mechanisms of injury? Are they traumatic or biomechanical/overuse?

• What physical issues might contribute to these injury mechanisms?

• What are the most common technical problems?

• What are the main components of the sport (e.g. jumping or landing, control of unexpected forces, symmetry of weightbearing, or control of more than one plane of movement)?

• How does the athlete generate and control force?

If issues are identified, appropriate action should be taken. This will fall into two categories:

1 The athlete has fixable biomechanical or motor control issues that can be addressed to prevent injury and enhance performance.

2 The athlete has unchangeable physical issues that require modification in technique, equipment or training methodology.

Although it seems logical that action will be taken, it is not necessarily the case. The sporting organisation may take one of a number of pathways in response to testing information. The passive pathway does not respond at the time to collected information. If enough data is collected over time, it may lead to the recognition of trends within the sport that may be acted upon, but often the information is merely stored as part of the monitoring process.

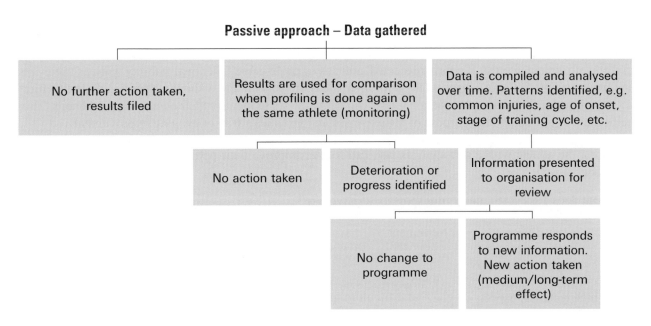

The active approach to profiling findings is to implement a direct intervention. This may be unidisciplinary or multidisciplinary.

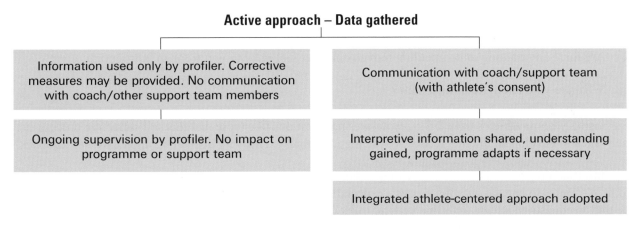

Sporting organisations are either *reactive* or *responsive* to profiling data. The *reactive* organisation suffers from non-integration of coaching, sports medicine and sports science personnel. Athlete screenings are conducted by sports medicine personnel, but these findings do not impact upon the training programme unless the athlete becomes injured. Communication between professions in this system is often impaired and athletes can become stressed by differences of opinion between the disciplines. In the reactive system, supplementary exercise is presented as injury prevention and as such is usually provided by sports medicine personnel. It tends to be perceived by the athlete as being separate and additional to his or her training programme. Compliance with injury prevention work is poor in this circumstance.

In a *responsive* sporting organisation, athlete screenings are followed immediately by meetings between professional personnel to discuss the impact on the training programme and the best route forward to ensure optimal training progress with the least risk of injury. A commitment within the multidisciplinary team to respect the opinions and expertise of others is necessary in order for this to work, as differences in opinion will naturally arise. Supplementary movement control work is presented as having the dual purpose of injury prevention and movement optimisation. It may be initiated by sports medicine personnel, but its principles will be carried throughout the training programme by all personnel. Because they are a part of normal training procedure, athlete compliance is maintained.

## Profiling and the Athlete

If you are trying to implement a movement efficacy programme for your sport, functional profiling can help to stimulate athlete interest. If poorly presented, athletes often perceive functional stability work as irrelevant and uninteresting. If the exercises selected for them are quite general and without a clear benefit, motivation will not improve. Using simple functional tests can help athletes to identify their own movement habits. This helps them to understand the purpose of the exercises and provides a way of gauging improvement.

Engaging the athlete with a self-analysis task can further improve their perception of the relevance of the functional testing.

1. What does a good athlete in your sport look/move like?

2. How is this different to your movement?

3. Why do you think that is?

4. Which technical aspects do you find difficult to improve?

5. Which technical aspects would you like to perform better?

6. Which technical aspects does your coach think are most important for you to improve?

7. Are there any training or competition movements that you are less confident about?

8. Are there any training or competition movements that feel risky to you from an injury point of view?

9. What are your strengths as an athlete?

Surprisingly, some athletes have difficulty answering questions like these, but this self-reflective process can help them to develop an internal feedback system rather than exclusively depending upon external feedback.

The information gathered from this type of questioning can be combined with functional assessment findings to help athletes to engage with the process, especially when test findings can be related to technique. It may be that an equestrian athlete finds that vertical trunk orientation is not as good over one leg on balance testing and that this relates to more difficulty on one rein than the other. A handball player drives much better off one foot than the other and on testing finds that he has more pelvic control on that side. A swimmer may find that her scapular stability is not symmetrical and that the weaker side is the same as the one that does not hold the water as well. A footballer who consistently lands poorly from contesting a high ball may find deficits in his trunk stability, or that he absorbs shock poorly in his hips and knees due to inadequate pelvic control.

Engaging athletes by illustrating relevance to their sport can help the athlete and coach to establish common goals and provide a meaningful language for discussion between strength and conditioning professionals, coach and athlete. If the tests highlight a weakness, some components of the athlete's programme will need to be modified to make sure they are corrected. It is therefore important that everyone involved understands the concept.

If you are a sports science, sports medicine or coaching professional, you may decide to analyse the role of profiling in your sport. Questions to reflect on include:

• Is profiling having an impact on your programme right now? If not, why not?

• How often is it performed in your system?

- Does the content of the procedure reflect the demands of your sport?

- Is relevant data communicated, and if so, to whom?

- Is data compiled for longitudinal analysis?

- How integrated and cooperative is your team?

- How does your system respond? Is it active or passive? Responsive or reactive?

---

### Clipboard Notes

An international women's netball team was experiencing a high injury rate and poor training compliance. The women were aged from 18–32, with varying training ages and international competition experience. The professional team included a coach, a strength and conditioning trainer, a physiologist and a physiotherapist.

Netball is a fast, multidirectional sport involving jumping, catching, attack and defence. Traumatic injuries of the knee and ankle are common. With the introduction of a new strength and conditioning coach, the training had taken a much greater emphasis on weightlifting, agility training and cardiovascular work. Injuries were occurring more frequently and conflict had arisen between the trainer and the sports medicine personnel. Player stress was rising and compliance with training was diminishing.

Functional sports-specific profiling was undertaken. Capsule functional assessments were performed, followed by progressively more task-specific movements relating to jumps and landings, change of direction strategies, balance and ball control. All professional personnel attended so that each could understand the implications of the findings to their specific disciplines. Fundamental stability, balance and control issues were identified.

The findings were discussed at a follow-up meeting. The coach now had insight into the physical reasons for some of the technical problems she had been working on; the strength and conditioning coach understood why his exercise selection was sound for the future but too advanced for the current level of control, and the physiologist understood that the periodised programme that she had designed would need to be modified. With a framework to establish common goals and a commitment to respecting the opinions of other professionals, the conflict was eliminated and an integrated plan made.

The players were given a five-week supervised remedial programme to work on movement control, stability, balance and mobility. Their awareness of good-quality movement in training and playing contexts was systematically increased, ready for integration back into their normal training programme. The strength and conditioning programme was adjusted to reflect the current level of the players rather than their assumed level. Maintenance exercises were integrated into coaching warm-ups and drills, and good movement principles emphasised in all aspects of training.

The result of the intervention was a dramatically reduced injury rate, improved training compliance and better technical performance[27].

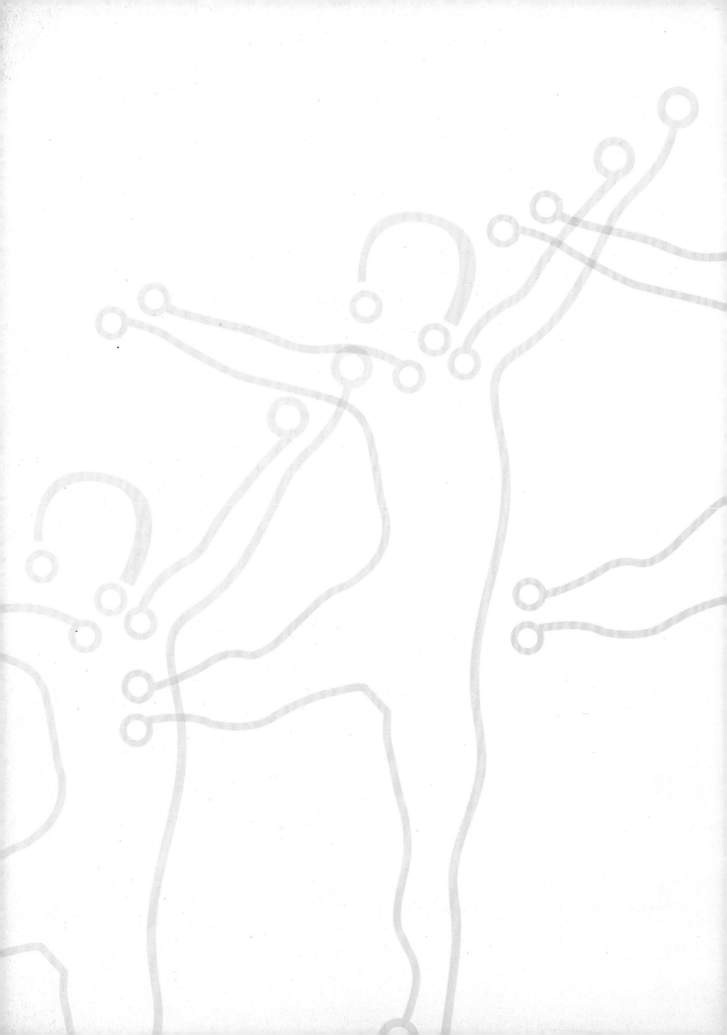

# Part Two
Developing Fluent Control

# Introduction

Developing fluent, controlled movement is like building a well-constructed house: you need to start with secure foundations. There are no short cuts if you want a structure that will perform well over time. For this reason, the programme in this section is systematic and progressive. Instead of presenting a general collection of exercises, it provides a pathway to follow, methodically developing abilities that lead to progressively higher levels of control.

The aim of the programme is to help you to move well. As discussed in Chapter 3, the control and movement of the upper, central and lower control zones are closely linked. Because of this, the relationships between the control zones are developed from the early stages of the programme and progressed together, rather than presenting separate upper, central and lower body programmes.

The programme is divided into four phases:

1. *Activation and awareness.* This is the most important phase but it is often mistakenly skipped over in favour of bigger, more exciting exercises. It creates the links between your brain and the muscles you are trying to activate using simple movements.

2. *Integration.* This phase progresses your new neuromuscular connections by teaching you to control your trunk against the movement of your limbs.

3. *Global coordination.* This phase develops Phase 2 skills into whole body movements and introduces multidirectional movement.

4. *Dynamic control and stability conditioning*. Optimising your movement ultimately requires more than one aspect of control. This phase improves your neuromuscular responses to dynamic control challenges when speed and coordination of your response is most important. It also introduces higher load demands requiring greater strength to maintain central axis control.

Do not bypass Phase 1. If you are serious about exploring new neuromuscular pathways, you need to activate your system first and familiarise yourself with some new movement habits. If you skip Phase 1 when these muscles are not a part of your normal functional motor patterning, the higher-level exercises will simply teach you to compensate in new ways.

Starting at Phase 1 does not mean that you are weak. Competitors at the highest level usually have to start at this point because their methods for compensating are so well established. The existing pathways between brain and muscle have been reinforced by thousands of repetitions. Establishing a new pattern is not always easy, so simple, focused movements are used to create new connections.

Even when you are able to progress to Phase 2, 3 and 4 exercises, keeping a small selection of Phase 1 exercises in your warm-up will ensure that you do not slip back into old patterns as the skill or load of the exercise increases. Phase 1 exercises focus your awareness deeply into your body, allow you to release unnecessary tension which may inhibit the stabilisers, and integrates the balance and sensory systems for low effort control. These exercises give you the opportunity to attend to the finer aspects of your movement, pick up control problems or asymmetries before they turn into injuries, and pre-activate patterns to prepare for sporting activity.

Your programme will eventually contain elements from each phase. You may find that your trunk control allows you to progress to Phase 2 quite quickly but that your balance needs more time at Phase 1 level. You may be able to perform Phase 4 mobility tasks but find Phase 3 stability exercises more relevant to your sport. You may also find that some exercises are particularly effective for you. You can retain these throughout your programme. All of this is appropriate as long as you have started at Phase 1 and worked your way forward.

When performing the exercises, aim for a perfect movement each time.

## Quality Control

As you fatigue, you start to use inappropriate muscles. When this happens, it is time to rest or change exercises. The aim is to establish a new pattern, so persisting with an exercise with a poor pattern is not productive. It is better to perform two sets of five repetitions well than to perform ten repetitions if the last four are poor. Remember that this is not a strength programme – it is a movement and control programme.

Be open to finding out something new about your movement. Awareness itself can lead to new physical possibilities. Many athletes have quite poor awareness of specific parts of their bodies but have experienced improvements by making new sensory connections. When performing the exercises in this programme, many athletes have mentioned that they have been given such exercises in the past but have not felt them working before. For these athletes, an increase in awareness and a greater attention to the quality of small movements have made the difference. It is not the exercise itself but the awareness with which you do it that matters most.

The following exercise outlines are therefore very specific. Don't just look at the pictures and think that you'll be doing the exercise correctly. *Read the instructions carefully*. If you follow the instructions, you will benefit from the exercises. If you just copy the pictures, you are likely to miss the key point that triggers the correct response. Be patient. These initial small movements are an opportunity to find something new in your body.

You might think "I can't feel anything!" but this is usually because you are accustomed to your more accessible muscles creating lots of obvious sensory feedback or noise. This noise gets worse as people try harder to create or control a movement, but if you pause and release some tension, often the necessary response becomes available.

The most important thing to remember is that although you should be focused, the movements should look effortless. This means that there should be no breath holding, facial grimacing, lip biting or tension. Breathe naturally. The aim is *efficient* movement which gives the best outcome for the least effort.

The best movers are not those who make a difficult thing look hard: they are the ones who make it look easy. You can be one of those people from the beginning, whatever your current level may be. Release your tension and make every motion as smooth and easy as you can.

## A Note on Equipment

Most of the equipment used in this programme is straightforward if used correctly, but Swiss Balls, sometimes known as fitness or stability balls, require a little background knowledge. These guidelines will help you to gain the full benefit of the exercises that use the Swiss Ball.

If the ball is inflated correctly, it will be firm but not hard. You should be able to sit on it with your hips and knees each forming 90-degree angles. Your hips should never be below your knees. Nor should you feel that you are perching on the front of the ball because it is too big.

Do not use a ball that is too big for you and then under-inflate it to make it smaller. You should have a sense that you and the ball are pushing against each other. When you push into it, it should push back. Working with a squashy ball will tend to switch off the deep stabilisers.

Size recommendations can only be general due to differences in people's body proportions and also the material that the ball is made of. Poor-quality balls tend to stretch due to the thinness of the material used, so a ball that fits you today can be too big next week. With a good quality ball the average person up to 5′7″ (170 cm) will find a 55 cm ball suitable, and for those up to 6′2″ (188 cm) a 65 cm ball will be suitable. If you are over 6′3″ (190 cm), a 75 cm ball will be preferable.

## The Art of Progression

Before you embark on your programme, it is worth understanding the often overlooked but important principles of progression. To achieve the release of unnecessary tension described in Chapter 4 and to ensure that you develop and maintain sound neuromuscular patterns throughout the programme, you need to start at the right level and progress systematically.

Progression is not just a case of trying something harder. That route is uncontrolled and can lead you back to just trying to cope, rather than taking you steadily forward. Tension patterns, compression and breathing problems emerge no matter how you try to suppress them when you are working beyond your capacity.

To take control of your progress, you need to understand that progression can broadly be brought down to the manipulation of two factors: load and skill.

### Load and Skill

Load encompasses any activities that require an increased muscular output from the body. It will include the amount of resistance that it must overcome; the range or distance over which it must work; the duration over which it must work, and the rate at which force must be generated. Skill involves anything that makes the task trickier, so this will include coordination, balance, stability and neuromuscular responses.

There are of course overlaps. Increasing speed when sprinting will require improved neuromuscular coordination, putting it into the realms of skill. However, with increasing running speed comes a change in muscle force output and the range of motion through which the muscles must contract, which falls under the category of load. Decreasing speed can make a task more of a control challenge (skill), but if you imagine a slowly descending squat, it can also greatly increase the perceived load on the muscles. Increasing or decreasing speed may then fall under either category.

The main principle is that wherever possible, work on either increasing skill or increasing load when changing an exercise or trying something new. Don't take on an exercise that is both more complex and heavier on the body at the same time. Put simply, either:

- maintain the load level and increase the skill component, or
- maintain the skill level required and increase the load.

Changing load and skill may not require big changes to an exercise. The simplest elements to manipulate are lever, base and plane.

The *lever* is the distance between two contact points for the body. The contact points for a kneeling press-up, for example, are the hands and knees contacting the floor. This is a much shorter distance than in a full press-up where the contact points are the hands and feet. The full press-up therefore has a longer lever. This increases load on the body and requires greater muscular effort to control the trunk and shoulders.

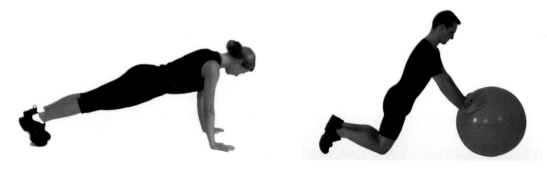

The *base of support* represents the surface area supporting the body and its centre of gravity. Feet wide apart constitutes a wide base which is very stable, whereas feet close together represents a narrow base. A narrow base requires greater balance and control so it requires greater skill.

*Planes of motion* can progress control in small increments. For example, adding single-sided arm movements in the transverse or coronal planes creates an unbalanced force on the body, challenging the rotational and side bending control of the trunk. The load change may be minimal, but the skill requirement is increased.

The diagram below illustrates some of the main methods you might use to progress.

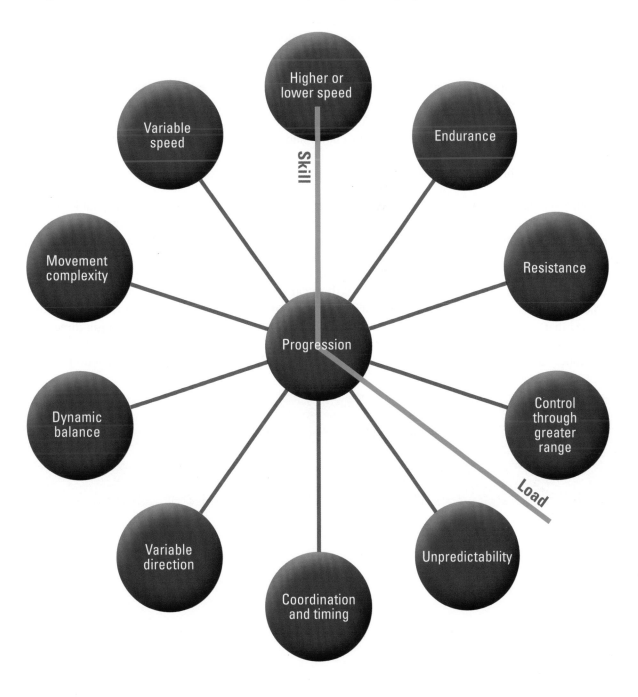

## Principles for Effective Programmes

From what we have already learned about movement efficacy, we know that multiple elements interact constantly to create and control movement. Involving many elements, or "modes" in the programme encourages this functional integration. The "three Vs" are simple programme principles which optimise motor learning, ensure a "multimodal" training experience, and increase the adaptability of the body.

Variation around a given exercise task, for example by changing plane, base, lever, eyes open/closed, load or speed, applies slightly different stimuli to the body. This creates an opportunity to expand the body's neuromuscular repertoire of responses and improve motor learning. Examples of this are demonstrated throughout the exercise library, for example as applied to trunk/upper control zone (OTT) and trunk/lower control zone (Lunge) in Chapter 7. Variation creates greater efficiency in the programme because multiple elements can be addressed by building upon an established skill.

Variety means that for any given goal, a number of different tasks will be used, each training a given behaviour, but through different strategies. For example, we might choose to work on CLA control, and choose a supine exercise (face up) like Greyhound (Chapter 6) to balance the anterior chain; in prone (face down) as in Ski Jumper (Chapter 7) to emphasise the posterior chain, and in standing as in Basic Balance (Chapter 6) to integrate CLA control with balance. Variety trains control responses to meet a wider range of functional positions and possibilities.

Variability develops robustness, which involves the body's ability to meet diverse or changeable functional and environmental demands effectively. Responsiveness to unpredictability, rapid change, and automatic reactions fall into this category. If you have only practiced the ideal scenario, you may not have developed the capacity to cope with the extra demand that real life applies. Wherever a skill is involved, mix up your variables – it challenges the nervous system to expand its spectrum of competence. Learn to hit a target from a range of distances and angles. Perform your skill under different heart rate or fatigue conditions. A very simple example is practicing a balance task with and without an acutely elevated heart rate – you might be surprised that your skill is not as robust as you thought. Mix up and vary speed, stride length, direction and acceleration/deceleration for running robustness. You are aiming to improve the body's capacity to adapt itself with subtlety and efficiency, calibrating itself automatically with minimal interruption to function.

**Key Point**

In order to create a comprehensive and systematic programme, take control of it through steady, intelligent progression and the three Vs where possible.

# 6 | Phase 1 — Activation and Awareness

The Central Control Zone
The Lower Control Zone
The Upper Control Zone
Activating Stability Relationships
Functional Mobility
Restoring Rotation

The exercises in this chapter are frequently overlooked as they seem deceptively small and simple. However, they invite you to notice and release unnecessary muscle activity while introducing some foundation control relationships. They make you pay attention to your habits, especially unnecessary tension patterns.

Phase 1 exercises are low load and low complexity, so you have the opportunity to increase your awareness of different body parts and ease out of old tension habits to create a relaxed, receptive platform for movement. Phase 1 incorporates simple exercises that make activation connections to key muscle groups, and coordinate muscle control relationships in each control zone. It also includes basic balance exercises and a selection of mobility exercises that complement the activation exercises. Use Phase 1 to establish your central longitudinal axis (CLA).

The actual number of repetitions and sets is relatively small, but each system is involved in more than one exercise. A variety of stimuli can enhance motor learning and transferability across more than a single exercise. The Phase 1 programme will be performed for two weeks in this form. It may be performed for longer, but after two weeks you would be expected to add Phase 2 elements. Phase 1 elements will continue to appear for pre-activation, or as part of warm-up or cool-down. Progressions for Phase 1 exercises have been provided so that you can continue to progress as you improve.

## The Central Control Zone

Gaining control of the CLA will be one of the most important elements to achieve early in the programme. In order to do this, Phase 1 CLA exercises start to develop awareness of the CLA while activating some of the key muscles that control it.

Of these, the most frequently discussed is transversus abdominis (TrA). There is often confusion regarding TrA, how it should feel, and whether it is working. As discussed in Chapter 3, TrA is a support muscle that responds automatically to the stimulus to move [43]. For this reason, we will be using simple movements initially to trigger a TrA response rather than trying to consciously activate the muscle without a movement stimulus.

TrA works at low levels for long periods in order to support our movements. We are generally not attuned to perceiving low levels of activation in our muscles. This is especially the case with TrA: because it is not a movement-producing muscle, our brain does not recognise its activity as readily as it does for the more familiar movement-producing muscles. We know how it feels to activate biceps: we can see it, make it perform a movement, and feel it contracting more and more as we increase the load on it. There is a strong, clear pathway between our brains and our biceps through regular, repetitive useage, so it is easy to recognise.

TrA will not give us that same type of feeling. We can't obviously see it contracting and if it is functioning normally, we don't normally notice when it is working. This can be frustrating when we are trying to exercise it, so we try to create a stronger, louder feeling around the area of the muscle to help us to hear it. This stronger feeling is actually other abdominal muscles working. This makes us feel strong in the trunk while we perform the exercise but doesn't make us move any better when we stand up. When you start to master these early exercises, you will notice a subtle sensation which is most easily felt deep in the lower abdomen, just above your pubic bones. It won't feel like a muscle contracting in the sense that you are accustomed to. It is more a sense of something securing your body position.

You are aiming for a sense of effortless control around your trunk and pelvic area. You should feel that it is easy to maintain your trunk position and move your arms and legs. This fools a lot of people into thinking that they are not doing anything, but this is not the case. Remember that the objective is to move effortlessly, not to strengthen an individual muscle.

The following exercises encourage TrA to activate, making you aware of the trunk control it provides. The exercises in Phases 1–3 focus on working your abdominal wall in a neutral position in order to secure your CLA. You may be accustomed to working your abdominals in curling actions, so this will be a different sensation. The initial exercises are easy awareness movements.

## ○ Ball Bouncing

This exercise teaches you to support your spine without buckling against vertical forces. This ability reinforces the CLA. Bouncing slightly amplifies the effect of gravity on your body, which stimulates a stabilising action in the small muscles located close to your spine.

**Bonus effect:** This exercise also introduces early neuromuscular knee training for post-injury or post-surgery where full weightbearing is not permitted.

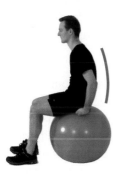 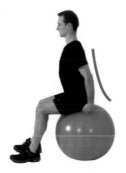 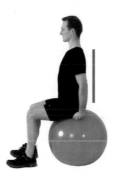

Sit on a ball with your feet and knees hip-width apart. Find your sitting bones with your hands. Slump your body and feel yourself roll off the back of your sitting bones. Straighten up and feel yourself roll over the front of your sitting bones. Now find the position where you are sitting straight down on your sitting bones. This is the pelvic position for all your seated work.

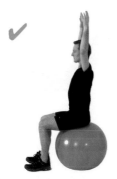 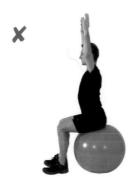 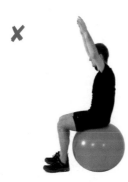

Stretch both arms above your head, feeling the stomach draw inwards in response to the arm raising movement. To initiate the bounce, squeeze your gluteals on and off in a quick pulsing action several times. Continue bouncing, making sure that you land each time directly on your sitting bones. If you do this, you will achieve the correct trunk response. If you land either with your pelvis tipped slightly forward or backward, you will use back extensors or hip flexors to stabilise.

Perform 6 x 30 second sets prior to other exercises to pre-activate the trunk stabilisers.

### Where should I feel it?

You should have a general sense of the lower abdominals working at a low, consistent level and a secure spine.

### What would a poor performance look like?

• Landing in a slumped position or with an over-arched back.

• Landing in a sideways-tilted position.

## ○ Greyhound

The Greyhound allows you to develop a secure CLA with low effort, and increases your awareness of your abdominal stabilisers. This is a great exercise when performed well, but it is usually performed with too much effort. This exercise teaches control of a lengthening response, which lays the foundations for elastic support strategy development.

There are two things to consider: first, you will be lying fully supported by the floor. Second, you will only be moving your limbs at a low-load level. The combination of these two factors means that you should not be using high abdominal effort. The question to ask yourself is: "How little effort can I use to perform these movements perfectly?" Most abdominal training is done to produce high force. TrA training aims to produce efficiency and economy of movement. This means the least effort for the best result. You are aiming for an elongated yet connected body with a freely and fully moving hip and shoulder.

If you have spent your athletic career performing high-force exercises for rectus abdominis and the abdominal obliques, you may have difficulty with this exercise at first. Don't reject it for that reason: this means that the Greyhound is something you need to do! It teaches you how to effortlessly maintain a neutral spinal position to support arm and leg movement without the need for superficial muscles to act as stabilisers. For this reason it can alleviate feelings of stiffness and restriction in the hips and shoulders. Many people will be able to move from Greyhound 1 to Greyhound 3 within several minutes. Greyhound 1 and 2 teach the basic pattern so that the Greyhound 3 exercise will be correct, but you do not need to spend much time on them. View them as a short warm-up.

### ○ Greyhound 1.0

Lie on the floor with your knees bent and feet flat on the floor. Start by releasing any unnecessary activity in the abdominals. To do this, rest one hand on your ribs and the other on your lower abdomen below your navel. Note your normal breathing pattern for a few breaths. Now gently inflate your abdomen, and then let the air seep out again. There is no need to squeeze the air out with your abdominals – it is unnecessary when there is no respiratory demand on you. Once you have done this return to your normal breathing pattern.

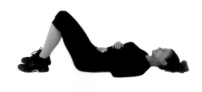

Now release any tension you may be carrying in your spine. Allow it to soften and relax into the floor.

Keep your hand on your lower abdomen just above your pubic bone and raise the other hand to the ceiling. Slowly take it over your head, focusing on allowing your spine and ribs to soften and lengthen along the floor. The movement impulse is out through the fingertips. Feel the abdomen drop from under your hand. Just like a greyhound, your abdominals have sunk towards the spine between your ribs and your legs. Maintain this dropped abdominal position, and with the least amount of effort possible, lift your arm back up to the ceiling.

**Note for therapists:** Instead of aiming to consciously activate TrA, take the alternative approach of actively inhibiting the muscular strategy you don't want (rectus abdominis, the external obliques and erector spinae) in order to stimulate the body to find an alternative automatic stabilising response to movement. The best results occur when people focus on releasing the spine instead of focusing on the abdomen.

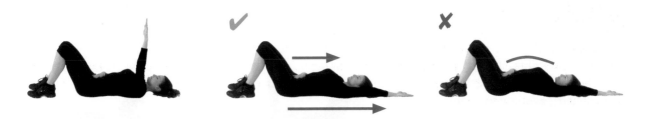

## What would a poor performance look like?

• Arching your back off the floor because you have not allowed your back muscles to release.

• Pressing the lower back down into the floor instead of lengthening it along the floor.

• Tensing or tightening the abdominal muscles instead of allowing them to drop down towards the spine.

Once you can feel the abdominals sinking and the sensation of the spine relaxing and lengthening along the floor, move straight to Greyhound 2.

### ○ Greyhound 2.0

Repeat the above action but this time, move both arms out over the head, all the time staying soft in the spine and lengthening the body along the floor. Maintain a secure pelvic position as an anchor and using the least possible amount of abdominal activity, bring the arms back up again.

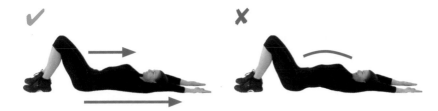

## Where should I feel it?

You should only feel a vague sensation very low in your abdomen. If your spine is relaxed on the floor and you are moving your arms without effort and without bracing your abdominals, you are doing a great job. If you make your abdominals feel like they are working hard, you are training yourself to use more effort than is necessary. This is the opposite of training efficiency. Keep aiming for smooth movement without effort.

Move to Greyhound 3 if Greyhound 2 is easily controlled without tension.

### ○ Greyhound 3.0(A): Increased Skill

Start with both arms up to the ceiling and both knees bent with feet on the floor. Perform a Greyhound 2 exercise to establish the correct action. Now combine this arm action with sliding one heel out along the floor, once

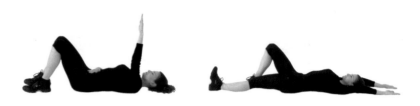

again focusing on lengthening the body along the floor. Press your heel out away from your fingertips to feel a deep stretching and narrowing around your midsection. Maintain this feeling of narrowness, and with as little effort as you can, smoothly bring your arms and leg back to the start position. Make sure you maintain an even pressure under both sides of your pelvis.

## Key Point

Pressing the heel away creates ankle dorsiflexion when you are at full stretch. This is particularly important for optimising the effect of the exercise on TrA.

| Reps | 10 reps alternating sides |
|------|---------------------------|
| Sets | 3 |

### ○ Greyhound 3.0(B): Increased Load

Start in the bent knee position as for the above exercises. You will not move your feet this time. Hold a two-kilogramme weight in your hands. With the philosophy of using as little muscle activity as possible, you will take the weight over your head, making sure that you focus on lengthening the spine along the floor. Maintain a secure pelvic position as an anchor and the sunken feeling in the lower abdomen while pulling the weight back up to the start position.

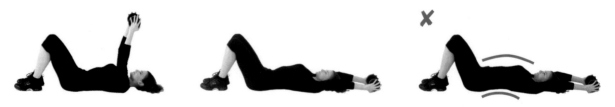

| Reps | 10 |
|------|----|
| Sets | 3 |

From this point, progress from stage to stage as you master each exercise.

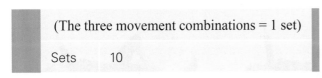

## Greyhound 3.1(A): Increased Skill

One set comprises three different movements. 1. Perform the Greyhound 3.0(A) exercise and come back to the start. 2. Then move the arm on the sliding leg side, lengthening this side of the body. Bring your arm and leg back in. 3. Now from the start position, move only the opposite arm to the sliding leg side.

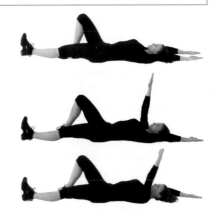

| (The three movement combinations = 1 set) |
| --- |
| Sets 10 |

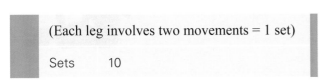

## Greyhound 3.1(B): Increased Skill

Start in the bent knee position as for the above exercise, with both arms raised towards the ceiling. As the left heel slides out away from the body and the left arm stretches overhead, the right arm will smoothly move straight out to the side. Maintaining a level pelvis and rib cage, bring the limbs back to the start position. Repeat the left leg slide, this time with the right arm stretching overhead and the left arm moving straight out to the side.

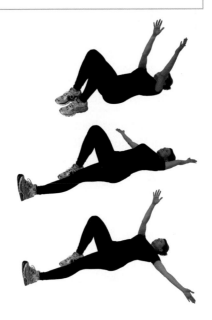

| (Each leg involves two movements = 1 set) |
| --- |
| Sets 10 |

## Greyhound 3.2: Supine Running

To increase the skill without load, and build coordination and endurance to this pattern, we will now progress to alternating arms and legs.

Start with your right arm straight over your head and your right leg straight. Your left knee will be bent and your left arm will be by your side with your elbow bent. Settle your breathing and reverse your arm and leg position, maintaining the length of your spine along the floor and a level pelvis.

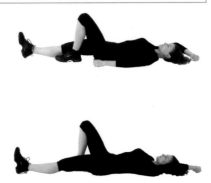

| Reps | 10 reps alternating sides |
| --- | --- |
| Sets | 3 |

## ○ Greyhound 4.0: Increased Load

Perform the Greyhound 3.1 exercises as previously outlined but instead of sliding your foot out along the floor, allow it to slide out and "take off" so that it is 10 cm from the floor at full extension.

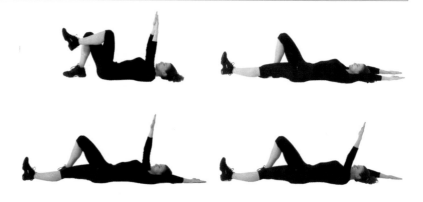

Choose one or two of the variations between Greyhound 3.1 to 4.0 to remain in your programme as clearing and preparing exercises. These are used in pre- or post-training, or on maintenance days. I call these cleaning your teeth exercises: routine, regular movements to ease away any tension habits that may have developed while keeping low-effort control technique online.

From this point on, the loading increases significantly.

## ○ Greyhound 5.0

Start in the knees bent position and support one knee with your hand. Maintain the long, relaxed spine and using as little effort as possible, raise the other foot. Put your foot back down.

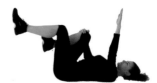

## ○ Greyhound 5.1

Start in the knees bent position and support one knee with your hand. Maintain the long, relaxed spine, and using as little effort as possible, raise the other foot. Now straighten this leg all the way out, releasing at the hip and maintaining your spinal position with as little effort as possible. Bring the leg back and replace it on the floor.

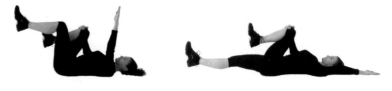

## ○ Greyhound 5.2

Athletes often start at Greyhound 5.2, but very few can initially manage this level of loading with the correct abdominal pattern. If you can't manage it well, do not spend time performing multiple repetitions of a poor pattern. Select a more appropriate level for the majority of your set and spend a little time in the middle of your set working on this new, more difficult level. Sometimes athletes are taught to place their hands under the pelvis to prevent their backs from lifting. This enables you to perform the movement but does not teach a correct pattern. Greyhound 5.2 is an example of a zone stacking exercise.

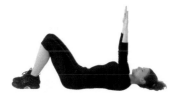 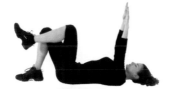 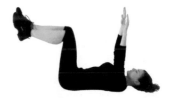

Start with your knees bent and your feet close to your body. Place one hand on your abdominals and reach the other arm towards the ceiling. Lift one foot off the floor until your knee points to the ceiling. Now try to lift the other foot without your abdominals popping up into your hand. Once you can do this, try it with both arms towards the ceiling.

### What would a poor pattern feel like?

• Your lower back tenses and lifts from the floor.

• Your abdominals pop up into your hand.

• Your hips feel locked in position.

## ○ Greyhound 5.3

Start with your arms to the ceiling and your hips and knees at 90 degrees as shown in Greyhound 5.2. Maintaining your hip and knee position, lengthen both arms over your head, allowing the spine to relax into the floor.

## ○ Greyhound 5.4

Perform Greyhound 5.3 adding the straightening of one leg out along the floor as the arms move over the head. Your fingertips and heel should be stretching away from each other and an inch or so from the floor before you bring the arms and leg back in with effortless control of your pelvis and spine. The 5.4 variation exerts a high control demand on the body, and many people cannot manage to sufficiently release the superficial abdominals as the leg extends. If performed with the deep dropping of the abdominal wall and full hip extension, it is a strong elastic support exercise. If the abdominal wall instead braces against the load of the limbs, it incorrectly becomes a suit of armour (protective) exercise.

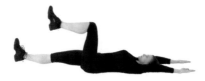

## ○ Seated Knee Lift — Trunk Control Against Hip Flexion

Many athletes experience the sensation of tightness in their hip flexors. Usually we would stretch a tight muscle, but what if stretching doesn't seem to help?

If your trunk stability is poor, you may use your hip flexors to improve control. Constant activity of the hip flexors in a stabilising role can cause the perception of tightness in the hip, but unless you improve your pattern, the hip flexors will continue to work in this way, making stretching ineffective. It also means that the hip flexors may not contract effectively through a full range. Your hip flexion action may actually be quite weak, especially if your trunk is not stable enough to provide an adequate fixed point for muscles to pull from. Even international-level competitors have had to start with this most basic of exercises to establish a normal relationship between the trunk and hip flexors.

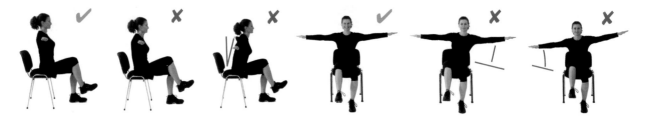

Sit on the front of a chair with both feet on the floor hip-width apart. Make sure you are sitting directly on your sitting bones. Lift both arms out to the side until they are level with your shoulders. This will help you to monitor your trunk position. Before moving, relax your breathing. Keeping your weight evenly pressing through both of your sitting bones, lift one knee and hold it in this position for 5 seconds. Your arms should not have moved and you should see no visible abdominal activity occurring. If you have kept your position correctly, your lower abdominals will be creating support for your hip at an appropriately low level. Check that you can still breathe by expanding your lower ribs. Your knee should be in line with your hip, neither outside nor inside that line. Your lower leg should hang straight to the floor without turning. If it doesn't, straighten it so that your foot will place itself precisely on the floor once you lower your knee.

### What would a poor performance look like?

- Your ribs draw downwards and inwards because you are overusing your oblique abdominals.
- Your trunk shifts sideways to counteract the load of the leg.
- Your trunk shortens on the lifting side.
- Your belly button turns towards the lifting leg.
- You collapse your trunk forward.
- Your knee is not in line with your hip and has moved either inward or outward.

| Reps | 10 per side |
| --- | --- |
| Sets | 2 |

### Progression

Sit on a wobble cushion and eventually a Swiss Ball to perform this movement. The challenge is far greater as you must keep your weight evenly distributed over the left and right sides of your pelvis. The distance between your armpit and your hip must remain the same on both sides during the movement so that only hip flexion is occurring.

# The Lower Control Zone
## GMax Activation

Coordination around the hip and pelvic area and the responsiveness of the gluteal group are intimately connected. Although many athletes practise strengthening exercises for this group, the key to improving their function is actually practising small, high-quality movements which unlock the pelvis from the spine and the hips from the pelvis. These movements are often new to the athlete and the increase in awareness that comes with them develops a relationship between movement and muscle. Very simple movements are needed at first.

### ○ String of Pearls Bridge

The String of Pearls Bridge is a simple movement that can help an athlete to restore mobility between the spine and the pelvis, unlock tight back muscles, and discover the relationship between the hip straightening movement and GMax. The aim here is re-patterning, and it is a little like balancing the treble and bass on your stereo system. We are not trying to switch one thing off and another thing on. Instead we are trying to increase activity in one area and decrease it in the other until we have a balance.

Start by lying on your back with your knees bent and your feet flat on the floor. Keep your feet hip-width apart and bring them towards your body. Placing your feet further from the body will bias the hamstrings, and we want to minimise this effect.

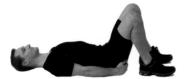 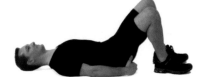 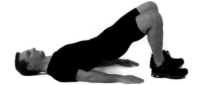

Relax your abdominals and start to tip your pelvis back towards you by pressing gently down through your feet. Your spine will peel from the floor like a string of pearls until your hips are straight but your back is still relatively relaxed.

Once you are in this position, you need to check which muscles you are using to stay up there. Feel across your lower back. If your spine feels like a deep valley between two hard ridges of muscle running down either side of it, it is likely that you are using a little too much back extensor (erector spinae) and not quite enough GMax. If you feel any discomfort in your lower back, it is also likely that you are using too much back extensor.

To rectify this, put your hands on your pelvis with the thumbs up and the fingers down. Drop your hips slightly and tip your pelvis a little more back towards you. Recheck your back – is the valley a little less deep? It is normal and desirable to have some back activity, but your erector spinae muscles should feel like gentle hills as you run your hand over them, not the Himalayas.

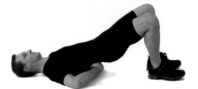 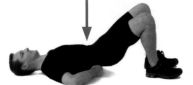 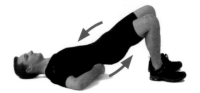

Notice that if you have tilted your pelvis a little you may find that your quadriceps feel stretched. This is an extra benefit in this position.

Once you are accustomed to feeling the difference between using GMax and using your back muscles, turn your attention to your hamstrings and adductor (inner thigh) muscles. Feel the muscles with your hands: are they firm or soft?

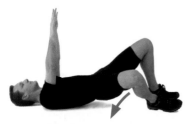

If you suspect that your adductor muscles are working too hard, maintain your bridge and move one knee outwards, maintaining your trunk position and a level pelvis. Move the knee back in and repeat with the other side The adductors must release to allow you to move your knee. You will sustain the position for the count of 10 and then return to the floor by slowly uncurling, placing one vertebra after the other on the floor. You do not need to use your abdominals to help, as this will decrease GMax's role.

**What would a poor performance look like?**

• Pushing hips and back straight up instead of rolling the pelvis into position.

• Using too much abdominal muscle to create a pelvic tilt.

• Hanging on with back muscles and hamstrings.

• Hanging on with adductors.

**Where should I feel it?**

You should feel your buttock muscles working.

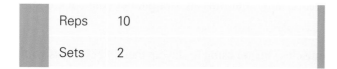

| Reps | 10 |
| --- | --- |
| Sets | 2 |

**Progression**

While holding the position, move one arm out to the side, ensuring that you keep your pelvis level. Bring it back up and switch to the other arm.

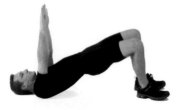 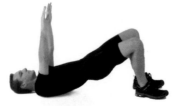 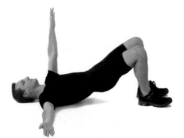

## Technical Note

Some people will worry that the spine is not held in a perfectly neutral position here. However, the aim of this exercise is to unlock a fixed relationship between the lumbar spine and pelvis in order to recalibrate the roles of erector spinae, gluteals and hamstrings. Many GMax-deficient athletes are dependent upon fixing their pelvic position with their back muscles to maintain stability, making it even more difficult to activate GMax and producing a feeling of lumbar stiffness. The String of Pearls Bridge teaches you to dissociate (independently move) your pelvis from your spine, gently mobilising your lower back. Improving this dissociative ability can help greatly with activation.

Although you have been instructed not to use your abdominals in this exercise, this does not mean that no abdominals are working! The muscles that you have direct control of at this time are more likely to be rectus abdominis and the abdominal obliques. If you relax these muscles, the deeper TrA can activate more effectively. Clinical experience has shown that actively relaxing the superficial abdominals also tends to encourage GMax to work more effectively in this exercise as it becomes the primary movement-producing muscle.

## ○ Hip Pops

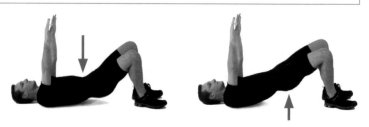

The ability to straighten the hip without overbending the spine is a critical movement for many sports. Without it, the contribution of GMax to the total power of the movement will be markedly reduced. Remember that GMax is a big, broad muscle and it is hard to compensate for the loss of its contribution. Hip Pops address awareness of the hip extension movement and inner-range activation of GMax.

Perform the String of Pearls Bridge as above. Once your trunk has reached the end point of the bridge, it will remain completely still throughout the rest of the movement: it will simply be carried up and down by the hip.

Place one finger on the crease of the hip and another directly opposite at the back of the hip on the same side. The two fingers should be pointing towards each other through the hip joint. This is your awareness focus. Move the top finger towards the bottom finger by softening the hips into a slight bend. Be conscious of this movement sensation. Now move the bottom finger towards the top finger, pressing through the feet, which encourages gluteal contraction to straighten the hips. Notice that the hips have moved but the spine has not bent within itself. Repeat 3 times before returning to the floor.

| | | |
|---|---|---|
| Reps | 10 |
| Sets | 2 |

**Progression**

Once you have the idea of the hip movement, perform it with both arms to the ceiling as shown above.

## ○ Hip Swivels

Pelvic rotation is a critical movement for normal efficient walking and running. This exercise teaches GMax activation in combination with pelvis and hip rotation. Start in the String of Pearls Bridge position. Put your hands under your buttocks. Keeping one side firmly up, let 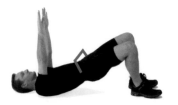 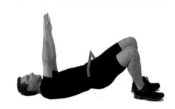 the other side smoothly drop down into your hand. This will look and feel as though your pelvis has rotated down on that side. Squeeze it back up by pressing through the foot on that side. Repeat with the other side.

| | | |
|---|---|---|
| Reps | 10 per side |
| Sets | 2 |

**Progression**

Once you have the idea of the hip movement, perform it with both arms to the ceiling as shown above.

## ○ Wall Squat

The Wall Squat takes this basic GMax activation and applies it to a vertical position. Having achieved an inner-range contraction of GMax, we want to link an awareness of hip bending with a neutral spine position while working GMax into a greater range of hip bending. This exercise is not intended to mimic a barbell squat in the weights room. Its postural position is vertical as opposed to tilted. Its priority is awareness and control of the neutral spine, independent hip motion with control through range, and eccentric/concentric GMax activity.

### ○ Wall Squat 1.0

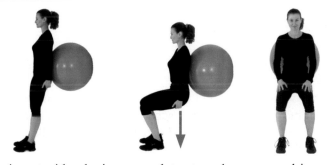

Stand with a Swiss Ball behind your back at waist level. Walk your feet forward to a comfortable point and lean back a little to allow the ball to accept your weight. Allow your hips to drop back towards the ball so that they are directly underneath your shoulders. Place your hands under your sitting bones. You will sit directly down into your hands, squeezing your glutes as you go. Pause when your knees are at 90 degrees and experiment with relaxing your glutes to make your quadriceps take more of the load and then switching the glutes back on to feel the load shared between the two muscle groups. Press through your feet into the floor and move straight back upwards again as if sliding up a pole.

### Common errors for this exercise:

1. You may not bend your hips as much as your knees so your shoulders end up behind your hips. If this happens, you will tend to use the muscles down the front of the hip and thighs but your glutes will not fire correctly. To correct this, place your fingertips into the crease at the front of the hip to remind your body to release the hip and allow a vertical alignment.

2. You may find that you knees move out of alignment with your hips and feet. Find a central point between the inner and outer borders of your feet and maintain your pressure here throughout the movement.

3. You may sneak your pelvis under the ball for extra support and sensory feedback. In this case, with your hands under your sitting bones, focus on the bones going straight down to the floor instead of back towards the wall behind you. If you feel that your weight is being supported more on one side than the other, lift this heel and perform the squat. Reducing the support on this side shifts more weight onto the other leg.

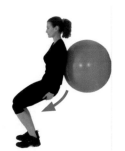
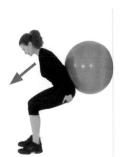
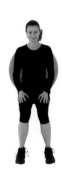

### Where should I feel it?

You should feel a shared load between thighs and buttocks, although you will feel the thighs more sharply.

Once you can perform 10 Wall Squats with good form, you can progress to the exercises overleaf.

## ○ Wall Squat 1.1 — Increasing Trunk and Hip Control

Start as for Stage 1 but this time take your arms above your head in a streamlined position. Repeat the squat but make sure that your sitting bones do not sneak backward, increasing your lumbar curve. It is much more challenging to keep the spine neutral in this position.

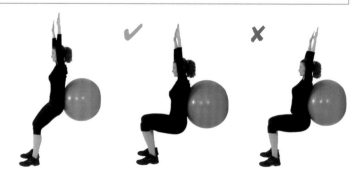

## ○ Wall Squat 1.2 — Trunk Control Against Moving Arms

Start with a Swiss Ball and a light weight in your hands. As you move down into your squat, take the weight above your head. Focus on keeping a consistent trunk position because it is easy to collapse into back extension with this exercise.

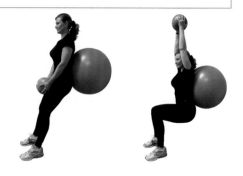

## ○ Wall Squat 1.3 — Increasing Coordination

Place your right hand on your left thigh. As you squat down, take the arm up and across your body, finishing above your right shoulder. Your knees and hips should remain pointing forward throughout the motion. This exercise can also be performed with a light weight or medicine ball.

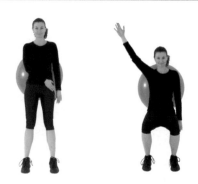

| Reps | 10 |
|------|----|
| Sets | 2 |

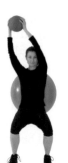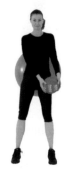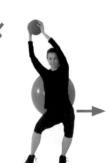

## GMed Activation

Gaining awareness and some basic endurance in GMed is helpful before trying to activate it in weightbearing.

### ○ Clam

Lie on your side with your top arm on the floor in front of you. Draw your knees and hips up, then push your top thigh forward along the line of your bottom thigh. Your top knee will overlap your bottom knee by about 5 cm. Notice that this pulls your trunk and pelvis into slight forward rotation.

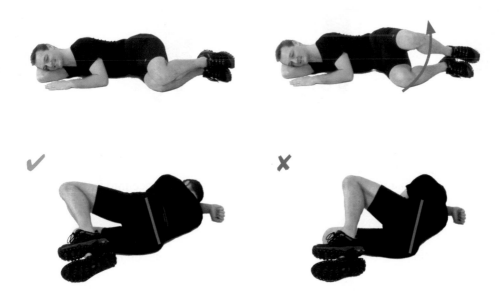

Maintaining a long, relaxed back, lift the top knee by pivoting between your feet and your hip joint. Keep your pelvis forward: it is easy to let it roll slightly backward to access stronger, more easily activated muscles. Count to 10. If you have performed the movement correctly, your top knee will land with the same amount of overlap that you started with.

| | |
|---|---|
| Reps | 10 |
| Sets | 2 |

**Where should I feel it?**

As you lie there, feel for a bony protuberance in the side of your top hip. You will feel the work just behind this bone, and you may feel it on the moving leg side or the supporting side.

**What would a poor performance look like?**

- Rolling the top hip back as you lift your leg.
- Lifting the top foot.

Once you have a basic GMed foundation, it is time to apply it to weightbearing.

## ○ Standing Knee Press

Stand next to a wall with feet together. Lift one knee and place it on the wall. First you need to focus on your stance leg. Place your hand over the bone at the side of the hip. Draw your body up over your hip. You should feel the hip bone under your hand move further underneath you. This is where it must stay throughout the exercise.

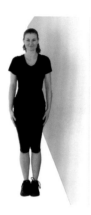 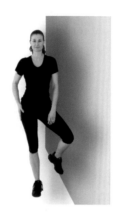 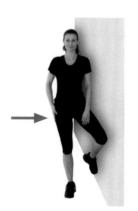 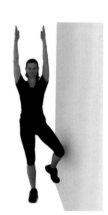

Straighten both arms up into a streamlined position. Press out with the knee into the wall, keeping the pelvis facing forward. Count to 10.

**Where should I feel it?**

Feel for a muscle working hard in the depression just behind the hip bone on the stance side.

| Reps | 5 each side |

# The Upper Control Zone
## Awareness Around the Scapula

If you need to improve your upper control zone, better awareness around your scapula can help you to feel the muscles in that area. We are not generally very aware of our scapula: we often don't relate well to body parts that we can't see or put our hands on easily. For sports such as golf, tennis and swimming, this movement also releases tension around the shoulder and neck and improves scapular mobility.

### ○ Hand Slides

Lie down on your side with your knees bent and your arms out in front of you with the palms together. Relax. You are aiming to move with the least possible amount of muscle tension. Slowly and smoothly slide your top hand forward over your bottom hand. Don't rush: you need time to feel what is going on. Notice how your scapula has moved over your rib cage, sliding forward and around in response to your hand movement.

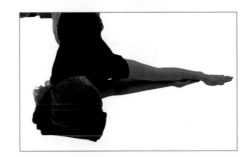

Once you have reached your limit, pause, make sure that everything is relaxed, and begin to move your hand back to the start position, again without letting your elbow bend. Your scapula will move back around your rib cage again, sliding towards your spine.

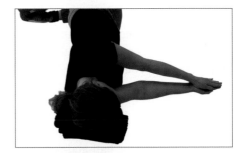

Repeat this movement again, but even more slowly. This time notice whether you are using muscles that you do not need. Notice your neck muscles and the muscles at the front of your shoulder: these are often overactive. If you notice tension anywhere, pause, relax, and then in your own time, continue on with your movement. You are aiming for effortless sliding of your scapula. Repeat as many times as you like, but at least perform 6 or 7 full movements.

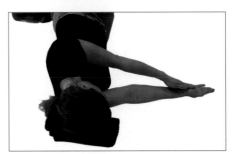

## ○ Diamond

As well as being a good quick test, Diamond works well as a simple exercise to activate lower trapezius and teach scapula-shoulder dissociation. It also targets the external rotators of the shoulder.

Lie on your stomach with your forehead resting on the floor. Place your arms in a diamond shape on the floor above your head so that your fingertips touch. Draw your scapulae slightly down towards your toes. Lift your forearms and hands off the floor and hold them there for the count of 5.

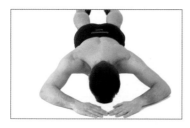 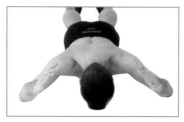

### Where should I feel it?

You will feel muscles working in your mid-back area.

### What would a poor performance look like?

• Tightening up the neck muscles: your upper trapezius and neck muscles should be completely relaxed throughout this exercise. If they are not, ask someone to tap you on either side of your spine at the level of the bottom of your scapulae. Aim to bring your scapulae towards the tapping finger before you lift your arms.

• Collapsing the front of your shoulders towards the floor as you lift your hands. To avoid this, just before you lift, be aware of the shape created between your arms and chest and the floor. Maintain that shape as you lift. If you collapse one shoulder it will move closer to the floor, distorting the shape. If this happens, focus on maintaining the ball-and-socket joint in a consistent place throughout the movement.

• Rotating the wrists and hands upwards: the hands should remain palm down with the wrists straight.

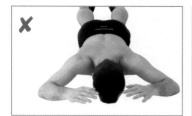 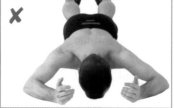

| Reps | 10 |
|------|----|
| Sets | 2  |

## ○ Windscreen Wipers — Active Shoulder Internal Rotation

As well as being useful as a test, Windscreen Wipers teaches you to control internal rotation of your shoulder joint while maintaining a stable scapula.

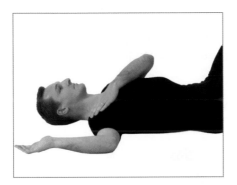 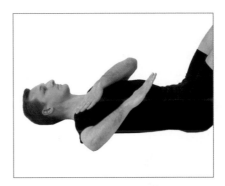

Lie down on your back with your elbow bent to 90 degrees, your upper arm level with your shoulder, and the back of your forearm and hand as close to the floor as you can without pushing.

Relax everything before you start. If you feel that your shoulder lifted closer to your ear when you positioned your arm, release it back down so that it is level with your other side. Place your other hand over the front of your shoulder. This hand will monitor the movement of the ball in the socket of your shoulder joint.

**Note:** if your pectorals (chest muscles) are tight, you may not be able to rest your elbow on the floor without your shoulder joint pushing up or forward. You must begin with your shoulder in an optimal position, so until you gain more muscle length, place a small, folded towel under your elbow to lift it slightly and take the pectorals off stretch.

Keeping your elbow secure on the floor, lift your forearm so that your arm rotates and your hand now points to the ceiling. Imagine this position as the zero position, with the floor being the 90-degree mark in each direction. This completes stage one of the movement. Keep moving in the same direction until you cannot continue without shifting your shoulder position. This completes stage two of the movement.

### Where should I feel it?

- You are aiming for a smooth, effortless movement, so it is not a question of where you should feel it, but where you shouldn't. There should be no sensation of tightness in your neck and no overstrain in your pectorals.

- You should be able to perform this movement without feeling your shoulder pushing upwards or rolling forward into your hand. If you detect the ball pushing into your hand, it means that it is losing its position in the socket by sliding forward.

| Reps | 20 |
| --- | --- |
| Sets | 2 |

## ○ The Sphinx

This basic movement will acquaint you with your serratus anterior muscle and give you an appreciation of a scapular motion.

Start on your stomach propped up on your elbows. Make sure that the elbows are in line with the shoulders and wrists, and that the arms are parallel to each other. Begin by sagging gently between your shoulders, then press your forearms into the floor to lift your upper body into a strong position with your neck in line with your spine. Hold for a count of 5.

You are aiming for your back to look smooth, with the scapulae pressed firmly onto the rib cage.

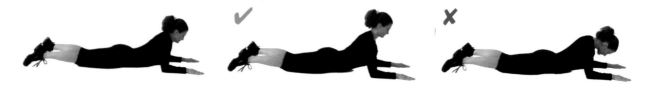

**Where should I feel it?**

This should not be hard work. You should feel general muscle activity around the back of your shoulders.

**What would a poor performance look like?**

Dropping the head or tipping it backward. Keep a long, neutral neck.

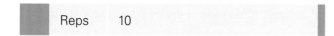

| | Reps | 10 |
|---|---|---|

# Activating Stability Relationships

## ○ Wall Press — Developing the CLA and Shoulder/Trunk Integration

The Wall Press is a good basic test of zone stacking and is also a foundation movement for coordination of the upper control zone with the central control zone. A former European junior champion in triathlon attempted this in the clinic and could manage only 5 repetitions before her TrA fatigued.

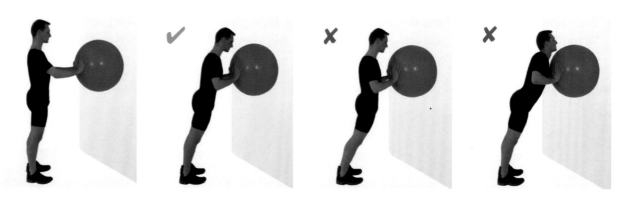

Place a Swiss Ball on a wall at chest height. Your arms should be straight and your body upright. Switch your balloon on to stimulate your abdominals to draw inwards and your shoulders to relax. Keeping this entire set-up consistent, press slightly into the heels of your hands and bend your elbows so that your body moves towards the ball. You should be looking into the ball if you have kept your head position. At the point where you are closest to the ball and about to press out again, you should especially focus on maintaining your lower abdominal position as it is tempting to let it relax and sag outwards.

**Performance points to note:**
- Long back of neck.
- Relaxed shoulders so that you can press from your upper control zone.
- Lower abdominals maintain a gentle inwards feeling.

**What would a poor performance look like?**
- Head tips back.
- Shoulders draw upwards.
- Back sags forward when the abdominals switch off.

**Where should I feel it?**
You are aiming for a strong secure feeling in your trunk and shoulders. Focus on feeling how your lower abdominals work to prevent your spine from sagging forward.

> **Note for therapists:** The best places to cue are at the base of the skull with a light upward pressure to prevent the head from rotating backward, and with fingertips just below the navel to provide sensory feedback for abdominals.

 | Reps | 10 |

If 10 repetitions are easy, progress to the Single Leg Wall Press.

### ○ Single Leg Wall Press — Shoulder/Trunk/Hip Integration and Rotational Trunk Control

Start in the set-up position as above, but lift one leg. Draw your body up over your hip so that your GMed is triggered and your spine is aligned vertically over your stance foot. Perform the press, making sure that your shoulders and pelvis stay parallel to the wall and that you do not lose your abdominal activation.

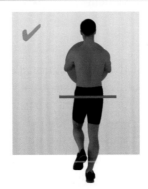
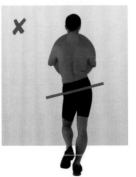

 | Reps | 10 each side |

## ○ Superman

This is another common and useful exercise when performed well but it is of little use if it isn't performed accurately. It coordinates the pelvis, trunk and upper body and increases awareness in all three control zones while activating muscles at low threshold. When performed well, it is an early elastic support exercise, integrating anterior and posterior chains.

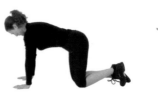 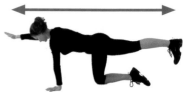

Start on your hands and knees with your head and neck in straight alignment with your spine. Hands should be positioned under shoulders, knees under hips. Draw your lower belly upwards and press your chest slightly away from the floor until your upper back is flat. Press straight out with one heel keeping your pelvis level, making sure that your supporting hip does not sag out to the side. Stretch out with the opposite fingertips so that you have a straight line from fingers to heel. Your chest and pelvis should be parallel to the floor.

Focus on this position feeling strong and secure as you really stretch your fingertips from your heel. Hold the position for the count of 5 and come back to the start position before switching sides.

**Performance points to note:**

- Head and neck in line with the body, not dropped down or rotated upwards. These head positions will switch off TrA and distort the scapular stability pattern.

- Chest pressed gently way from the floor to maintain a secure scapula.

- Heel, not toe, pressing out so that a strong straight line from the trunk through the hip is achieved.

- Feel that TrA is tucked up towards the spine.

- Pelvis level, not rotated or sagging out through one hip (as shown in Chapter 5, Superman).

---

**Variation 1**

Start in your basic Superman position with opposite arm and leg outstretched. Move your arm out to the side, then under your body and straight out in front again. Your trunk should remain still throughout the movement.

**Variation 2**

Increase the speed of dynamic control. Perform the Superman as described above but this time snap your arm and leg out into position and then hold for a moment to ensure that you have hit the target position. Bring your arm and knee back under your body. Keeping your back neutral, repeat this quick, accurate movement.

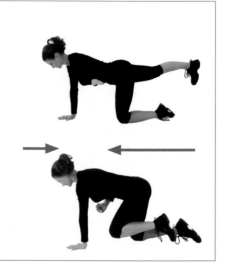

---

Once you can perform 10 repetitions each side, move on to Hovering Superman.

## ○ Hovering Superman

Take up the Superman position and then lift your knees from the ground. Maintain your balance and press one heel out behind you until your leg is level with your back. Lift your opposite arm and maintain your position for a count of 5.

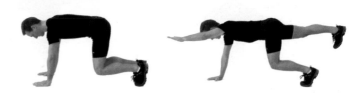

Add Variations 1 and 2 as outlined on the previous page.

## ○ Basic Balance

The purpose of the Basic Balance exercise is to connect the foot to the hip, decrease unnecessary muscle activation so that your limbs can move freely, and increase low-effort stabiliser activity. When the eyes are closed, Basic Balance exercises can help to integrate the vestibular and sensorimotor balance systems. This is important when you cannot depend on your vision as your primary balance system. If you need your sight to judge an opponent's movement, track a ball, or cope with variable lighting conditions, this type of training will help. If you have to move over uneven surfaces, decreasing dependence upon your vision and increasing the responsiveness of your sensorimotor system will help you to avoid injury.

Stand in your balloon posture. Lift one leg and move both arms directly above your head. Relax any gripping action around your ankle and soften the foot so that it can listen to the floor accurately. Lift your body up over your hip to ensure that you are activating GMed and reduce any tension that you may be holding in your trunk.

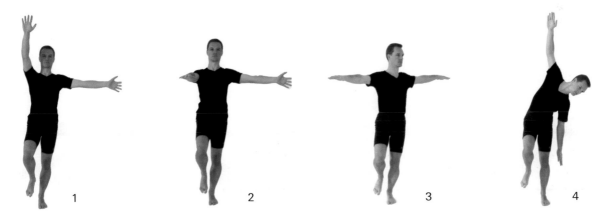

1. Move one arm down to your side and back up.

2. Take both arms to the front and move one to the side, repeating the same action with the other side.

3. Bend the stance knee and turn your trunk one way and then the other.

4. With arms outstretched, bend your upper body to one side so that one arm points upwards and the other one downwards.

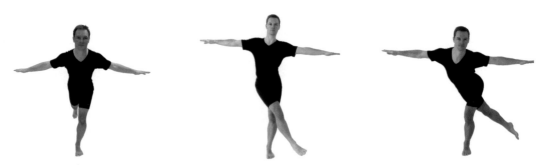

5. Move the other leg forward as far as you can, back as far as you can, to the side and across your body diagonally.

Once you can do this, practice the same routine with your eyes closed. This can be progressed on to a balance board for an increased challenge.

**Progression**

To ensure that you are not using excessive tension around your stance knee and to increase the dynamic element, gently and repetitively bend your stance knee in a rhythmic pulse throughout the entire sequence.

## ○ Star Hold — Global Stability Connecting the Hip, Trunk and Shoulder

Lie on your side with your feet together and your body in a straight line. Press up onto one hand, creating a straight body line. Reach the other hand to the ceiling. Make sure your hips are straight. Hold for a count of 10. If this is easy, start in the basic Star Hold position, and raise the top leg up.

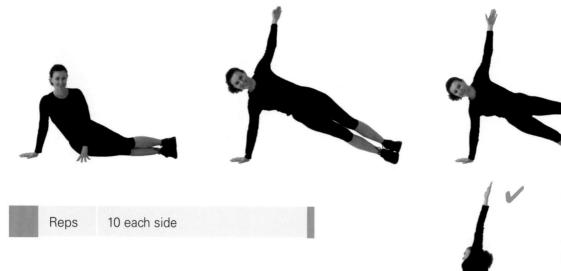

| Reps | 10 each side |
| --- | --- |

**Where should I feel it?**

You may feel your shoulder muscles or the sides of your trunk and hip.

**What would a poor performance look like?**

Allowing the hips to drop, or bend and move backwards.

# Functional Mobility

The following exercises combine stability and mobility. This helps to teach you good movement habits and encourages the body to support itself effectively while releasing tight muscles.

## ○ Straight-up Hamstring Mobility

Sit on a chair with one foot on the front of a Swiss Ball. Sit up onto your sitting bones. Push the ball away with your foot until you feel a stretch in the back of your thigh, knee and calf, maintaining your trunk position. Move the ball in and out 4 times and on the last one, hold for a count of 10.

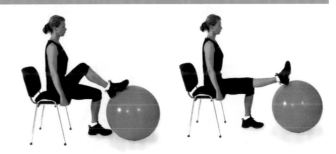

**What would a poor performance look like?**

Letting the back sag as the foot moves away from you.

## ○ Wind-up Stretch

This stretch increases mobility between the leg and the trunk.

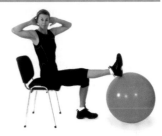

Take up the same position as above, pushing the ball out until you feel a stretch in the back of your leg. Staying up on your sitting bones, put your hands on your head and turn your trunk one way and then the other. One way should feel tighter and the other should feel looser. Slowly rotate your chest from left to right 4 to 6 times.

## ○ Floor Press

This simple technique combines trunk control with shoulder mobility.

### Variation 1

Lie on your back with your knees bent. Take one arm over your head, palm facing upwards. Keep your elbow straight and your arm close to your head. The other arm stays by your side, palm facing downwards. Prevent the back from arching by lengthening the spine and press both hands into the floor for the count of 5. Swap arm positions and repeat.

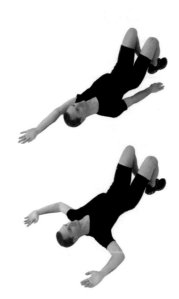

**What would a poor performance look like?**

• Arching the back off the floor; allow it to relax and lengthen.

• Bending the elbow; this will decrease your shoulder mobility.

### Variation 2

Lie on your back with your shoulders and elbows at 90 degrees resting on the floor. Your back must remain relaxed on the floor. Press down into the floor with both elbows and wrists for the count of 5.

## ○ Standing Leg Swing

This movement develops a fluid, straight leg movement pattern on the foundation of a stable trunk and pelvis, and a secure CLA.

Lift and position yourself on one leg. Stand tall and swing the other leg fully back and forth, allowing your arms to move normally. Your trunk should remain vertical and your leg should swing in a straight line. Your pelvis should remain in a constant position throughout the movement.

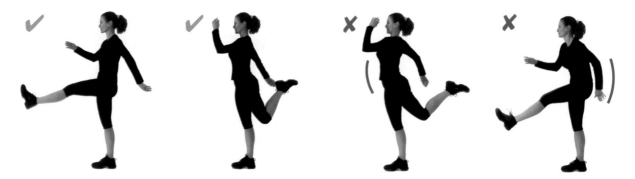

**What would a poor performance look like?**

• The pelvis tips forward and backward instead of staying level as the leg moves.

• The trunk tips sideways to stay balanced.

## ○ Rotational Leg Swing

Once the Standing Leg Swing has been achieved, the transverse plane can be added. This is relevant particularly for kicking sports.

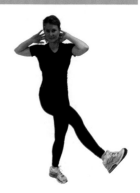

**Variation 1**

Begin by standing on your left leg and swinging your right leg. Keeping your head facing forward, move both arms to the right as the leg swings forward, turning your whole upper body. To maintain lengthening, press out into the floor with your foot.

**Variation 2**

Place your hands behind your head, with elbows wide. As you swing your right leg, turn your shoulders to the right, maintaining your CLA. This time allow your head to turn with your upper body.

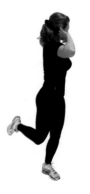

# Restoring Rotation

Rotation occurs throughout the body and is essential for normal movement. The body needs to rotate in a spiral from the feet to the top of the neck, and the spine needs to counter-rotate to decrease spinal stress and increase movement efficiency.

## ○ Thigh Slides

This is an easy "feel good" mobiliser of the mid-back. Sit comfortably upright with your hands on your thighs. Making sure that your head stays facing forward, slide one hand forward and the other hand back towards you, allowing your shoulders to turn fully into the movement.

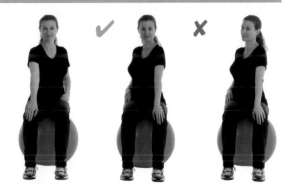

## ○ Knee Creepers

Small movements make big differences. You may have used this technique as a test in Chapter 5 but it can be used as an easy pelvic mobility exercise to encourage symmetrical pelvic rotation, as needed for walking and running.

Sit comfortably upright with your hands on your knees. Keeping your weight even on both sitting bones, slide one knee forward and the other back. This motion causes a rotation of your pelvis and lumbar spine. Smoothly and easily, reverse directions so that your pelvis and lumbar spine rotate the other way.

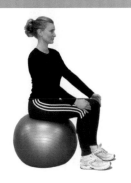

## ○ Pelvic Rotation Over a Fixed Foot

The combination of pelvic rotation and weight transference is necessary for tennis players, golfers, footballers and baseball players, but some people have a mobility awareness block around this area of their body.

Stand with your arms relaxed. You are going to turn your body to the left, allowing your right heel to lift so that your foot can pivot to allow your pelvis to freely rotate over your left foot. Letting your arms swing freely, turn to the right, lifting your left heel to allow your pelvis to rotate. Increase your awareness by noting which way your weight is moving when you rotate.

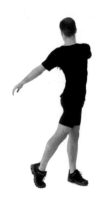
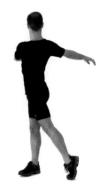

If one side feels a little restricted, hold the rotational position and smoothly shift the pressure inwards and outwards under the sole of the foot on this side. You should feel the restriction ease after a few repetitions.

The following exercises were inspired by the movement philosophy of Moshe Feldenkrais. They should be performed slowly to allow you time to notice your own movement.

## ○ Total Body Rotation

This movement restores mobility to a stiff mid-back, as well as increasing mobility deep in the hip. It integrates the rotation from the foot to the top of the neck. If you used the Total Body Rotation test in Chapter 5, this technique addresses any restrictions you may have found.

Stand with your feet hip-width apart. Turn and look behind you, noting a spot that you can comfortably see. Do not strain yourself. Turn back around the other way, noting a spot that you can comfortably see.

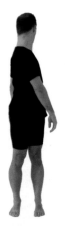
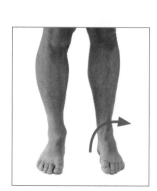
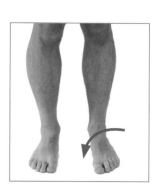
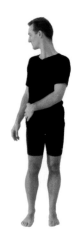

Once you have noted how much motion is available, turn your attention to your feet. Note the pressure changes in your feet as you turn. It should follow the same pattern: as you turn to the left, the left foot pressure moves towards the outer part of the foot and the right foot pressure moves to the inner part of the foot. In other words, the pressure moves in the direction of the turn.

Decide which direction is more restricted. Turn in this direction and stop when you have reached your comfortable limit. You should have your weight on the outside of that foot. Keeping your body in the same position, focus on smoothly shifting the pressure under your foot from the outside to the inside surface. If you place your hand up around the top of your thigh, you will notice that the foot motion is causing your thigh to rotate. You may notice as you continue that you feel the movement deep in your hip.

Once you have completed 10 smooth pressure shifts with your foot, keep your weight on the outside of the foot and turn in the opposite direction. This will feel strange because it is not your normal method for moving. Perform several turns with the weight maintained on the outside of your foot and then come back to standing normally on both feet. Retest your movement by turning in the direction of the original restriction, allowing your feet to move normally. You should find that you move much further.

You can also benefit from working with the other foot. As you turn to the left, experiment with changing the pressures under the right foot. Always recheck your movement after performing this self mobilisation.

## ○ Counter Body Rotation

Counter body rotation around the CLA is the basis for efficient gait, whether walking or running. Restrictions in pelvic rotation decrease your ability to absorb shock and they increase stress on lower body structures. Good pelvic rotation engages small muscles around the spine to increase stability in your lower back. This movement aims to increase awareness and mobility in your spine.

Lie on your side with your hips and knees bent to 90 degrees. Pause before beginning the movement. Slowly slide your top knee forward over your bottom knee. As you smoothly draw it back, again focus on maintaining a long, relaxed spine. The most common error is tightening the lower back muscles as you slide the knee back. Focus on keeping the lower back the same length throughout the movement. If you do this, your CLA is being maintained and the correct muscles will be working. Repeat this movement several times, aiming to make the forward and backward movement as pure as possible.

Once you have mastered this, add counter rotation from the shoulders. As you slide your top knee forward, move your top shoulder backward fully, opening your chest towards the ceiling. Slowly reverse the movement, drawing the top knee back toward the hip and allowing the top shoulder to rotate fully forward. Make the movements slow, smooth and easy. Repeat 10 times each side.

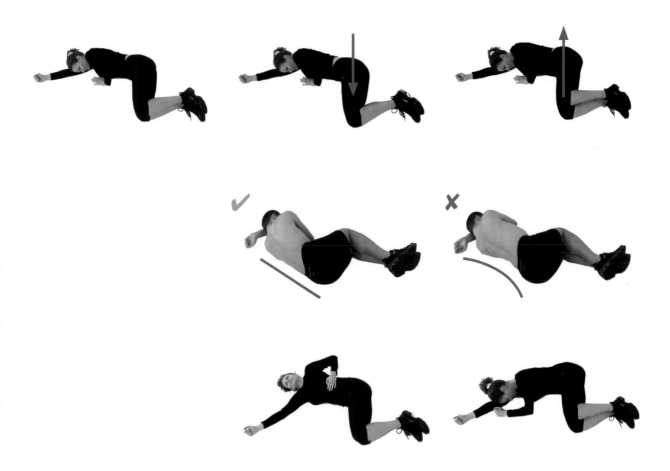

**Clipboard Notes**

An elite badminton player with recurrent hip pain was assessed and found to have poor trunk and pelvic stability. He was an immensely strong-looking player with highly developed quadriceps and hamstrings, and he regularly performed a heavy strength programme in the gym. He depended upon his adductor group to compensate for poor GMax/GMed activation, and had frequently presented with adductor strains in the past. His lack of central control had eventually taken its toll and he sustained a serious injury to his hip joint.

Despite his elite status, this player found the Wall Squat 1.3 extremely difficult even with a one-kilogramme weight. His hips would move sideways as the weight moved across his body and he was unable to control this. The String of Pearls Bridge helped him to find and activate his GMax in order to improve his pelvic control.

The player also found the Wall Press very difficult as he had no appreciation of a neutral trunk position and no TrA activation to maintain control. His spine would sag into extension as he approached the wall. Ball Bouncing and Greyhound exercises taught him how to control his trunk with low effort.

Once the athlete had learned to secure his CLA and to activate his trunk and pelvic stabilisers, he was able to progress through Phases 2–4, integrating what he had learned into his on-court training so that new movement habits became his natural way of moving.

Stories like this are common: athletes are allowed to compensate, and if they are achieving success their faults are interpreted as individual style. Small movements are rarely tested, bypassed in favour of exercises more in keeping with the athlete's elite status. However, big, dramatic movements are built on a collection of smaller elements, and if these elements are missing, problems will eventually emerge. In this case, a talented and high-achieving athlete was rendered unable to train or compete for an extended period due to a long history of uncorrected motor control problems. Like so many other athletes, he benefited from the basic movements provided in Phase 1, and was able to progress through to Phase 4 by building his stability in a systematic manner.

# 7 | Phase 2 — Integration

Central Longitudinal Axis Control
Integrating the Trunk with the Upper Control Zone
Integrating the Trunk with the Lower Control Zone
Balance
Mobility

Having activated some key relationships, you now need to coordinate your control zones to work effectively together. Phase 2 exercises will show you how to add variation to key exercises and to progress the foundations achieved in Phase 1. Progression involves a change in either load or skill, steadily increasing physical capability in a systematic way.

## Features of Phase 2 are:

**1** The stabilising of one body part against the movement of another.

**2** A higher level of challenge to CLA stability.

**3** Control of body weight against gravity.

**Remember your basic guidelines:**

- balloon posture

- relaxed face and jaw

- listening feet

- normal breathing

- a performance objective of effortless control

As mentioned in Chapter 6, the quality of each movement is the most important factor to consider. Once your system fatigues, it may be impossible to continue to perform an exercise correctly. Although a guide to the number of repetitions and sets is given for the exercises, you may need to adapt these to your ability. It is more productive to perform 2 sets of 5 repetitions and perform each one perfectly, than to perform 10 repetitions with poor form. Unless otherwise specified, 2 sets of 10 repetitions will be sufficient for each exercise.

If you decide to perform 2 sets of an exercise, use the break between the sets to perform a different exercise that uses different muscle groups. For example, a set of Over the Top which addresses anterior chain muscles can be alternated with a Suspension Bridge which addresses posterior chain muscles.

# Central Longitudinal Axis Control

## ○ Single Leg Bounce

This exercise has been used for many sports to train symmetry of weight distribution over each leg. It quickly exposes trunk control issues and highlights control preferences between sides of the pelvis. This is equally important to correct whether your sport requires you to stand or sit.

Sit on a ball with your feet and knees a little closer than hip-width apart and find the position where your weight is going straight through your sitting bones. Take both arms above your head, feeling the stomach draw inwards in response to the movement. Now peel one foot off the floor, keeping your weight evenly distributed across both sides of your pelvis.

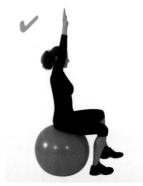

Begin bouncing, taking care to land directly onto your sitting bones. Your task is to maintain a constant neutral pelvic position as you bounce.

| Reps | 5 each side |
| --- | --- |

## What would a poor performance look like?

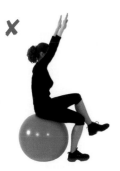

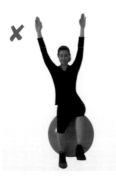

Your pelvis creeps forward on the ball so that your spine slumps.

Your pelvis moves sideways in the direction of the lifted leg.

### ○ Pelvic Bouncing Lateral Tilt (BLT)

Rowers, paddlers and riders need both stability and controlled mobility around their lumbopelvic areas. The stable Single Leg Bounce is extremely important for balance and symmetry, but to further develop controlled mobility, the following "displace and recover" exercise can be added.

### Step 1

Before attempting this exercise, check that you are able to perform the Pelvic Side Tilts (test 5.2), Chapter 5. This ensures that you have the available range to work with.

### Step 2

Begin a basic Ball Bounce with both feet on the floor and your arms stretched vertically. Then tilt your pelvis to land more on one sitting bone for one bounce, and recover to the centre for one bounce, before tilting the pelvis the other way and recovering back to the centre.

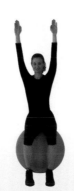 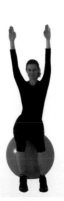 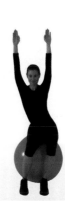

### Step 3

Now you can progress to the Single Leg BLT, aiming for consistent control.

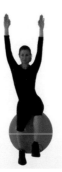 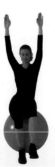

## Integrating the Trunk with the Upper Control Zone

An ideal exercise programme provides a wide range of control challenges for the body, and variation around a central task is an efficient way to diversify the physical element being trained. The next few pages illustrate how to diversify and progress a basic exercise by changing the plane and the range of motion to be controlled, and the coordination requirements, from upper on central control zone to integration between all three control zones.

### ○ Over the Top

Over the Top (OTT) is a key exercise for a number of reasons. It trains the shoulder and trunk as a functional partnership, and as it requires load bearing through the arms, helps to stimulate rotator cuff activity. As a trunk exercise, OTT trains control in a neutral trunk position, which reinforces the central axis. Most of the OTT elements train zone stacking.

Kneel behind the ball with your hands on it. Roll over the ball, walking with your hands on the floor until your thighs rest on the ball. Find your balloon posture by lengthening the back of your neck and allowing your lower abdominals to move up into the Greyhound position. Your head should be level with your spine looking straight down at the floor with the back of the neck long.

Maintaining a strong, straight body line, push your body back over the ball. Imagine that you are opening the angle between your arm and your trunk as your body moves away from your hands. Your body will remain level, and your back will not sag downwards. To pull forward, imagine closing the angle between your arm and your trunk.

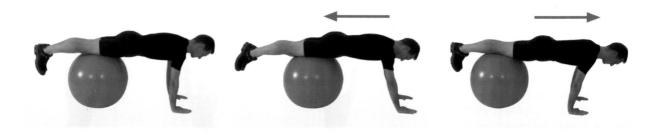

### Key Point

Starting with the ball too far down your legs will make you use your hip flexors and superficial abdominals to maintain the spine's position against gravity. Start with the ball under your thigh. Some people find it effective to point their toes and press them away from the crown of the head. This will often trigger an automatic response from the abdominals, which lift towards the spine. Others find that bending the ankles and pressing the heels away helps their spinal position. Experiment with both and select the option that lifts and lengthens your spine.

**What would a poor performance look like?**

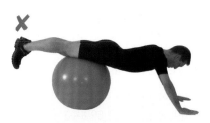

- Your spine sags towards the floor, compressing your vertebrae. Focus on lengthening your spine by pressing the top of your head away from your tailbone. This helps you to draw your lower abdominals up with low effort to support the neutral spinal position.

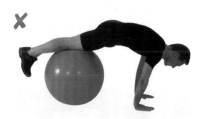

- Your trunk bends as you pull forward. Focus on the movement being generated by your arms as you maintain a straight trunk instead of using hip flexors and superficial abdominals.

- Your shoulders collapse or move towards your ears. Maintain your neutral head position, lengthen the back of your neck, and lift your chest a little so that you feel stronger in your shoulders.

## ○ OTT Progressions

Once OTT is established, the following variations can be mixed into the set to achieve slightly different effects.

### ○ OTT Circles — Altering the Control Plane

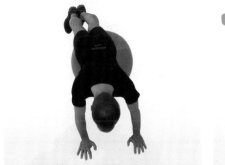
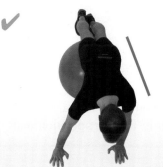
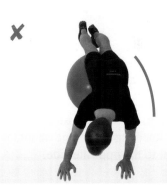

Set up as for OTT. Keeping your body absolutely straight, move your trunk in a circle over your hands. Do not allow the pelvis and trunk to move out of line.

### ○ OTT Press-ups — Increased Upper Zone Control: Moving the Upper Limbs on a Stable Trunk

Set up as for OTT. Using the ball as a fulcrum, bend your elbows and tip your trunk downwards. As your head moves downwards, your feet will move upwards. Press straight up to the start position.

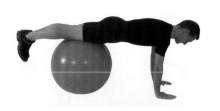
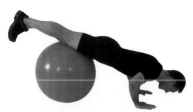

○ **OTT Squat Thrust — Hip Mobility and Trunk Proprioception: Moving the Lower Limbs on a Stable Trunk**

Set up as for OTT. Push backward, but as you pull forward, draw your stomach into your spine and bring your knees under your body. Take your legs back down to the start position.

The most important part of this exercise is the return to the start position. If your body awareness around your trunk area is not good, you will either stop short of the neutral start position with your hips slightly bent, or you will move past the neutral start position by relaxing your abdominals and letting your spine sag. As you come down, think about stretching the top of your head away from your feet so that you generate the right amount of trunk tension to control the movement.

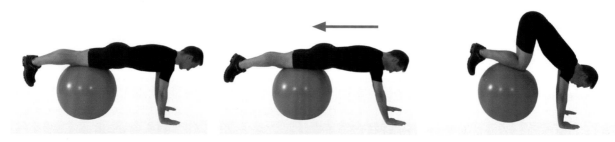

○ **OTT Twisting Squat Thrust — Increasing Lumbopelvic Control Through Rotation and Flexion**

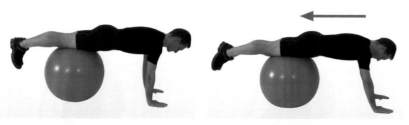

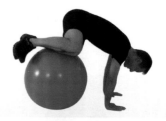

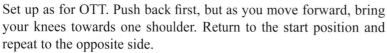

Set up as for OTT. Push back first, but as you move forward, bring your knees towards one shoulder. Return to the start position and repeat to the opposite side.

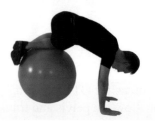

○ **OTT Scissors — Maintaining the Axis with Pelvic Rotation**

Set up as for OTT. Press your right thigh down into the ball and pass it under your left thigh so that your pelvis turns to the left. Slowly reverse the movement and repeat it to the other side.

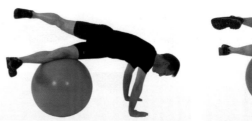

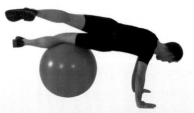

## ○ OTT Single Leg Squat Thrust — Increased Hip Control and Rotational Trunk Control

Set up as for OTT and perform a normal straight squat thrust. On your next repetition, press back as you normally would but as you come forward, use only one leg, allowing the other to straighten behind you. The supporting knee should come through straight in line with the hip joint. Do not let it drift towards your midline. This would indicate either inadequate trunk control or poor hip control.

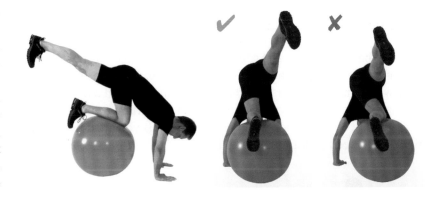

## ○ Upper Zone Stabiliser

This exercise was originally developed as part of the rehabilitation of an Olympic weightlifter. It has since been used as a training exercise for a variety of athletes who have high upper limb demands in their sport. It is interesting to note that an untrained person with normal upper limb to trunk integration would find this exercise relatively simple but an elite athlete with poor integration and well-developed compensatory strategies will struggle with it. The correlation between shoulder pain and poor integration is high.

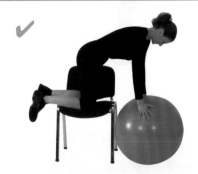

Kneel on a chair with your hands on the ball. Position your knees under your hips and your hands under your shoulders. Stay long through the back of your neck. Keep your weight through your hands and move the ball in small circles and back into the centre again. You should feel your abdominals contracting in response to the ball's movement.

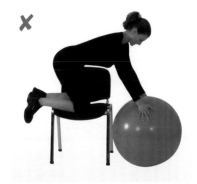
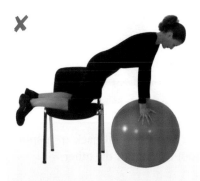

**What would a poor performance look like?**

- Reducing the load on your arms by shifting your weight backward.

- Moving your shoulders towards your ears.

- Collapsing your chest so that your scapulae wing off your rib cage.

Perform 4 x 60 second sets

## ○ Pull Backs

So far we have addressed integration of the upper and central control zones in pushing motions. This exercise introduces integration for pulling motions.

Stand in balloon posture and soften your hips and knees. Your stretch band should be attached to a fixed point in front of you at the same height as your elbow. Grasp the stretch band with both hands and make sure you start with light tension on it. With relaxed shoulders and a long spine, pull the stretch band towards you with one hand, keeping your wrist straight as you pull. Allow your chest to broaden as you pull. Slowly release your arm forward and pull back with the other hand. If you are doing this correctly, you will feel your abdominals working to keep your trunk in alignment.

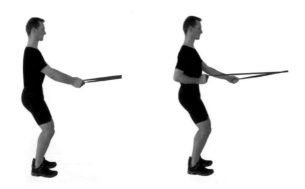

**Progression**

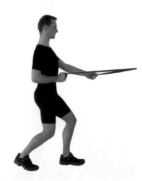

Perform the pull back in a split stance with one foot in front of the other.

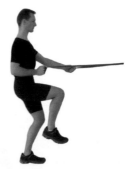

Perform the pull back on one leg with the knee slightly bent. This movement can be performed using pulleys as an alternative.

## ○ Press-ups

Once you have achieved a controlled Wall Press, higher loads can be introduced by altering the body angle. The OTT Press-up is a good bridge between the Wall Press and a Press-up off the floor as it assists you in keeping your trunk controlled. Once you can perform this exercise without difficulty, you can progress to the following exercises.

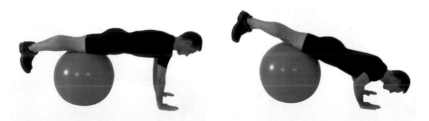

Press-ups off the floor are good general exercises that can be done anywhere. However, it is easy to do them poorly when you don't have basic trunk and scapular stability. Focus on maintaining a long neck and trunk throughout the movement.

### ○ Press-ups: Level 1

Take up a position on hands and knees and walk your hands out until your body forms a straight line from your knees through to your ears. Lengthen from the back of your neck down to the base of your spine and press your chest slightly away from the floor.

Keeping your trunk alignment controlled by drawing your lower belly upwards, bend your elbows and lower your chest to the floor.

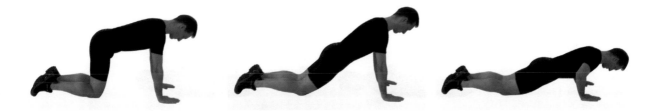

**What would a poor performance look like?**

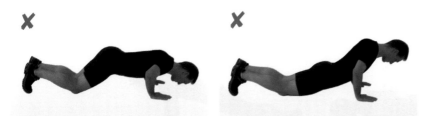

- Dropping your head or tightening the back of your neck.

- Letting your lower back sag forward.

- Bending your hips.

## ○ Press-ups: Level 2

Take up a plank position with your hands on a bench. Lengthen through the back of your neck, straighten your hips and draw your lower belly up to your spine.

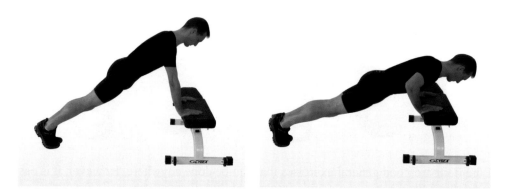

Lift your chest a little by pressing the bench away from you. Bend your elbows and move your chest towards the bench without losing your trunk alignment. Keep the back of your neck long and in line with the rest of your body.

## ○ Press-ups: Level 3

For practical purposes, this level is listed here as a progression, but it is actually a Phase 3 exercise.

Lie on your stomach with your hands placed at shoulder level. A wide hand placement will target your chest muscles more and a narrow hand placement will target your triceps more. Straighten your knees so that they lift off the ground and lengthen the back of your neck.

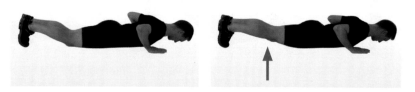

Lift your lower belly up towards your spine and press up off the floor so that your trunk hovers in a straight line just off the floor. Continue to press up until your elbows are straight. You should have a straight line from your ear through your shoulder, hip and knee to your ankle.

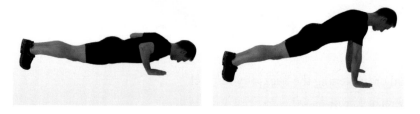

Lower yourself to hover just above the ground and repeat.

# Integrating the Trunk with the Lower Control Zone

## ○ Ski Shifts

This exercise progresses the Natural Squat to train effective weight transference and pelvic control. The key is to maintain alignment between your upper and lower body. If you lose this alignment, you will place your pelvis in a position that knocks out your GMax and GMed.

Begin with your feet apart and arms crossed in front of you. With awareness of your foot pressures, drop into a balanced Natural Squat. Keeping your shoulders and hips vertically aligned, move your weight onto one foot so that you can feel a connection all the way from that foot up to the hip. If you cannot feel that connection, you have either moved your chest across and left your hips behind, or moved your hips across without your shoulders.

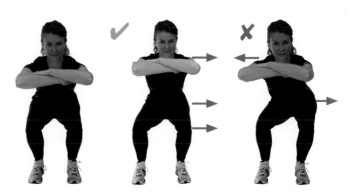

While in this position, oscillate in and out of knee bending, creating a pulse of force between your foot and hip. Make these movements smooth and as low effort as you can. After 5 or 6 pulses, move back to the centre and press back up to standing. Repeat to the other side.

## ○ Vertical Leg Drive

This is a strong progression from Ski Shifts.

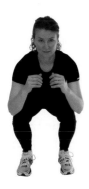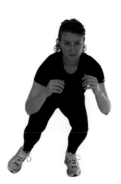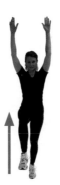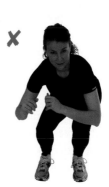

Begin in the Natural Squat as above, and guide your body weight over one foot. Make sure that your hips and shoulders are in line. Bring your attention to the weightbearing foot and make sure it is long and broad, listening to the floor. Now press firmly through it and drive all the way up into a fully vertical position.

> ### Key Point
>
> If you do not strongly feel your gluteals, you either have a tense foot or you did not achieve pelvis–hip alignment.

**Clipboard Notes**

A fit, committed trainer presented at the clinic with knee, foot and Achilles tendon issues. He had been struggling to find symmetry in his squat and habitually loaded one leg more than the other. He had a long-term habit of functional rigidity in the feet, with poor intrinsic foot function and a tendency to collapse his knee inward.

On performing the Vertical Leg Drive exercise he tended to rush, trying to get to the finish position where he could stabilise by fixing through his hip and legs. His knee collapsed inwards and his feet continued to grip.

The key to unlocking the pattern was to slow down the process, asking him to pause at the bottom of the movement and release his foot before continuing. When the foot relaxed, the pattern was perfect, with smooth, accurate vertical force and no hint of knee or hip instability. He actually had the capacity to perform the task competently but needed to release his tension to access that control.

## Lunges

The lunge is a fundamental movement for developing the lower body/trunk relationship, specifically the support behaviour. It is often included in training programmes and is commonly performed without adequate accuracy. As with any element of a strength and conditioning programme, you are not only aiming to strengthen a muscle, but to strengthen a total pattern. There is no point in performing this exercise for repetitions and sets if the basic form is not established. You will not reap the benefits of the exercise.

When assessed carefully, fundamental control faults can be observed in athletes of all levels, even when they perform regular lunges in their routines. Depending upon their sport, these faults correlate with inefficient force generation, poor foot placement in running, injury, lack of symmetry and dynamic balance problems.

The listening foot, central axis control and GMax-GMed activation established in Phase 1 are necessary to perform an effective lunge. It may even be necessary to start below the level of the Static Lunge as outlined in Chapter 5 in order to establish the correct pattern. Some athletes particularly struggle to generate GMax activity once the muscle moves out of inner range, especially if the muscle is working eccentrically, i.e. lengthening as it contracts. Decreasing the loading on the leg with the pre-lunge options below can help them to learn a correct pattern.

### ○ Supported Lunge

Having gained some lateral pelvic activation and having learned through the Wall Squat to cleanly bend and support the hips, we can now begin to gain control of one side of the pelvis at a time.

Repetition of lunges when fully weightbearing will not necessarily bring about the necessary changes. However, when loading is slightly reduced, the body is often able to learn a new pattern and relinquish an existing, less effective, one. Then the loading can be increased again.

The Supported Lunge is an extremely useful tool to start transitioning from control in even weightbearing (bilateral) to control on one side (unilateral) in the lower control zone. It provides just enough support to be able to feel the correct motion and activation without provoking an athlete's compensation strategies.

Begin in the same position as for a Wall Squat, then bring one foot back under you to rest on its toes. The front leg is the working leg. Your pelvis will be level, and your knee aligned with your hip and ankle. As with the Wall Squat, you are aiming to take your sitting bones straight towards the floor by bending your hip and knee, stopping when your knee angle is 90 degrees. Your knee should not move past your ankle. If it does, start with your foot slightly further forward.

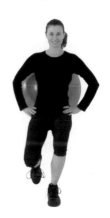

Place one hand under the sitting bone of the front leg and the other in the crease of the hip. This ensures that you will sit straight down towards the floor and cleanly bend the hip. This in turn stimulates GMax to activate. Press into the floor with a wide, relaxed foot and slide back up again. Your hips should stay straight and level throughout the movement.

The lunge can cause problems in all three planes. The instructions above address the sagittal plane, and once this is achieved well, then the coronal and transverse planes can be addressed.

---

**Training Tip**

Imagine you have a car headlight on the front of each side of your pelvis. You can even curl your hands and place them on the front of each pelvic bone to help feel this. You must keep your headlights straight and level.

Do your headlights dip down to the floor? This will be a sagittal plane collapse. Bring them back to level by releasing and lengthening your spinal muscles and easing your tailbone in the direction of the floor.

Do your headlights turn to one side? This is a transverse plane collapse. Bring them back so that the beam from your headlights is straight ahead.

Do your headlights tilt to the side? This is coronal plane collapse. The hip often drifts out to the side, the knee drifts inwards and the opposite shoulder can tend to drop. First see if you can adjust the headlights to level and maintain them through the movement. If you are finding that difficult, there is a good alternative cue.

Place your hand on the outside of the front hip. That hand's job is to ensure that the hip moves straight down towards the floor instead of drifting sideways. Stretch the other arm up to the ceiling. This gives a vertical orientation to the trunk to keep it positioned straight over the pelvis. With the hands in this position, move smoothly down into the Supported Lunge.

The headlights and hand cues are equally useful in the full weightbearing Static Lunge.

## ○ Supported Single Leg Squat

Logically it would seem that this exercise is more advanced than the Static Lunge; however, athletes who are struggling to control the Static Lunge have often mastered this exercise first.

Stand with one foot behind you resting on a chair and take a hop forward with your supporting leg. Ensure that your front knee as it bends maintains its alignment with your ankle and hip, that your sitting bones are moving straight to the floor, and that your supporting hip does not creep sideways. If your knee moves forward past your foot, you either need to hop further forward or focus more on a downward movement of your pelvis rather than a forward movement.

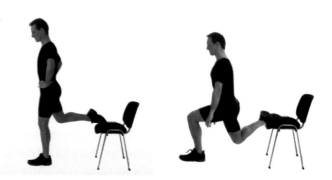

## ○ Static Lunge

Stand with one foot in front of the other, hip-width apart. Raise your back heel. Put your arms straight out to the side. Maintaining a vertical trunk, carry your body straight to the floor.

**Note:** Your body weight should not be moving forward so your knee will not end up in front of your ankle. Keep your "headlights" level and facing straight ahead.

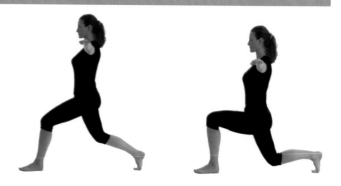

**Progression**

Adding a variety of stimuli can improve control far more than simply repeating the same movement. Manipulating the influence of the eyes, inner ear and sensory systems and learning to control one body part while another moves will help you develop more transferable balance and stability.

**Variations**

- Decrease your dependence on vision for balance and increase the role of sensory feedback from your body by performing the lunge with your eyes closed.

- Increase the complexity of the lunge by adding rotation in the transverse plane.

○ Static Lunge — Rotational Transverse Plane

Hold a light medicine ball or weight in your hands in the Static Lunge position, left leg forward. As you lower yourself to the floor, move the ball to one side by turning your shoulders. Keep your head looking straight ahead and keep your pelvis facing straight ahead. Maintain your knee alignment.

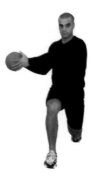

Challenge your balance systems further by performing a rotational lunge and allowing your head and neck to turn with your shoulders as you move the ball across your body.

## ○ Static Lunge — Coronal Plane

Start with the medicine ball above your head. As you move down into your lunge, take the ball over your head to one side. Your pelvis and knee should remain straight. Start by keeping your trunk upright and simply moving the ball across. As you become more comfortable, you can start to gently curve your upper spine sideways with the ball. Do not allow your hips to move in the opposite direction to the ball.

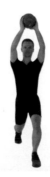
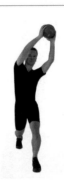

## ○ Stretch Band Lunge

Use a stretch band to increase resistance.

A partner will loop a length of stretch band around your chest and stand to the side of you. As you perform the lunge, your partner will gently pull the band and you must try to maintain your trunk in an upright position against this resistance. Your partner can change positions around you to vary the direction of resistance.

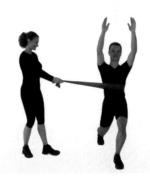

You can improve your trunk and pelvic neuromuscular responses by challenging your control with sudden changes in resistance. To achieve this, repeat the lunge with your partner, increasing and decreasing the resistance through the band at random intervals.

## ○ Static Lunge — Unstable Surface

You can challenge your balance and stability by making your support surface unstable. This instability causes you to wobble, which in turn stimulates you to speed up your control responses in order to maintain your balance.

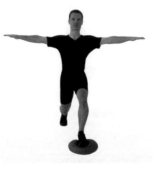

Place a wobble cushion under your front foot. Make sure that you keep your weight on the front foot as you perform the Static Lunge. It is tempting to shift your weight to the back foot.

If your Static Lunge is secure, you may choose to progress on to the Dynamic Lunge.

## ○ Dynamic Lunge

Having established the necessary motor pattern for the support strategy in the Static Lunge, you can now move onto the more proprioceptive and neuromuscular challenge of the Dynamic Lunge. As we explored in Chapter 5, the Static Lunge makes sure that the necessary muscle activation pattern is present for support. The Dynamic Lunge makes sure that this happens in time to provide that support as the body moves over the ground.

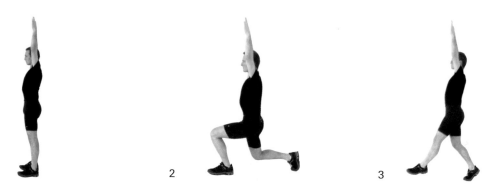

1. Start with your feet together and your arms straight above your head. Having your arms above your head accentuates the trunk control demands of this exercise. It may be useful to hold a light pole to help you to monitor yourself.

2. Step forward into the lunge, maintaining a neutral spine and knee–pelvis alignment. Your trunk should be carried by your pelvis, neither collapsing forward nor backward. Your hip smoothly moves downward on foot contact.

3. Push strongly off the front foot to come back to the start position.

**What would a poor performance look like?**

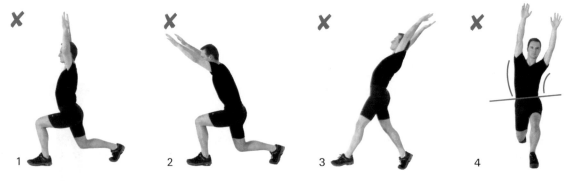

1. Your back sagging into a deeper curve as you move forward. This loss of your CLA puts your spine in a weak position.

2. Collapsing forward with your arms and trunk.

3. Using your arms and trunk to push backward instead of using your legs. The alignment from your shoulders to your hip should stay vertical throughout the entire movement.

4. Tipping your trunk to the side as you step forward. This can be due to pelvic or trunk stability problems. To keep your trunk upright and symmetrical, perform the lunge holding a light pole above your head with straight arms throughout the movement. Focus on keeping the pole level.

## Variation 1

Perform the Dynamic Lunge with your eyes closed to decrease your dependence on vision to keep your balance.

## Variation 2

Add a plane of movement. This can be performed in two ways for rotation.

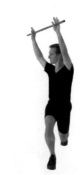

*Method 1*: Hold a light pole above your head with straight arms. As you step forward onto your left foot, turn the pole and your head to the left. Reverse the movement to come back to the start position.

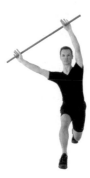

*Method 2:* Hold a light medicine ball or weight in your hands. As you step forward onto your right foot, take the ball to the right. Keep your head looking straight ahead and keep your pelvis facing straight ahead. Don't let the knee move out of line.

## Variation 3

To challenge control in the coronal plane, start with the pole to learn the pattern and then use a medicine ball above your head. As you step forward, move the ball across to one side making sure it does not pull your pelvis out of line.

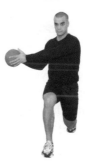

## Variation 4

As with the Static Lunge, you can challenge your system further by turning your head as you perform a rotational Dynamic Lunge.

## Variation 5

Withstand external resistance applied by a training partner through a stretch band around your chest, then try to maintain control as your partner increases and decreases the resistance through the band at random intervals.

## Variation 6

You can challenge your balance and stability by making your support surface unstable. Stepping forward onto a wobble cushion may not be completely safe as cushions tend to slide easily on the floor. However, if you have access to a Bosu unit, place it against a wall (ideally a mirrored wall) and lunge onto its surface. Aim to maintain your alignment for each repetition.

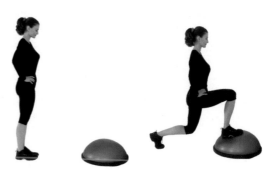

## ○ Step-ups

The Step-up teaches you to control forces between your foot and your hip and lays the foundations for strong propulsive action. This is essential for anyone who has to produce forces directed through one side at a time, e.g. in running, jumping, Nordic skiing and cycling.

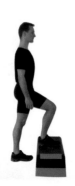 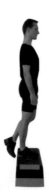 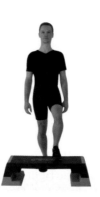 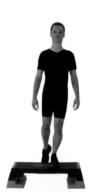

Start with your foot on a low step. Put your hands on your hips and make sure they are level. You may have to actively relax the hip on the working side to let it drop level with the other side. Press down into the step, feeling that an increase in pressure through the foot can be contained between the step and your hip as if it is a closed system. If you lose control of the pressure or allow it to "seep though a puncture", your hip will move upwards or backwards or your knee and foot will roll inwards.

To ensure that you can contain the forces between your foot and your hip, maintain this connection and rock your weight onto the foot and back off it again. Every time you move your pressure onto the leg, ensure that the forces are absorbed in the sagittal plane by the knee and ankle bending and that the pelvis stays completely level. Once you have performed this several times, continue on through the movement, pressing through the step with your trunk carried vertically until you are standing on the step with your hip and knee straight.

Keeping your hips level, control the movement all the way back down.

The down phase is as important as the up phase as it trains eccentric control. You will feel your quadriceps contract easily but you may have to feel the GMax muscle with your hand to make sure it is contributing to the movement. As you master this movement, you can increase the height of the step until it is the height of a normal weights bench. Then increase your speed to make the movement more explosive.

---

### Training Tip

Become aware that your hip is moving up and over your foot. GMax must actively straighten the hip for this exercise to be effective. If you tip your trunk forward, GMax does not have to activate, so float your trunk upright.

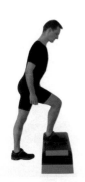

## What would a poor performance look like?

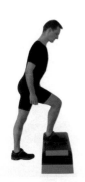 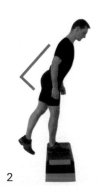 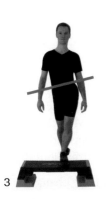 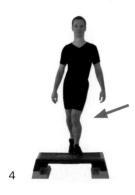

1. Trunk tipping forward. This enables you to avoid using GMax.

2. Knee straightening before the hip. This indicates an overdependence on the hamstrings.

3. The pelvis is not level throughout the movement. This flags a gluteal insufficiency.

4. The knee falls inwards. This is indicative of poor gluteal control of the femur (thigh bone).

Once you have recognised the feeling of keeping your forces between your hip and your foot with no "seeping", you can add the arms to the movement. If you begin with your left foot on the step, you will have your right arm forward and your left arm back. Your arms will switch positions as you step up.

### ○ Space Invaders

This is a great exercise for building hip abductor strength and endurance on a foundation of trunk support. You should feel it most in GMed on the sides of your pelvis.

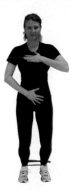 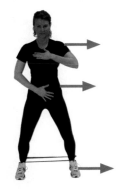 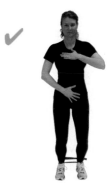

Tie a length of firm stretch band into a small loop and step into it. When starting this exercise, you can place the loop just above your knees. As you become stronger, you can place the loop above your ankles. Stay upright with your hips and knees bent in the Vertical Hip Release position. Keeping your central axis vertical, press your left leg out to the side, moving your whole body with it. In essence, you are pressing your whole body out against the resistance of your right leg.

Maintain the pressure through the centre of your right foot, otherwise your knee will be drawn inwards. Once you have placed your left foot firmly on the floor, keep the left knee straight by maintaining the pressure through the centre of the foot and slowly lift the other foot across, placing it so that there is still a small amount of tension in the band.

Repeat 10 times in one direction, then 10 times in the opposite direction

Perform 3 sets in each direction

## What would a poor performance look like?

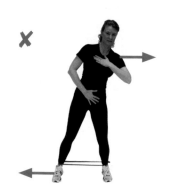

- Tipping the trunk sideways away from the direction of movement. This enables you to avoid using your GMed. You will not benefit from this exercise if you let your trunk tip. To avoid this problem, watch that your head and shoulders remain level throughout the movement.

- Shifting your hips backward. This changes the muscle group that produces the movement. Make sure that you keep your hips lined up under your shoulders.

- Allowing your knees to buckle inwards. Keep your knees in line with your hips and ankles.

## ○ Suspension Bridge

In this exercise, the first priority is establishing a balance in the posterior chain between GMax and the back extensors. Usually people focus their effort so hard on keeping their pelvis up that they arch their backs and overuse their back extensors. The procedure below establishes coordination between the back and pelvic muscles for an effective exercise position.

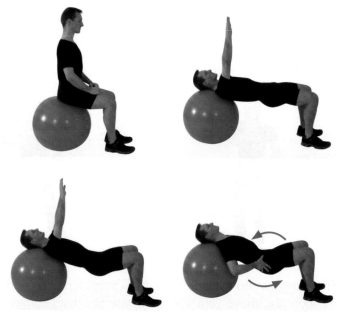

Start by sitting on a Swiss Ball. Sink your lower belly in and maintain a neutral head position while walking out with your feet, until your head and shoulders are resting on the ball. Make sure your feet are directly underneath your knees and that your hips, knees and ankles are in line.

Now feel the muscles in your lower back. If you have large ridges of tight muscle on either side of your spine, it is likely that you are overusing your back muscles and under-using your GMax. To rectify this, place your hands on your pelvis with your thumbs up and fingers down. Drop your hips slightly and turn your pelvis back towards you as if it was a large wheel. Relax and then repeat this motion until you can feel your GMax creating the movement. Feel your backmuscles again: the ridges should feel less prominent. You are not trying to eliminate your back muscles altogether but to create a balance between the two muscle groups. Your GMax should be doing most of the work, however. Don't worry if you need to start with your pelvis tilted backwards in order to reduce your back muscle activity. Once your brain works out how to support the pelvis more effectively against gravity, you will be able to move into a more neutral position. Once you have achieved this basic position, a range of variations can be practiced, each with a slightly different action. The following pages illustrate how to introduce challenges in each plane.

### ○ Coordinating Foot Movement with Pelvic Stability

Move into the Suspension Bridge. Check your back muscles and position your pelvis to maximise your GMax activation. Lift your left heel and your right forefoot. Slowly switch your foot position so that you are performing alternate heel and toe raises. Maintain your hip position by connecting through your feet into the floor and maintaining a squeeze in the gluteals.

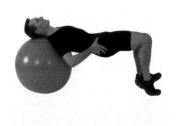

Perform 6 alternating foot and heel lifts to form a set and then walk back up the ball to a seated position. Then walk back out into the Suspension Bridge position and repeat the set before trying another variation.

### ○ Pullover — Sagittal Plane Control, Integrating Arms, Trunk and Pelvis

Move into the Suspension Bridge position with a light weight in your hands. Press the weight upwards and then slowly take it over your head, allowing your body to lengthen with your abdominals drawing in. This is effectively a Greyhound exercise in Suspension Bridge position. Maintain your neutral trunk position, visualize your pelvis as your anchor, and draw the weight back up to the starting position.

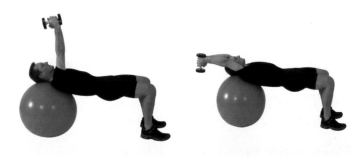

**Variation**

Take the weight over in a slightly diagonal direction from one hip over to the opposite shoulder.

**What would a poor performance look like?**

The most common error is to arch your back in response to the weight (a collapse in the sagittal plane).

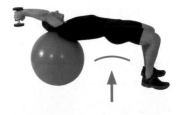

### ○ Transverse Plane Control

Begin in the Suspension Bridge position with both arms to the ceiling. Maintaining a level pelvis and level rib cage, move one arm straight out to the side until it is level with your body.

If this is easily controlled, add a light weight to the moving hand.

**What would a poor performance look like?**

If you are unable to stabilise your trunk in the transverse plane, your ribs will roll towards the moving arm or your pelvis will rotate in the opposite direction in an attempt to counterbalance the movement.

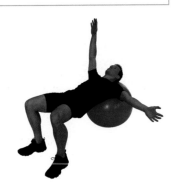

## O Sway — Coronal Plane Control with Weight Transference

This extremely useful exercise teaches you to maintain your trunk alignment in the coronal plane and triggers GMax and GMed to accept control of the pelvis as you transfer your weight.

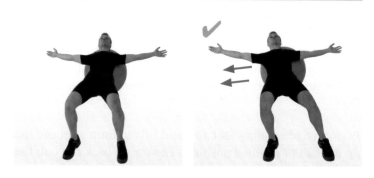

Move into the Suspension Bridge position. Now move your feet further apart so that you have a wide base. Take your arms straight out to the side. Visualize a straight line down the centre of your body.

Keeping this straight central line, move your body over the ball to one side. Pause for a count of 3 and return to the centre. Move to the other side.

**What would a poor performance look like?**

Moving your chest and your pelvis separately so that your straight central line becomes a curve. You must keep your armpit and hip in line to benefit from this exercise.

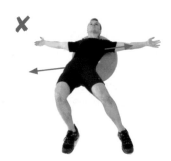

## O Medicine Ball Side Connector

This exercise challenges the central and lower control zones to stay connected during coronal plane lengthening.

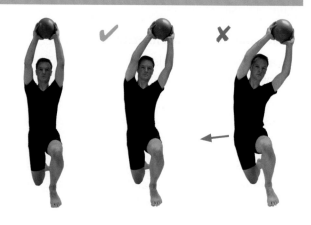

Begin in a half-kneeling position with the front knee aligned with your hip and ankle and your pelvis level. Press the medicine ball upwards allowing your trunk to lengthen. Keeping your "pelvic headlights" straight and level, move the medicine ball to one side with a sense of upwards lengthening. This will help prevent a sideways collapse as the ball brings the trunk into a gentle sideways curve.

Bring the ball back up to the centre again.

## ○ Medicine Ball Square Rotation

Sometimes an athlete's trunk control strategies are so dominantly "suit of armour" that when they try to rotate their upper body, their lower body is pulled out of alignment. This can cause stress through the groin, hip, knee and ankle.

Where the Medicine Ball Side Connector exercise trains zone connection, the Medicine Ball Square Rotation trains independent movement of one zone on another so that functional mobility is restored. This movement is therefore fundamental to the spiral elastic strategy.

### Key Point

In order to have functional mobility, it must first be available. Check your available mobility with the Seated Thoracic Mobility test from Chapter 5, and warm-up the movement before starting.

Begin in the Vertical Hip Release position with weight evenly distributed between your feet. Keeping your "pelvic headlights" and your knees pointing forward so that your whole lower control zone is square to the front, turn your shoulders and move the medicine ball around the body. Return to the start position.

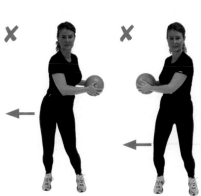

**What would a poor performance look like?**

• The knees turn away from the direction of rotation.

• The pelvis turns along with the upper body, placing rotational stress on the knees.

• The spine tightens and shortens into extension instead of maintaining its length.

## ○ Ski Jumper

Previously known as Titanic, the name of this exercise was changed as a new visualisation cue was found to be successful. Think of the ski jumper at the moment of launch into flight. The body alignment is thrust from a folded position to one that is straight and long. This is the same sense that we want for this exercise.

This exercise develops the posterior chain control of the CLA, teaching the hips to drive from flexion to extension on a neutral spine. It coordinates the relationship between back extensors and GMax, creating a sense of secure control around the lower back and pelvic area.

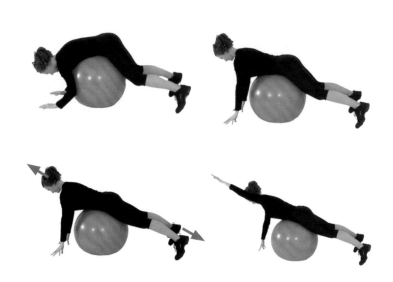

With your feet against a wall, place a ball under your pelvis. Allow yourself to bend forward over the ball with hips and knees bent. Press up with your hands until your elbows are straight. Your shoulders will remain at this height. Make sure that your nose is facing the floor so that your head and neck are in neutral. Keeping your heels on the wall, press the crown of your head as far from your heels as you can. The movement is not upward but outward. This will straighten your hips and knees. Notice that this movement has pressed the front of your hips firmly forward into the ball, as if you were going to squash something between your hips and the ball.

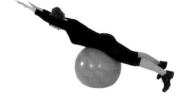

Once you have achieved this position, your back muscles should feel firm but not strained. Your GMax is responsible for keeping your hips in position. Now stretch one arm forward, feeling your TrA pull upwards. Bring it back down and reach out with the other arm. This should feel the same on both sides.

5 repetitions on each side make a set. Perform 2 sets

To progress, hold both arms in front of you and count to 10

---

### Clipboard Notes: Ski Jumper Transference

A number of weightlifting coaches have now adopted Ski Jumper as a movement initiation exercise prior to teaching the Medicine Ball Clean exercise. It lays the foundations for the athlete to learn how to coordinate their hips with their spine, feel the driving impulse through the body and learn timing and activation in a safe and supported way.

## ○ Floor Bridge

The Floor Bridge coordinates GMax with your back extensors to balance out your posterior chain, and increases trunk control.

Lie on your back with a Swiss Ball under your legs. Keep your arms on the floor and make sure that the ball is as close to you as it can be. Press forward and down with your thighs so that you smoothly roll your hips up off the floor. The ball will roll slightly out away from you until your hips and knees are straight. Pull your toes back towards you by bending your ankles. Relax your ribs slightly towards the floor to take any strain off your lower back muscles. Count to 10 and return to the floor.

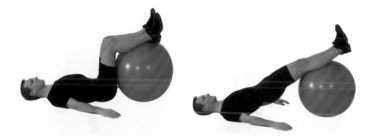

This instruction contrasts with the usual method for performing this exercise, which is to lift your pelvis off the floor. If you try to forcefully lift your pelvis off the floor, you will feel your back muscles and hamstrings working hard. The movement itself separates the pelvis from the rest of the body. This is not the purpose of the exercise. You are trying to coordinate better balance and timing between your back muscles and GMax. For most people, this means decreasing the amount of superficial back muscle used and increasing the contribution of GMax.

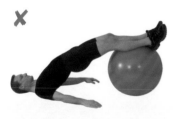

To feel the difference, perform the exercise as a rolling action as first described. Feel your back muscles and GMax and how the motion flows through the whole leg. Return to the start position. Now try to lift your pelvis strongly off the floor. Feel your back muscles and GMax. You will most likely find that the lifting technique uses a great deal more back muscle than the rolling technique and this is not the pattern you are trying to achieve.

To progress the Floor Bridge, start with your arms up to the ceiling. Move into the bridge position and keep your trunk straight as you move one arm out to the side. Bring it back up and move the other arm. Different directions of arm movement will challenge your balance and stability. Move one arm over your head and bring it back up. Move an arm across your body starting from the opposite hip and crossing over and above your head. Add a small weight in one hand to challenge your control with an unbalanced load.

# Balance

## ○ Wobble Cushion Steps

Stand on your left leg on the wobble cushion. Step forward into a partial lunge with the right leg and then push yourself back to the start position on your left leg. The working leg is the one on the wobble cushion. Focus on lightly and quickly regaining balance as you transfer your weight. Repeat this movement at different angles, adding a step to the side, backward or diagonally.

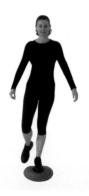 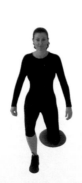 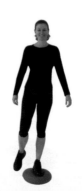 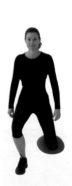

## ○ Standing Leg Swing Balance

Perform the Standing Leg Swing functional mobility exercise from Phase 1, but this time as you swing your leg forward, move smoothly up onto your toes and maintain your balance for a count of 2. Sustain the sense of an upright, floating spinal position as it is easy to let your back sag in this position. As you swing your leg back, let your heel come back to the floor.

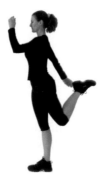 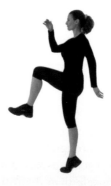

## ○ Compass Balance

Stand on one leg with a relaxed, "listening" foot. Imagine that you are standing on a compass, with north in front of you and south behind you. Bending at the hip and knee and keeping your knee in line with your hip and ankle, bend to touch the floor with your hand in the north position. Stand up again by pressing out through your foot. Keep your chest up as you bend at the hip and knee. Using the same hand, touch the floor at east, west and south, standing up between each movement. You should feel your GMax working to help you control your hip and thigh as you perform this exercise.

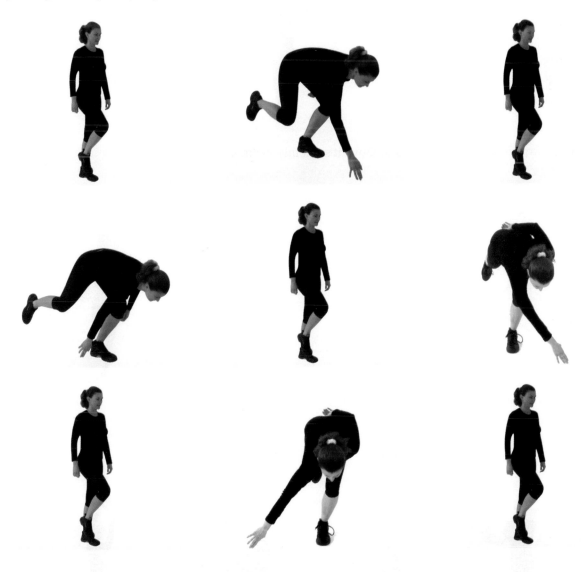

### Key Point

A foot that rolls inwards takes the knee with it. It is easier to maintain your knee alignment if you focus on maintaining foot pressure in the centre of your foot.

## ○ Single Leg Balance with Medicine Ball Movements

Holding a medicine ball in both hands, stand on one leg with your knee and hip slightly bent and your foot feeling broad and relaxed. Move the medicine ball with the following variations:

### ○ Variation 1

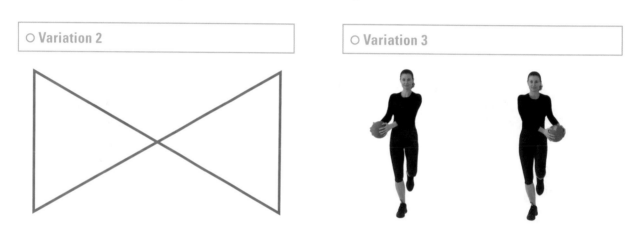

Hold the ball straight above your head and move it smoothly in circles.

### ○ Variation 2

Start with the ball above your head. Move the ball through the shape indicated in red.

### ○ Variation 3

Keep your pelvis facing forward and rotate your upper body, moving the ball to the side.

### ○ Variation 4

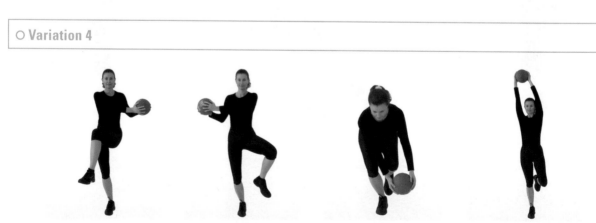

Lift your knee a little higher and take it across your body so that your pelvis and chest rotate in opposite directions. Soften your hip and knee and move the ball down to one side, then straighten your knee and push the ball up to the opposite side.

## ○ Balance Board Squats

Stand with your feet wide apart on a balance board. Keeping your trunk upright, sit down into your hips. Keep some tension in your GMax throughout the whole movement. Press back up again using GMax to support the movement.

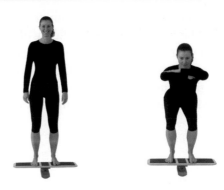

# Mobility

Just as we are learning to develop stability relationships between different parts of the body to reflect the way the body normally functions, we can also develop mobility relationships. The following exercises lengthen chains of muscle rather than single muscles to integrate balance and stability with mobility. They are a challenging but enjoyable part of a cool-down.

## ○ Triangle Pose

**S*tep 1:*** Stand with your feet facing forward and wide apart. Draw yourself up into the balloon posture which will lengthen your neck and help you to align your pelvis under your shoulders. Turn your right foot 90 degrees outwards. Turn your left foot slightly inwards. Your right heel should be in line with the arch of your left foot. Your pelvis and chest will face forward throughout the movement. Breathe in and raise both arms out to your sides with your palms down.

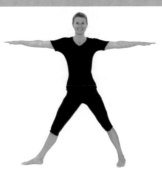

***Step 2:*** Keep your chest open and as you breathe out, reach as far as you can to the right. Once you have reached your limit, tip your trunk sideways so that your left hand points to the ceiling and your right hand slides down the inside of your front leg. Keep lengthening through the top of your head.

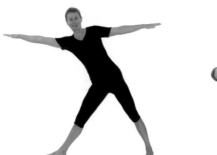
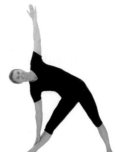

Breathe normally for 5 to 8 breaths. Inhale and come back up to the Step 1 position.

### Where should I feel it?

Depending upon where you are most restricted, you may feel the stretch down the side of your trunk or down the inner thigh of your front leg.

When you first try this pose, your hips may try to move backward as you tip your trunk. Try to keep them in line with the rest of your body. If your hips move backwards, your chest will tend to rotate towards the floor. Focus on the chest spiralling upwards.

## ○ Extended Warrior Pose

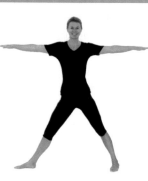

***Step 1:*** Stand with your feet facing forward and wide apart. Draw yourself up into the balloon posture, which will lengthen your neck and help you to align your pelvis under your shoulders. Turn your right foot 90 degrees outwards. Turn your left foot slightly inwards. Your right heel should be in line with the arch of your left foot. Breathe in and raise your arms out to your sides with your palms facing downwards.

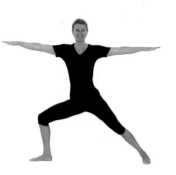

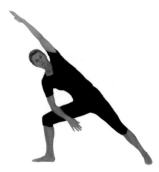

***Step 2:*** Breathe out and bend your front knee to 90 degrees, making sure that your knee does not fall inwards. Tip your trunk sideways, resting your right arm on your front leg and stretching your left arm over your head. Focus on your chest spiralling upwards and keep your hips forward to maintain your body alignment. Your left arm should remain level with your left ear. Lengthen from your left fingertips to the outside of your left foot.

Breathe normally for 5 to 8 breaths.

Step 3 is a separate pose; however it is easily combined with the Extended Warrior Pose.

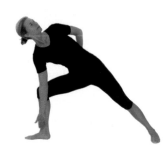

***Step 3:*** Rest your left forearm behind your back and slide your right arm down past the inside of your right knee. Press your left shoulder back and spiral your chest upwards. Use counter pressure through your right arm to prevent your right knee from falling inwards. This will feel like you are opening the right hip. Inhale and move back to the Step 1 position.

**Where should I feel it?**

You will be stretching all the way from the shoulder to the hip and you may also feel a pull in your inner thighs.

## ○ Revolving Lunge

***Step 1:*** Step forward with your right foot and position yourself in a wide lunge with your front knee at 90 degrees. Both feet will point forward. Straighten your back knee and stretch both arms upwards.

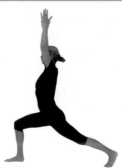

***Step 2:*** Turn your trunk to the right. Reach your right hand to the ceiling and your left hand to the floor, lengthening your body from the top of your head to your back heel. Breathe normally for 5 to 8 breaths. Breathe in and return to the Step 1 position.

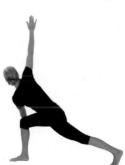

### Where should I feel it?

You will feel the stretch on the front of the thigh of your back leg, and you will feel the twist in your trunk.

## ○ Hip and Spine Twist

This exercise can be broken down into two separate components, depending upon where your restrictions are. Then they can be combined into a stretch that connects the thorax and pelvis.

## ○ Mobilising the Hip

***Step 1:*** Sit upright with your knees bent, ankles crossed and knees falling out to the side. Lift your left leg and cross it over your right leg so that the sole of the left foot is on the floor to the right of the right leg.

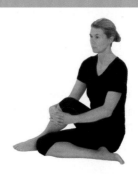

***Step 2:*** Wrap your arms around your left knee and draw your spine and your leg together so that your spine lengthens all the way from the floor. Stay in this position for several breaths and then relax.

### Where should I feel it?

This position will cause a stretching sensation at the back of the hip if this is where you have a restriction.

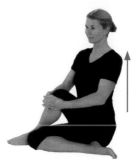

## ○ Mobilising the Spine

***Step 1***: Sit upright with your right leg straight. Lift your left leg and cross it over your right leg so that the sole of the left foot is on the floor to the right of the right leg.

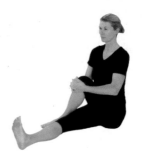

***Step 2:*** Lengthen your spine from the floor and turn your chest to the left, bringing your right arm to the outside of the left thigh. Bend your right elbow and point your hand to the ceiling. Use this arm to help you to keep lengthening and turning your chest.

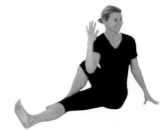

**Where should I feel it?**

This position will strongly stretch across the buttocks as well as mobilising your trunk.

## ○ Lengthening the Hip and Spinal Connection

***Step 1:*** Sit upright with your knees bent, ankles crossed and knees falling out to the side. Lift your left leg and cross it over your right leg so that the sole of the left foot is on the floor to the right of the right leg.

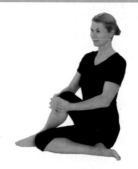

***Step 2:*** Lengthen your spine from the floor and turn your chest to the left, bringing your right arm to the outside of the left thigh. Bend your right elbow and point your hand to the ceiling. Use this arm to help you to keep lengthening and turning your chest.

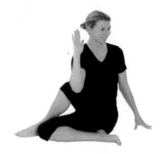

# 8 | Phase 3 — Global Coordination

Global Coordination
Progressive Upper Body Loading
Combination Stability, Mobility and Balance Sequences

Now that you have activated the balance and control mechanisms and integrated the upper and lower control zones with the trunk, you can consolidate these skills with more global, whole body movements.

Features of Phase 3 are:

**1** Whole body movement.

**2** Dynamic rotational control.

**3** Multidirectional movement.

**4** Increased loading.

**5** Moving between high and low body positions.

**6** Pushing and pulling.

Remember your basic guidelines:

• Balloon posture.

• Neutral trunk is maintained with your lower abdominals drawing in.

• Pelvic and knee alignment is controlled by your gluteal group.

• Normal breathing.

• Relaxed face and jaw.

• Performance objective of effortless control.

The cue for your hips and knees is now to imagine them as coiled springs, bending smoothly and softly with elasticity. As the loading starts to rise in the exercises, it is important to remember to have a relaxed face throughout the movements.

# Global Coordination

## ○ Medicine Ball Clean

The purpose here is to learn kinetic chain coordination in the lower limb, trunk and upper limbs and also to develop a strong pattern for hip extension on a neutral trunk. This pattern is essential whether you have to power yourself forward or upwards. This is an ideal movement to train the correct patterns if you are planning on introducing power cleans into a training programme.

Start with a medicine ball in your hands and your feet apart. Keeping your head and chest upright, drop your sitting bones into a Natural Squat with your feet flat. Press out with your feet into the floor and draw the medicine ball up your body until you are standing straight with your arms stretched upwards and the ball above your head.

When your arms are at full stretch, you should feel that your lower abdominals have scooped into the Greyhound position and your GMax is squeezing your hip straight. This combination should make you feel very secure around your lower back area.

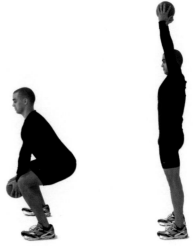

## What would a poor performance look like?

- Moving the ball upwards with straight arms. This tends to stimulate you to bend your spine backwards instead of lengthening it upwards in neutral. Instead, focus on drawing the medicine ball up your body.

- Swinging your hips forward using momentum instead of using your GMax to straighten your hips. The movement should be upwards for your whole body, so don't focus on pushing your hips forward, as this increases spinal extension and doesn't target GMax.

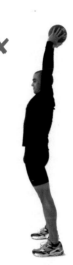

Loss of the CLA due to poor spinal control.

## Variation

Once you have established this pattern, it can be combined with a single leg drive. The exercise starts as above. As you approach the lowest point of the squat, begin to press out into the floor with the leg that you will be driving through. Maintain this steady pressure as you complete the downward phase and drive up to the stance position. This creates the connection from foot to hip and greatly improves the timing of the gluteals. Keep your balance for a moment and return to the start position.

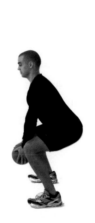

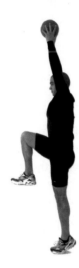

## Progression

For greater explosiveness and balance, perform the single leg drive version of the Medicine Ball Clean, but this time allow the drive to lift you off the ground to land on one leg. Maintain your balance for a moment before repeating on the other side. To really challenge yourself, land only on your toes and keep your balance.

One repetition of this exercise comprises one double leg clean, one on the left leg and one on the right leg

Repeat 10 times to complete the set

## ○ Medicine Ball Sweep

This exercise trains the same mechanisms as the Medicine Ball Clean, but adds extra lateral pelvic control.

Start with your feet together and a medicine ball in your hands. Step sideways to the left into a squat and move the ball down towards your left foot, keeping your head and chest up. Push back up and across strongly through your legs so that you end up standing on your right leg with your arms stretched above your head. Feel the Greyhound sensation in your abdominal area and a strong hip pressing the floor away. Pause and hold this position for a moment before repeating it to the other side.

### Progression

For an increased balance and lateral pelvic control challenge, perform the sweep, but as you push back up and across, focus on exploding off the ground. Land on one leg and pause to focus your balance in perfect alignment.

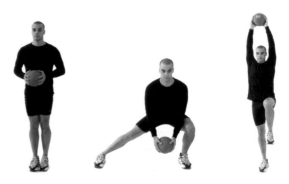

### What would a poor performance look like?

- Dropping the chest and head forward to avoid the muscular effort of controlling a deep hip bend. To gain the benefit of through-range GMax activation, focus on taking your tailbone to the floor in the squatting phase.

- Failing to hold a straight body line from the medicine ball down your body to your supporting foot at the end of the movement. Make sure that you feel the weight of the ball dropping directly through your trunk to your foot: if you watch yourself in the mirror, an imaginary line from the ball to the floor should not fall either side of your foot.

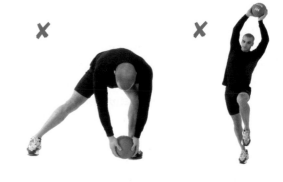

## ○ Medicine Ball Spiral

Before performing this exercise, warm up with the Total Body Rotation movement described in Phase 1. This will help you to rotate your pelvis over your foot smoothly and safely.

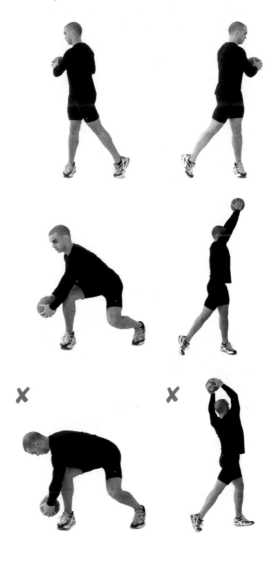

Stand with a medicine ball in your hands and your feet apart. Soften your hips and knees and lengthen your spine. Turn your body to the left, allowing your right foot to pivot and your pelvis to turn over your left foot. Reverse the motion and turn to the right.

Once this motion is established, deepen the hip and knee bend as you turn to the left and straighten your legs as you turn to the right. Your spine should maintain the same shape throughout the movement. If you can control this stage, add greater contrast with your arm movements by moving the medicine ball downwards as you lower your body and sweeping it upwards as you lengthen yourself. Focus on maintaining a neutral spine throughout the movement.

### What would a poor performance look like?

- Dropping the chest and head forward to avoid the muscular effort of controlling a deep hip bend. To gain the benefit of through-range GMax activation, focus on taking your tailbone to the floor in the downward phase of the movement.

- Keeping the back heel fixed to the floor. Remember to release the heel as you turn.

- Allowing the spine to collapse into an arch when the arms reach upwards.

## Pulleys

Pulleys offer a great deal of versatility for whole-body integrated movement requiring shoulder, pelvic and trunk stability. The exercises can be adapted to emphasise any plane of movement and can combine high-low, left-right, push-pull and rotational motion. Pulley work is an ideal method for working with elastic support, as most of the exercises included here work on connected zones moving against each other.

If you do not have access to a pulley system, the movements can be learned using stretch band at first. It should be remembered that with elastic equipment, the resistance becomes greater at the end of the movement, whereas pulleys can deliver more consistent resistance throughout the movement. Do not start with high resistance. This will simply teach you how to brace yourself using excessive effort. You should select a resistance level that is challenging but allows you to remain fluid in your movement.

## ○ Straight Pulley Push

Stand with the pulley behind you set at shoulder height and the handle in your right hand. Lift your elbow so that it is level with your hand. Start with your feet together and your hips and knees slightly bent. Your free hand will be stretched out in front of you. Your movement will involve the opposite arm and leg.

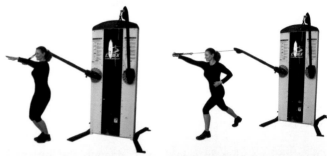

Maintaining a neutral trunk position, step forward with your left leg and push your right arm forward strongly, pulling back with your left arm as your shoulders turn to the left. Your pelvis and knee should be facing straight ahead.

### What would a poor pattern look like?

- Relaxing your abdominals and allowing your spine to collapse into a deeper curve. Maintain a firm trunk throughout the movement.

- Allowing your pelvis to tip sideways. Aim for a level pelvis throughout the movement.

- Allowing your knee to drift inwards. Maintain an open hip and central foot pressure.

## ○ Trunk Incline Pulley Push

Some sports require a neutral trunk in a forward-tilted position. A sprinter driving out of the blocks or a sprint canoeist reaching forward to catch the water represent this body position. The Pulley Push can be adapted for this position by using the same technique, but the movement objective is driving the trunk out of the pelvis. This cue is helpful in preventing collapse of the trunk in this angled position.

Start with the pulley set one hole below shoulder height. As you drive forward, you are aiming for a straight line from your hand through your body to your back foot. To achieve such a position, you need your TrA to be tucked up in the Greyhound position.

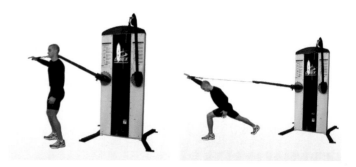

## ○ Trunk Rotation Pulley Push

Start with your feet at a 45-degree angle from the pulley column. The pulley is set at shoulder height. Take the pulley in the hand closest to the column. Place this hand on your chest with your elbow horizontally in line with it. Bend your hips and knees so that they feel like loaded springs.

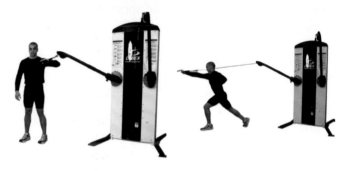

Keeping your trunk long, light but firm, drive forward onto your front leg, turning your pelvis and pivoting your back foot so that both feet are facing in the direction of the push. Turn your chest as you move and punch through with your arm. Your focus should be in that order: legs, pelvis, chest and arm. Control the movement back to the start position.

## ○ Pulley Pull

Set the pulley midway between hip and shoulder height. Stand in a Static Lunge position with your left leg and right arm forward and the pulley in your right hand. Your left arm is pulled back with the elbow bent. Without turning your hips, pull the handle straight back, switching arm positions as your shoulders turn right.

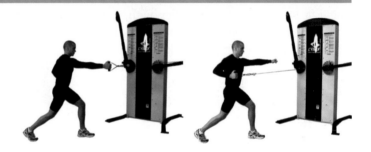

**Progression**

Perform the same movement standing only on your left leg with the hip and knee slightly bent.

## ○ Pulley Pull Drive

This exercise is good for developing hip extension timing and coordination with shoulder rotation. Practise the Lunge Drive (Chapter 5) to establish the correct movement.

Start in the Static Lunge and arm position as above. As you pull back with your arm and turn your shoulders, drive up onto your stance hip. Your end position is tall and upright over your front leg with your hip and knee straight.

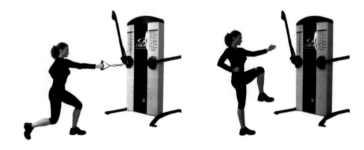

## ○ Trunk Incline Pulley Pull

This exercise is used to integrate upper limb pulling with a lengthened trunk position.

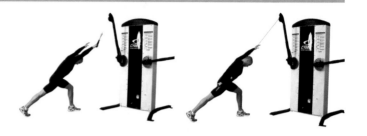

Set the pulley at head height. Start in a Static Lunge position with your trunk inclined forward and both arms stretched overhead. Your body will be a straight line from your fingertips to your back heel. Make sure that your knee is in line with your ankle and that you have engaged your front GMax. Hold the pulley in one hand. Maintaining a straight body alignment, pull your arm straight down, feeling the connection between your arm pull and your abdominals.

## ○ Cross Body Pull

Stand at 90 degrees to the pulley with your left shoulder closest to it and your feet slightly apart. Your hips and knees should be slightly bent. The pulley should be set as high as it can be. Take the pulley with both hands and lengthen your body to prepare for the movement.

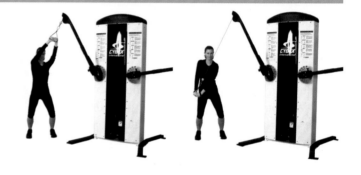

Pull down and across to the right side of your body. Keep your trunk feeling long throughout the movement and the impulse moving out through your feet into the floor.

**Note:** You will lose the benefit if you allow your body to compress as you pull down.

**Variation**

Once you have established this movement, start with your feet together and hips and knees straight. Lift your right knee as you pull down. Keep the front of your body long and open, resisting the temptation to overuse your superficial abdominals.

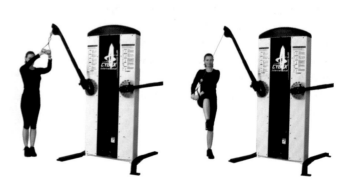

# Lunge-Based Variations

## ○ Standing Stretch Band Leg Drive

This exercise is good for developing strong propulsive movement of the body over the foot.

Start in the Static Lunge position with opposite arm and leg forward. A partner will place a length of stretch band around the front of your hips to provide resistance for you to push your hips against. Lengthen your trunk. The main movement muscle is GMax.

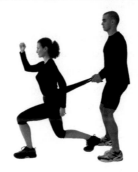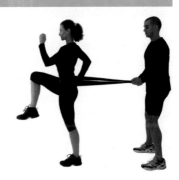

Drive your body forward and up onto the stance leg, lifting the opposite knee and switching the arm position. Hold this position for a moment and then repeat. Make sure you fully lengthen up through the back of your neck, through your trunk and out down the back of your leg. If you are compressed in the trunk or leg, it is easy to balance with a combination of the hamstrings and quadriceps rather than the more effective blend of gluteal and deep abdominal muscles.

## ○ Standing Knee Lift Drive

This exercise coordinates strong hip flexion with stable pelvic support.

A partner will loop a length of stretch band around your ankle and hold it with light tension close to the floor. Take up a Static Lunge position with this leg backwards.

Drive forward onto a straightening front leg and bring your back knee through to hip height. You should end up with your trunk erect and your stance hip and knee straight. When you first start this exercise, perform one movement and pause in the knee lifted position. Once you become proficient at it, repeat the exercise at increased speed without the pause. You must make sure that your leg returns to the same spot behind you each time.

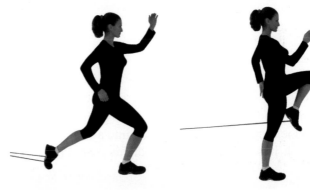

## ○ Compass Lunge

This version of the Static Lunge develops multidirectional control from the pelvis to the foot and dynamic balance for the trunk.

Stand with your feet together and imagine that you are in the centre of a compass with north in front of you. All of the movements will be performed with one leg as the moving leg, no matter which direction you move in. Allow your fixed foot to pivot naturally as you introduce side and angled movement. Relax your arms. To increase the demand on your trunk stability, the sequence can be performed with your arms stretched above your head.

The North Lunge: This is a straightforward Dynamic Lunge as outlined in Phase 2.

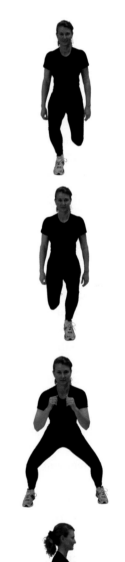

The South Lunge: Take a large step backwards and drop your back knee towards the floor. Keep your trunk vertical.

The East Lunge (right leg version): Keep both feet facing forward and take a large step to the right, dropping your body into a wide squat position. Keep your trunk vertical as it is easy to tip forward in this position. Focus on opening at the hips.

The West Lunge (right leg version): Pivot on your left foot, bring your right leg across your body and step into a normal lunge. Push strongly through your front foot and pivot on your left foot to come back to the start.

The Northwest Lunge (right leg version): Step diagonally forward across your body to the left, allowing your back foot to pivot. Your shoulders continue to face forward as your pelvis and lower body turn.

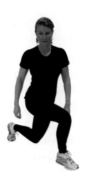

The Northeast Lunge (right leg version): Step diagonally forward to the right, allowing your left heel to lift and turn with the movement. Your feet will be pointing slightly away from each other. This will keep your pelvis facing relatively forward so that your hips open.

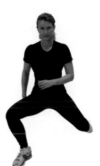

The Southeast Lunge (right leg version): Step diagonally backwards to the right, allowing the hips to open. Your back knee will be pointing diagonally backwards and your front knee will be pointing forward.

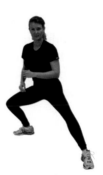

The Southwest Lunge: Move the right leg behind the body to the left, keeping the shoulders facing forward. Before trying this motion, ensure that you have sufficient lower leg rotational mobility using the Listening Foot exercise in Chapter 4.

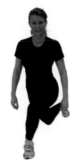

**Variation 1**

Move continuously between lunge positions without touching the ground with the moving leg in between each motion. You will be continuously controlling and balancing your body dynamically through motion.

**Variation 2**

Perform the entire sequence with eyes closed.

## ○ Progressive Lunge

These movements are often performed in warm-ups with little attention to form. They should not be taken so lightly. If you cannot perform a Dynamic Lunge with perfect form, you will not be able to control a Progressive Lunge. Poor movement habits can develop if this is not addressed. The aim is to hold your form through a series of steady, rhythmic, alternating deep lunges across a space.

A Progressive Lunge is actually a combination of a Dynamic Lunge and a Lunge Drive. It therefore requires both support and propulsion behaviours in the lower control zone (see Chapter 3).

Timing your arms can be tricky at first. If you start with your right leg forward in a lunge position, your left arm will start forward. Switch arms as you drive up into the single leg stance. Keep your arms still as you drop into the left lunge, and again switch on the upward drive. Never switch arms on the downward lunge phase.

### Variation 1: Long-Lever Trunk Control

Perform a series of alternating Progressive Lunges with your arms above your head. You should be able to maintain a steady neutral trunk that does not tip forward, backwards or sideways. Your pelvis should remain level and your knee always in line with your hip and ankle.

### Variation 2: Rotations

Start with a medicine ball in your hands and your feet together. As you step forward with your right leg, move the ball to the right, turning your shoulders with it but keeping your head facing forward. Step straight through onto your left leg, moving the ball to the left and turning your shoulders to the left.

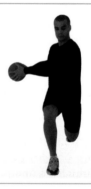

### Variation 3: Figure 8s

Start with your medicine ball in your hands and your feet together. As you step forward with your right leg, loop the medicine ball down to the right and around in a circle so that as you prepare to step forward on your left foot it crosses the centre of your body, ready to loop down to the left as you step forward. The shape of one complete left and right sequence looks like a figure 8 on its side.

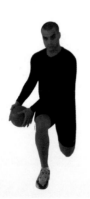 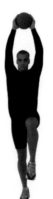 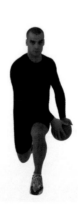 

## Variation 4: Trunk Inclines

As you step forward, incline your trunk so that you have a straight line from your hands to your back foot. Think about lengthening your trunk so that it feels streamlined.

Drive forward onto your front leg and pull your arms down strongly as your trunk moves vertically. Focus on bringing the hip forward under the trunk to achieve a vertical line. If you focus on straightening the trunk, it is most likely that you will arch your back as you recover.

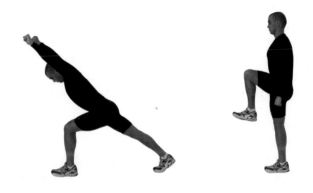

## Swiss Ball Exercises

Phase 3 exercises increase global body coordination and higher global control loads. Your performance objective is still effortless control. Release as much tension as you can while maintaining your alignment, and continue to breathe normally.

### ○ Swiss Ball Pendulum

This exercise trains trunk rotation with pelvic stability.

Assume the Suspension Bridge position. Your shoulders and head will be supported on the ball and your feet positioned slightly wider than hip-width apart, directly under your knees.

Bring your hands together above your chest. Keeping your elbows and shoulders locked in position, turn your shoulders and arms to the right, pushing the ball under you in the opposite direction. Keep driving the right side of your pelvis up with your GMax as it is most common to collapse this side.

Control the rotation back to the start position and perform the turn in the opposite direction. Take care not to lose the fixed point by dropping the hips.

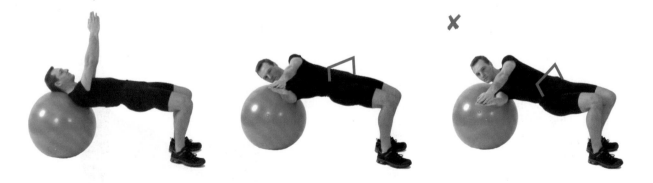

## ○ Swiss Ball Body Spin

This exercise trains smooth pelvic rotation with control of the trunk in a neutral position. This is a zone stacking exercise which teaches you to initiate rotation around your axis from the feet and hips.

Start with the ball under your hips and your feet apart against a wall. Lift your lower abdominals a little, straighten your elbows to lift your shoulders, and squeeze your hips forward into the ball. This position emphasises a balance between the back muscles and GMax to maintain the trunk position.

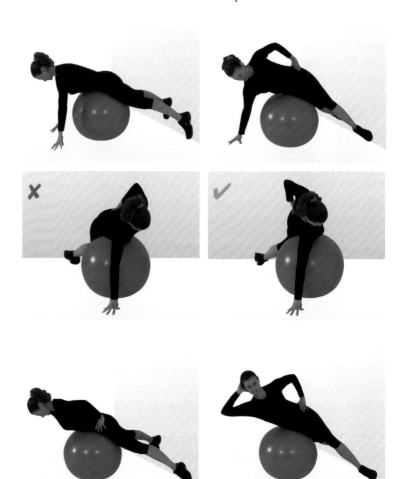

**Introductory movement:** Turn your left foot slightly outwards. Place your right hand on the floor and your left hand on your left hip. To gain an understanding of the movement without load on the trunk, turn your hips to the left, using your right hip to move the ball to the left. Allow your feet to pivot in response to the movement. Your whole body should be facing to the left. Return to the start position and repeat the movement in the other direction. Your hips remain in line with your trunk at all times.

**Body spin:** Turn your left foot slightly outwards. This is your fixed point. Place your left hand on your left hip and your right hand behind your head. Pulling from the left foot, drive the right side of your pelvis into the ball and slide it under your body so that your pelvis turns to the left. Allow your feet to pivot as you move. Keep your trunk straight and control the motion back to the start position.

**Advanced Version**

Perform the same hip drive action with both arms straight above the head. This creates a long lever for the trunk so the loading is far higher.

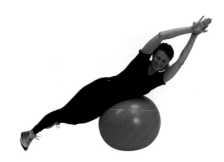

## ○ Swiss Ball Press-ups

This is a zone stacking exercise which integrates shoulder girdle and trunk.

Start in a kneeling position with your hands on the ball. Draw yourself up into a balloon posture. This alignment must be maintained no matter what angle your trunk is positioned in.

You may initially need to place the ball against a wall. Tip forward so that your weight is supported by the ball. Keeping the back of your neck long and your hips straight, bend your elbows to bring your chest towards the ball and then straighten them.

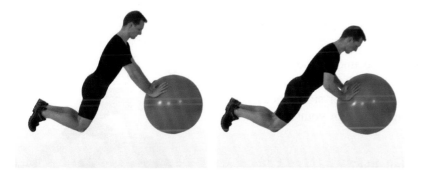

**What would a poor pattern look like?**

• Dropping your head or tightening the back of your neck.

• Bending your hips.

• Letting your lower back sag towards the ball.

• Bunching your shoulders towards your ears.

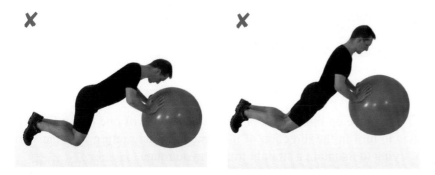

All of these errors involve compressing or shortening the body. Focus on lengthening from the top of your head to your tail to achieve the position that will most effectively activate the correct muscles for the movement.

## ○ Incline Plank Knee Drive

This is a zone stacking anterior chain pattern exercise involving smooth hip flexion.

Support your body with your hands on a bench and your feet on the floor. Straighten your body by lengthening from the back of your neck to the base of your spine and drawing your lower belly up. Lift your chest slightly by pressing away with your hands to make sure that you are engaging the muscles around your scapulae.

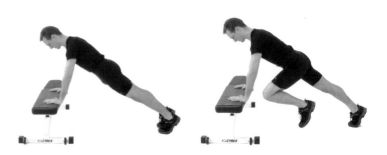

Without moving your trunk, bring one knee under your body in a straight line. Your body should remain completely still apart from this leg. Return it to the floor and repeat with the other side. Focus your awareness on feeling long, strong and light through your centre, with clean, smooth leg motion.

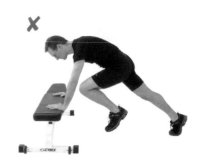

### What would an incorrect movement look like?

Your spine should not bend as you bring your knee in, or arch as you straighten your leg back out.

## ○ Twisted Floor Bridge

This exercise trains you to maintain a strong central axis around which to rotate your pelvis.

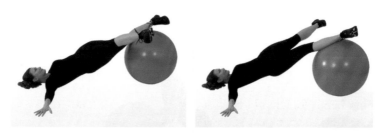

With your arms out to the side on the floor, move up into the Floor Bridge position. Lift one leg and pass it over the other one, allowing your pelvis to turn in the direction of movement. Slowly return it to the start position. Repeat in the other direction, trying to maintain a straight trunk as you rotate.

### What would an incorrect movement look like?

- Loss of control of your CLA will cause your back to collapse into an arch or a side-bend and your pelvis will not be able to cleanly rotate around the axis. You are no longer in lumbar neutral and no longer training the muscles that protect your spine during strong rotation, such as in kicking a football.

- You lose control of your supporting hip and sit down as the leg moves across, blocking pelvic rotation.

## ○ Walking Drills

Walking Drills are commonly used by track athletes in their warm-ups but are useful for many athletes to train symmetry, balance and stability through the supporting leg. You are aiming for perfect balance over your stance foot.

Start with both arms stretched above your head and your feet together. Step forward, contacting the floor with your heel. Roll over the foot up onto your toes, lengthening your body through to your fingertips as you draw your other knee up to waist height. Pause in perfect balance and repeat on the other side.

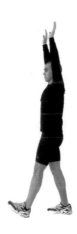

**What would a poor pattern look like?**

• Allowing the hands to drift to one side. This indicates a body alignment problem associated with a stability issue. It causes a collapse on one side of the body which in turn prevents the hip stabilisers from functioning properly. If you are not sure whether your hands are drifting, hold a light pole as you perform the drill. The pole should remain horizontal throughout the movement. If it tips downwards on one side, focus on pressing that side upwards as you move.

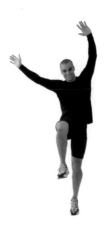

• Failing to drive up onto the toes smoothly and in balance.

• Keeping the knee or hip bent. You should be working muscles to extend your joints from your feet through your ankles, knees and hips.

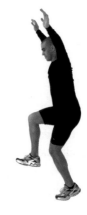

# Progressive Upper Body Loading

## O Handstand

Just as the press-up is a useful body weight strengthening exercise with the arms positioned in front of the body, the Handstand can be used to strengthen with the arms in an elevated position. Lower trapezius and serratus anterior are generally active if the position is performed well.

### O Handstand: Preliminary Level

This level helps you to become accustomed to supporting yourself in an inverted position. Kneel on a bench and place both hands on the floor with your head hanging down. Press yourself away from the floor to stabilise your shoulders. Keeping one arm firm, lift the other for a count of 5 before switching sides.

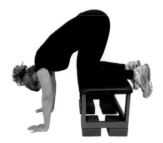 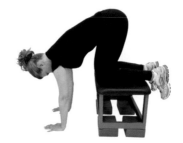 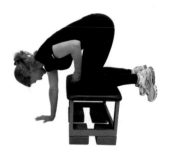

### O Handstand: Basic Level

This level demands greater trunk control and allows you to become more comfortable supporting your body weight with your arms.

Facing away from a wall, place your hands on the floor and walk your feet up the wall. Lengthen your body and firm up your trunk as you press yourself away from the floor. Sustain the position for as long as you feel comfortable and then walk back down the wall.

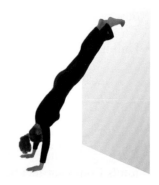

### O Handstand: Standard Level

This level requires full shoulder range and sufficient strength.

Facing the wall, place your hands on the floor and flick your legs up so that your heels rest on the wall. Lengthen your body and firm up your trunk as you press yourself away from the floor. Sustain the position for as long as you feel comfortable and then return to the start position.

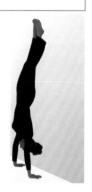

## ○ Handstand: Advanced Level

Once you have the strength to maintain a full Handstand you can introduce an inverted press-up. Maintain your firm trunk position in the Handstand and start with small elbow bending and straightening movements. The amount of movement can be increased as you become stronger. Do not try to go for a large range of motion at first – bending the elbows is easy but straightening them may not be!

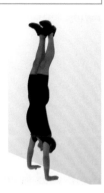

# Combination Stability, Mobility and Balance Sequences

## ○ Aeroplane Sequence

Step forward with your left leg into a lunge.

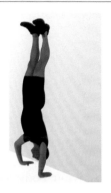

Drive your body weight forward onto the left leg, straightening your hip and knee and drawing your right knee up.

Maintain this position and move up onto the toes of your supporting leg, keeping your balance.

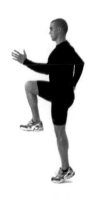

Bring your heel back down and with your hands behind your head, turn left and right with your shoulders without moving your pelvis.

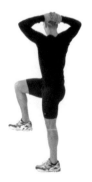
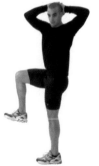

Then move your arms to the side and press your right knee outwards while keeping your pelvis facing forward.

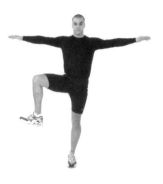

Bring your knee back across your body so that your pelvis rotates but your chest is still facing forward. Bring your leg back to the front and tip your trunk forward as you press your heel out behind you. You should have a straight line from your head to your heel.

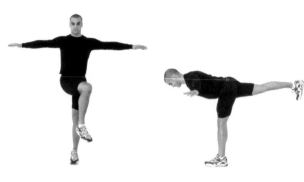

Starting with your arms out to the side, turn your chest so that your left arm is pointing to the floor and your right arm is pointing to the ceiling.

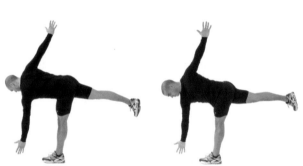

Turn your chest in the opposite direction. Recover to a straight position and, in one motion, bring your trunk back to vertical with your knee held high in front of you. Return to standing with your feet together.

## ○ Star Sequence

Lie face down on the floor with your hands under your shoulders and your elbows tucked in. Your toes will be turned under.

Straighten your knees so that they lift off the ground and draw your lower abdominals up towards your spine.

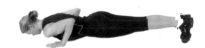

Keeping your elbows in, press up so that your body hovers in a straight line just above the floor. Count to 5. Now press fully upwards into a plank position, keeping the back of your neck long and your hips straight. Count to 5.

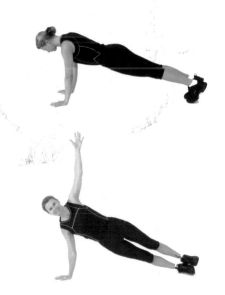

Maintaining the support in your right arm, turn your body onto its side with your left arm up towards the ceiling. This is the Star position. Keep your hips up and your shoulder pressed away from your ear. Do not let your hips drift backwards. Count to 5.

Lift your top leg and count to 5.

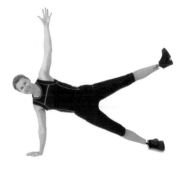

Keeping your balance, circle your top leg up and back and allow your pelvis to rotate so that your toes can touch the floor behind you. Stretch your top arm over your head so that your whole body lengthens. Count to 5.

Reverse the movements, working back from Star to plank to floor press.

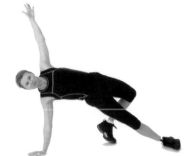

# 9 | Phase 4 — Dynamic Control

Medicine Ball Exercises
Upper Body Loading
Dynamic Control
Swiss Ball Exercises
Full Flexion Pattern Development
Stability Reactions
Mobility

Now that you have activated the systems, integrated them with each other so that your upper and lower body connect through your trunk, and learned to control different planes of motion, these skills need to evolve from conscious focus to automatic response. In order to do this, you will be distracted with a catching task or a speed demand to control. You don't have the same time available to prepare for each movement, and some of your focus will be diverted from yourself to your task. Now is the time for the movement and postural habits that you have developed to move from being the main focus to being the underpinning foundation for movement that they should be.

This is also the time to introduce general conditioning exercises for global stability and control of the trunk as it moves out of the neutral position. These higher-loaded exercises require both local and global stabiliser activity.

## The characteristics of Phase 4 exercises are:

**1** Control of movement at increased speed

**2** Control of movement when distracted

**3** General global stability conditioning

## Medicine Ball Exercises

Once you have established the medicine ball techniques, you can use them as intensely as you like. They are relatively low-load exercises compared with weight training so they can be used in high-repetition sets. The aim is to integrate the legs, trunk and arms. You are therefore aiming for fluid, well-coordinated movements. Many athletes over-stress the muscles of their shoulders because they do not transfer the power of their legs and trunk to their arms. Others over-stress their lower backs and groins because they do not freely move in their hips when dynamically challenged. The following exercises work on improving common patterns. These exercises work on improving a variety of common patterns.

### ○ Side Squat Tosses

Side Squat Tosses encourage elastic, explosive, multi-joint movement in the legs, central axis control and consistent GMax activation in both the eccentric phase (the muscle working as it lengthens) and the concentric phase (the muscle working as it shortens).

Begin standing with the medicine ball in both hands. Toss the ball up and to the side, and side skip to catch it in a deep wide squat. Absorb the motion in your hips keeping your trunk upright. Spring back up as you toss the ball in the other direction. Repeat the side-to-side movement with a steady rhythm 10–15 times.

You might start with small ball tosses but as you gain confidence, challenge yourself to toss the ball higher and wider.

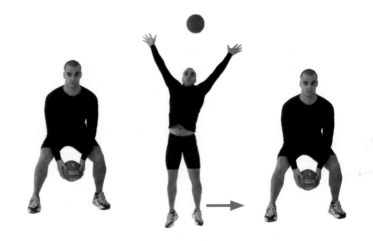

### What would a poor pattern look like?

Many athletes do not use their GMax effectively, so they do not bend their hips sufficiently. They bend their hips to a certain point and then tilt their trunks forward when they are trying to lower their centre of gravity. If they do this, they overtrain their hamstring and adductor muscles, and these muscles do not provide sufficient support for the hip. To avoid this, focus on suppleness in the hips to allow you to bend smoothly. This helps you to keep your trunk upright and puts GMax in a position where it can work more effectively.

## ○ Toss and Stretch

This adaptation of Side Squat Tosses increases the demand on your dynamic trunk control. It also requires coordination of the feet with the pelvis in response to the movement to encourage fluid, natural control.

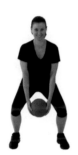 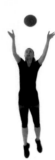 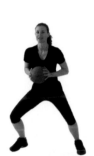 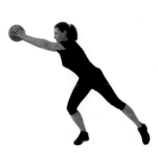

Begin standing with the medicine ball in both hands. Toss the ball up and to the side. Side skip to catch the ball and take a further step with your outside leg into a deep side lunge. Allow the heel of your back foot to lift and pivot so that your pelvis can turn as you catch the ball and push it away from you in the direction of movement. Your spine should be neutral in shape, and you should feel a line of tensile connection between your back foot through your trunk to your hands.

Pull the ball back into your centre and toss it into the air in the opposite direction. Side skip and step to catch and reach in the opposite direction.

Once you understand the elements of this movement, try to make it as smooth and continuous as possible. Don't use a medicine ball that is too heavy to start with, and maintain a neutral spine throughout the movement.

**What would a poor pattern look like?**

- This is a smooth, integrated movement from the feet to the hands. Poor performance is usually the result of a failure to release the back foot and turn the pelvis in the direction of movement. This effectively blocks the movement and causes the spine to bend and the arms to disconnect from the rest of the movement.

- Allow your lower body to turn naturally and focus on really stretching your arms and trunk out of your pelvis.

> **Training Tip**
>
> The combination of Greyhound (Chapter 6) and Ski Jumper (Chapter 7) creates the foundation for this reaching movement. Both teach you a long strong position for the trunk, integrating anterior and posterior chains.

## ○ Overhead Tosses

Overhead Tosses provide an increased trunk control challenge and integrate upper body action on a stable trunk and pelvis. It is relevant for any athlete involved in over-arm activities, whether it is a footballer taking a throw-in or a volleyball player serving. This is a linear elastic development exercise, which should be built on the foundation of a great Greyhound exercise.

Stand with your feet together in front of a wall with a medicine ball in your hands. Soften at your hips and knees. Step forward with one foot and toss the ball firmly against the wall. Focus on standing up to the movement. As you release the ball, your front hip should stay forward, and the trunk will move over it as you release the ball.

The biggest challenge with this exercise is maintaining a neutral trunk. As you take the ball over your head, make sure that your back doesn't bend backwards with it. You should feel your lower abdominals drawing in to support your spine as you raise the ball.

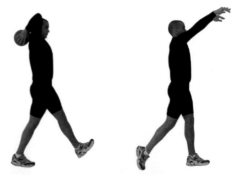

### What would a poor pattern look like?

Many athletes lose the benefit of the exercise by allowing their hips to move backwards as their trunk moves forward. They are effectively collapsing their trunk, losing their fixed point for force production and decreasing their power. Stand up tall as you throw and keep a forward focus for your whole body.

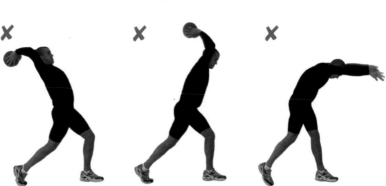

### Variation

To add diagonal motion, start with the medicine ball over your left shoulder and toss it firmly at the wall when you step through with your right foot. Switch to the opposite diagonal and repeat.

## ○ Quick Rotations

Quick Rotations require a strong central axis, a stable pelvis and an accurate rotation motion. Your challenge is to use your local stabilisers to maintain an upright trunk while your oblique abdominals generate force. This is a spiral elastic development exercise.

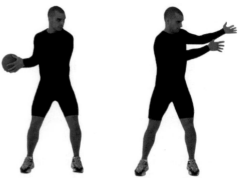

Holding a medicine ball, stand side on to a wall with feet apart and hips and knees softly bent. Your trunk position should be relaxed and upright. Whilst keeping your pelvis still, move your medicine ball away from the wall, allowing your shoulders to turn and your trunk to "wind up". Quickly rotate your trunk back towards the wall and release the ball.

Catch the ball as it rebounds and follow its momentum back into rotation away from the wall. Make sure that your trunk doesn't tilt forward. Your pelvis will remain in a consistent position throughout the movement. Quick Rotations can also be performed in a Static Lunge position.

## What would a poor pattern look like?

Poor technique will show up as a tendency to allow the rotation to pull the spine into forward or backward bending. Aim to keep your trunk upright and try to keep the ball's movement parallel with the floor.

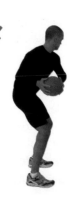
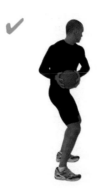

> ### Training Tip
>
> The most common error in this exercise is to use too heavy a medicine ball. If you do this, the body tends to lock together and turn as a block, which trains zone stacking, or, if the ball is way too heavy, the suit of armour strategy. Spiral elastic support development requires thorax to pelvis separation, so select a weight that allows smooth, speedy rotation of the upper body.

## ○ Follow Through Rotations

This exercise integrates pelvic rotation and weight transference into the rotational movement.

Holding a medicine ball, stand side on to a wall with feet apart and hips and knees softly bent. Your trunk position should be relaxed and upright.

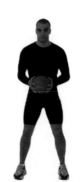
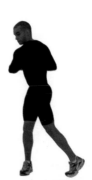
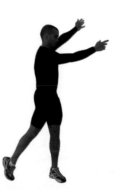

Swing the medicine ball away from the wall, allowing your weight to transfer onto your back leg and your pelvis to turn slightly away from the wall.

As you swing the ball through strongly, allow your weight to transfer onto your front foot and your pelvis to turn towards the wall. Release your back heel to allow the foot to pivot. As you catch the ball, allow yourself to rotate away from the wall again.

## What would a poor pattern look like?

Poor technique will show up as inadequate hip bending and a tendency to allow the rotation to pull the spine into forward or backward bending. Aim to keep your trunk upright and keep the ball's movement parallel with the floor.

## ○ Stepping Rotations

Having worked on isolated trunk rotation control and pelvic integration, the lower body can be added to complete the movement chain.

Stand side on to the wall a little further away than for the previous exercise. Start with your feet together. Side-step strongly towards the wall to initiate the throwing movement. Continue to rotate the pelvis and trunk over your front foot before releasing the ball. Make sure you release your back heel in order to let your pelvis rotate freely. One side will feel natural and the other side will not. Practice a few movements without the medicine ball to make sure the movement sequence is established before loading it.

You can vary your arm position. Arm options are:

1. Arms start low and rise to waist height as you rotate to release the ball.

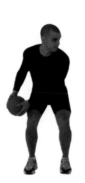
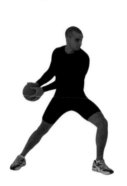
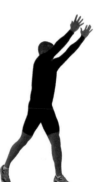

2. Arms start at shoulder height with the palms facing towards the wall.

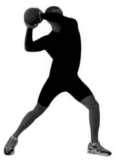

3. Arms are maintained at waist height throughout the movement.

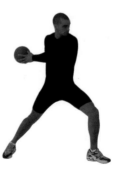

**What would a poor pattern look like?**

If you don't allow your back heel to release and turn as you move, your movement becomes blocked and you will try to throw the ball using your arm instead of using the momentum generated from your lower body and trunk. Releasing the ball should feel like a whip cracking. It should not feel like you have to use a great deal of shoulder strength.

## ○ Lunge Bounces

This exercise increases force production and focuses on integrating your arm action with your trunk and lower body. Start with your feet together and a medicine ball in your hands. As you begin to step forward into a lunge, raise the ball above your head, keeping your trunk neutral. As your front foot contacts the floor, firmly throw the ball into the floor.

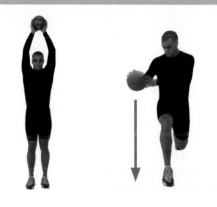

**What would a poor pattern look like?**

Allowing your spine to extend as you take the ball over your head means that you have lost trunk control and disconnected your arms from your trunk and lower body.

## ○ Standing Quick Throws

This exercise coordinates the trunk and the upper limbs with a light plyometric stimulus.

Stand with knees and hips softly bent, a long neutral spine and weight grounded through relaxed feet. Remember to keep the back of your neck long in the balloon position.

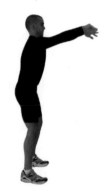

Take a light medicine ball at chest level and throw it at the wall with both hands. Catch and repeat rapidly. Feel how the abdominals and gluteals create a secure pelvis and spine.

**Progression**

Perform the same exercise on a single leg, maintaining a firm pelvis and trunk. Keep your pelvis level and your knee in line at all times.

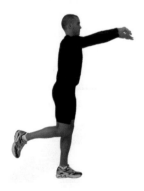

**What would a poor pattern look like?**

Your trunk should remain upright during this movement. Some athletes try to stabilise with their back muscles instead of the abdominals by pushing their hips out behind them and deepening the curve in their spine.

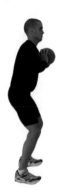

# Upper Body Loading

## ○ Plyometric Press-ups

Plyometric Press-ups can be introduced at a variety of resistance levels. All of these variations are examples of zone-stacking development.

### ○ Standing Plyometric Press-ups: Level 1

For young athletes and those who do not have sufficient scapular stability and upper-body strength to perform full Press-ups with good form, a Standing Plyometric Press-up can be performed to increase the speed of stabilising reactions.

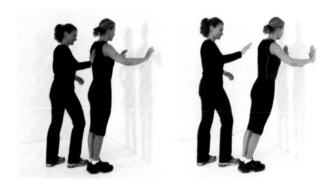

First you need to be able to perform a good Wall Press. Then ask a partner to place a hand on your back between your scapulae. This will give your partner a marker for where to keep their hand throughout the exercise. Start to perform your Wall Press. As you move back out to the start position, your partner will provide a barrier to your movement, pushing you back to the wall each time. You must keep your form regardless of the speed you select. Your trunk must remain neutral, your head and neck relaxed, your chest open and your shoulders down.

**What would poor technique look like?**

• Your pelvis is moving separately to your chest because you have lost your trunk stability.

• Your shoulders are creeping up towards your ears.

### ○ Plyometric Press-ups: Level 2

Take up a press-up position with your hands on a bench. Lengthen through the back of your neck, straighten your hips and draw your lower belly up to your spine. Lift your chest a little by pressing your hands away from you. You must be able to perform an incline press with good form before attempting the plyometric version. To do this, simply bend your elbows and move your chest towards the bench without losing your trunk alignment. Keep the back of your neck long and in line with the rest of your body. Once you can do this, increase the speed and force of the upward press so that your hands lift off the bench between repetitions. Your trunk should stay in neutral throughout the movement.

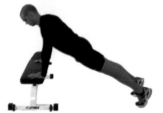 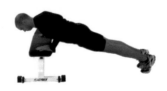 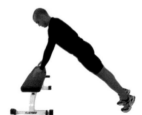

**What would poor technique look like?**

• Your hips are higher than your chest because they are bent.

• Your hips are sagging below the line of your body because you are not using your abdominals.

• Your shoulders are creeping up towards your ears.

## ○ Plyometric Press-ups: Level 3

This exercise targets shoulder and trunk stability while practising zone stacking. This means that your head is held in a straight line with your spine and with your nose pointing to the floor, your chest is open and your neck long, your hips are straight and your lower abdomen is drawn up towards the spine. Once you can do this, push forcefully off the floor so that your hands lift off.

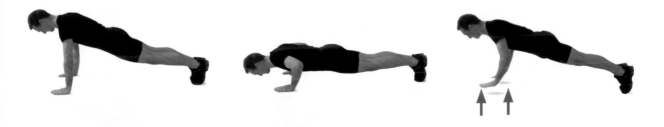

## ○ Spiders

This exercise targets shoulder and trunk stability.

Perform your press-up to the left of a low step or block. Then place your right hand on the block and perform a press-up. Place both hands on the block and perform a press-up. Drop the right hand to the floor beside the block and perform a press-up. Focus on keeping your head and neck in line with your trunk at all times throughout the movement. Maintain straight trunk alignment.

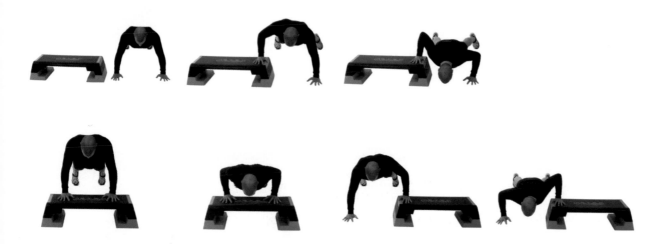

# Dynamic Control

## ○ Multidirectional Catching Lunges

This exercise introduces distraction, so the control that you have developed in Phases 1–3 must now become more automatic.

Stand with your feet together. Decide which leg you will use to lunge onto. Have a partner toss a tennis ball so that you must lunge to catch the ball, and push back up to stand on your other leg for balance. Repeat with the ball being thrown at different angles and depths.

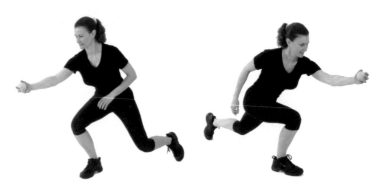

Maintain a long, strong, trunk position, no matter where the ball is thrown. It is easy to collapse your trunk for low balls, but aim instead to deepen the bend in your hips and knees to maintain a better trunk position. You are aiming to challenge your body to control larger ranges of motion and to be strong at different muscle lengths.

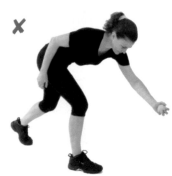

**What would a poor performance look like?**

Failure to bend at the hip and knee.

**Progression**

Perform the same exercise with your supporting leg on a wobble cushion or foam pad to increase the balance challenge.

## ○ Pendulum Lunges

This exercise introduces the new skill of controlling the body weight over a pivoting foot.

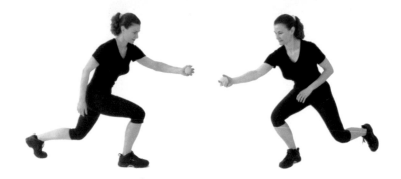

Start with your feet together facing a partner. Your right leg will be your main lunging leg for the first set. Your partner will throw a ball to your left side. You need to pivot on your left forefoot and rotate your pelvis into a lunge to catch it. Throw the ball back as you push back out of the lunge and pivot on your left foot to catch the ball in a lunge on your right side. The movement is a continuous swing from side to side.

## ○ Multidirectional Jumps and Landings

Control of landings requires dynamic balance, pelvic stability and trunk control. If your trunk shifts off-line each time you land, it will increase the stress on your lower limb joints. You will therefore aim to keep your trunk in a relaxed, upright position above your pelvis for each landing.

Before performing this exercise, you need to have established an elastic, controlled landing on both feet. Aim to minimise the sound of your landing to encourage your hips and knees to bend and absorb impact.

Start with your feet slightly apart. Your aim is to create an elastic jump with quiet landings. Jump upwards and land on one leg, softly absorbing the landing force through your hips and knees. Make sure that your trunk is central and upright and that your knee and pelvic alignment is straight. Hold your balance for a moment.

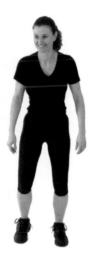 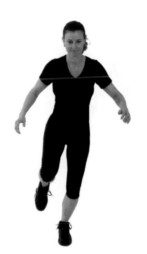 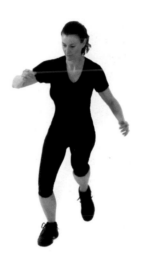

Once you can control a soft, light and elastic single leg landing, vary the direction of your jump so that you have to control forward, sideways and angular momentum with stability, alignment and balance. Hold each landing for a count of 3 before repeating.

**Variations**

Once you have mastered this, you can vary it in two ways. Research indicates that vision plays an important role in landings [102] but athletes are often visually distracted at the time of landing. So, (1) you can either increase the balance challenge by performing the jump with your eyes closed, or (2) add distraction by having a partner toss you a ball to catch just before you land.

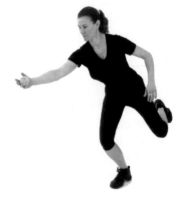

## ○ Side Leaps

The relationship between pelvic stability and trunk position has an effect on change of direction speed. As we learned in Chapter 3, athletes can overshoot with their trunks as they try to control lateral momentum, allowing their shoulders to move beyond the pelvis as they land with the outside foot. This puts the hips in a disadvantaged position to push from and makes quick changes of direction difficult. Athletes who change direction effectively start counter-moving their trunks slightly even before their outside foot contacts the ground.

GMed and GMax contribute to the pelvic foundation that places your trunk for effective direction change. In earlier phases, these muscles have become accustomed to functioning, and now they need to learn to support both a strong sideways push and also to control lateral momentum.

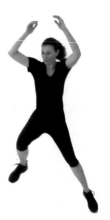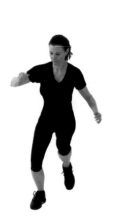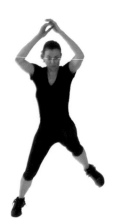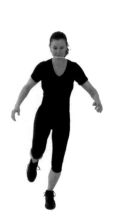

Stand on one leg with your body upright. Soften your hips and knees and leap up and out to the side, aiming to lengthen all the way from the trunk down to your toes on your push-off side. Land softly on the opposite leg, making sure that your trunk does not tip past your pelvis, that your knee is aligned, and that your pelvis is level. Immediately push back in the other direction, aiming for the feeling of being a rubber ball bouncing as you absorb the landing and immediately take off again.

Once you can do this, mark two lines a metre or more apart, depending upon your height, and leap lightly on a forward diagonal, progressing up the lines. Repeat the exercise moving backwards. You can add a jump height element, as well as jump breadth, by placing hurdles between the lines.

## ○ Mini Trampoline Leaps

Your stability will be tested further by jumping onto a slightly unstable surface in this exercise. Make sure that your mini trampoline is secured and will not slip. Stand far enough away from it that you will need to leap rather than step onto it. Ensure that you can perform the basic movement before adding distraction. You will jump from three directions.

**1** Start with a straight leap from behind the mini trampoline. As you land, soften your knee to absorb the force and keep your pelvis level, your knee aligned and your trunk central. When your form is perfect, ask someone to throw a ball to you just before you land. They can throw it slightly to the side or make you reach high or low to catch it.

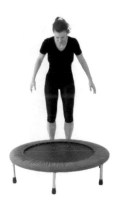 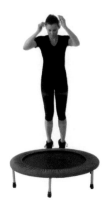 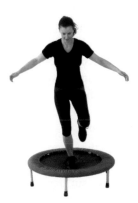

**2** Stand to the side of the mini trampoline. Push strongly up and across from your outside leg and land with the other leg on the mini trampoline. Your landing should be soft and controlled with no overshooting of your trunk. Once you can do this, add the catching task.

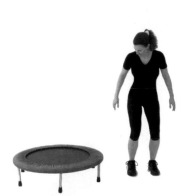 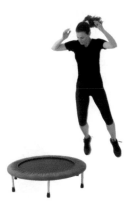 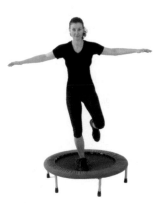

**3** Start midway between the first two start positions with both feet facing forward. Push strongly off the outside foot and land with the other foot pointing in the direction of movement. Your trunk should not collapse forward as you absorb the landing into your hip and knee. Once this is achieved with good form, add the catching task.

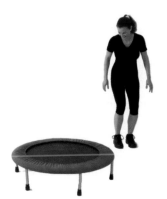 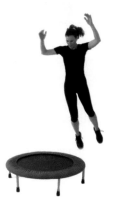 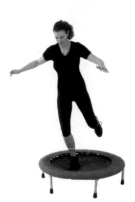

## ○ Low and High Balance

This exercise combines stability, balance and control in the pelvis and lower limb with mobility and control in the trunk.

Stand on one leg. Have a partner toss a ball for you to catch high and to the side, or low and to the side. Keep good alignment of your knee and pelvis, bending smoothly at the hip and knee to catch low balls.

**Progression**

Perform the exercise on a foam pad or a mini trampoline to add the challenge of a less stable supporting surface.

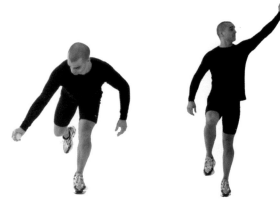

## ○ Box Jump onto a Single Leg

This exercise combines an explosive jump with stability, balance and momentum control. Prior to performing the single leg version, make sure that you can perform a jump landing with two feet on the box. Make sure you absorb the landing and forward momentum by landing lightly with soft, springy hips and knees.

Jump off both feet and land on one foot on the box, absorbing the landing elastically in your hips and knees and maintaining trunk, knee and pelvic alignment. To generate more power from your legs, perform the movement with your hands behind your head.

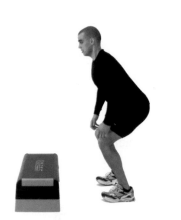
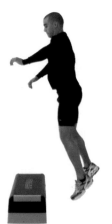
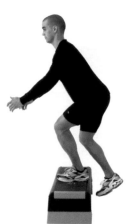

## ○ Stair Bounding

Having mastered the basic step-up, you can now progress to rapid alternating Stair Bounding. Depending upon your height, you will climb two or three stairs at a time.

Imagine a ball-bearing bouncing off a piece of glass – it sharply pings off the surface. This is how you will contact each step. Your aim is to be as light and fast off each step as you can. You should feel elastic and powerful.

Keep your trunk upright and push strongly through your legs to propel you up the stairs.

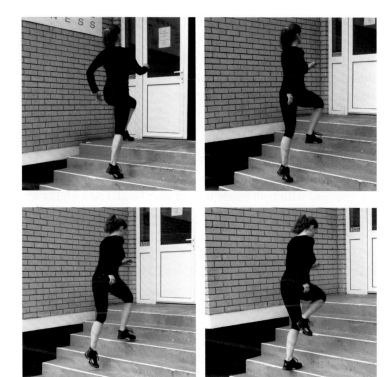

Bending forward will decrease the effectiveness of the exercise.

## Swiss Ball Exercises

Phase 4 exercises continue to increase global body coordination and higher global control loads. Do not allow yourself to make it look or feel difficult. Your performance objective is still effortless control. Release as much tension as you can while maintaining your alignment and continue to breathe normally.

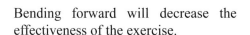
### ○ Swiss Ball Side Raises

This exercise aims to strengthen the trunk's side flexors and coordinate them with hip stability.

Lie sideways over a Swiss Ball with your feet on a wall. Place your uppermost foot forward and your lower foot back on the wall. This prevents you from sitting back into your hips. Arrange your body so that it is directly on its side and lengthen your trunk over the ball. Support your head with one hand and place the other on your uppermost thigh.

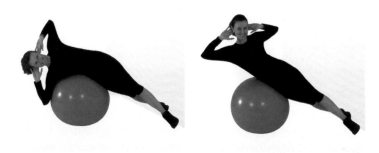

Keeping your body in this plane, slide your hand in the direction of the wall creating a side-bend to your trunk.

## What would poor technique look like?

It is easy to allow your hips to bend so that they move behind the line of the shoulders. Keep a straight body line.

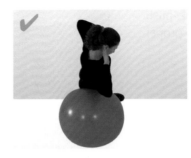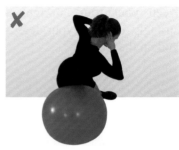

### Advanced version

This exercise lends itself well to increasing load by increasing the length of the lever. For the next level, perform the exercise with both hands behind your head. For a higher level, again stretch both arms out over your head.

## ○ Swiss Ball Full Press-ups

If you have not tried this exercise before, place the ball against the wall. Once you are familiar with it, you can move the ball away from the wall.

Support your weight in a press-up position with your hands in a comfortable position on the ball. Keep your head position neutral and your hips straight with your lower abdominals in. Bend your elbows and move your chest towards the ball. Press back out again.

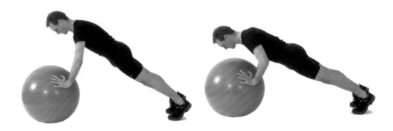

### Progression

Perform the same movement with one leg lifted behind you.

### What would poor technique look like?

- Dropping your head.
- Bending your hips.
- Dropping your hips so that your back sags.
- Letting your shoulders creep up towards your ears.

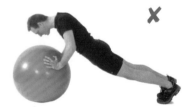

## ○ Swiss Ball Elbow Circles

Support your weight on the ball with your elbows and forearms parallel and take up a plank position. Maintaining a neutral head and trunk posture and drawing your lower abdominals upwards, move the ball in circles using only your arms.

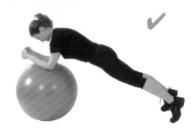

The same exercise can be performed with straight arms. This is called a **Ramp**. If the Ramp is too easy, perform it with one leg lifted from the floor.

**What would poor technique look like?**

- Dropping your head.

- Bending your hips.

- Dropping your hips so that your back sags.

- Letting your shoulders creep up towards your ears.

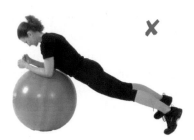

## ○ Elbow Support Knee Drive

Once you can perform the Phase 3 Incline Plank Knee Drive without difficulty, you can increase your global stability demand by introducing a Swiss Ball. Place your elbows and forearms on the ball so that they are directly under your shoulders and parallel to each other. Straighten your body out with your feet in line with your hips. Lengthen from the back of your neck to the base of your spine, drawing up your lower body. Lift your chest slightly to create a strong shoulder position. Without moving your trunk or the ball, bring your knee under your body in a straight line. Do not lift your hips as your knee moves under your body.

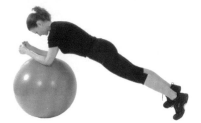
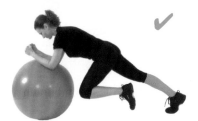
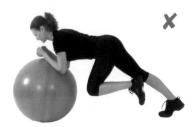

## ○ Single Leg Squat

Start in the basic Wall Squat position with the ball behind the curve of your lower back. Make sure your feet are slightly forward and positioned closer than hip-width apart. Bend your knees and hips slightly.

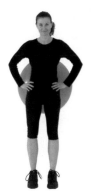
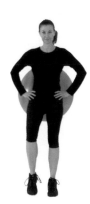
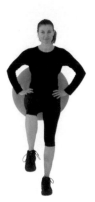
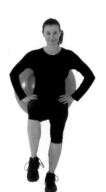
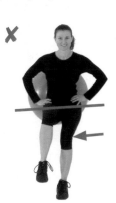

Focus on the GMax of the side that is going to support you. Lift the heel of the other foot off the floor so that you only have light toe contact, making sure you can support the position with your hips level and your knee in line with your ankle. You may need a small amount of toe support to keep your alignment. It is better to do this than to perform full Single Leg Squats with poor form. If you are able to maintain your alignment, take the supporting toe off the floor and continue the squat movement. Do not move past 90 degrees at the knee.

## ○ Swiss Ball Hamstring Curl

This exercise trains your symmetry and control of a central body line with a posterior chain bias; concentric and eccentric hamstring strength and trunk control.

Start on your back with the Swiss Ball under the soles of your feet. Your arms will be on the floor to increase your base of support. Press your feet down into the ball to lift your hips. Your GMax will work to keep your hips up. Roll the ball out away from you until your legs are straight. Aim for a straight movement. Keeping your hips up, pull the ball back towards you again.

Once you can achieve 10 of these without difficulty, cross your arms over your chest and repeat the movement. You should focus on a straight movement and straight body line.

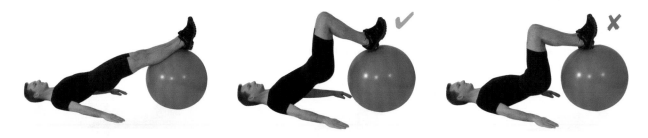

### What would a poor performance look like?
If you are not using your GMax, your hips will move up and down as your legs move in and out. Try to keep a consistent hip height.

## ○ Kneeling Ball Balance

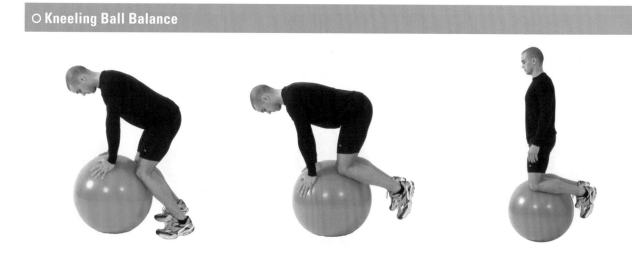

This exercise targets trunk and hip stability.

Put your hands and the front of your lower legs on the ball and rock forward until your feet come off the floor. Bring your knees underneath you and straighten your hips so that your trunk is upright. Use your GMax to maintain a straight hip position and the balloon posture cue. Do not hook your feet onto the ball for support.

**Variations**

1. Take both arms over your head. Move one arm down to the side and back up and repeat with the other side.

2. Take both arms out in front of you. Move one to the side and move it back and repeat with the other side.

3. Take both arms to the side and turn your shoulders one way and then the other.

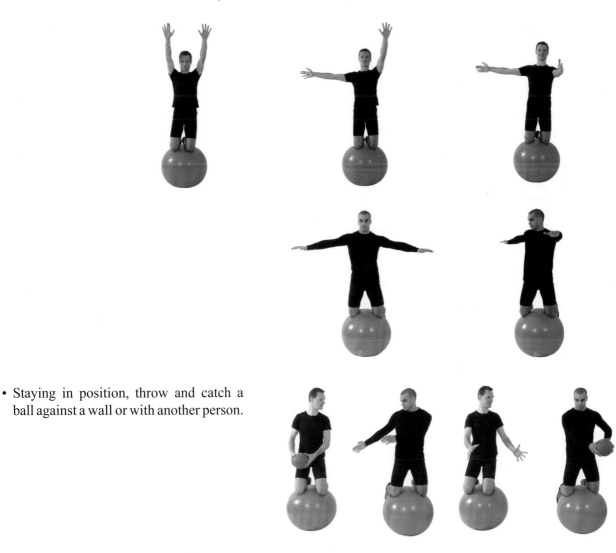

- Staying in position, throw and catch a ball against a wall or with another person.

- Work in pairs. Link arms with a partner who is also kneeling on a ball. Both of you lengthen your bodies so that your hips are straight. Keeping your arms straight, pull one of your partner's arms towards you and push the other away. This will create a rotational pressure on your partner's trunk. Your partner's job is to resist this pressure and create a counter pressure.

  In pairs again, work on side-bending control by pressing one arm down and pushing the other arm up. Your partner resists this pressure and provides a counter pressure.

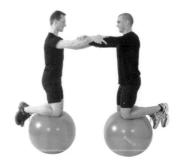

In all of these exercises, you should feel connected from your shoulders to your knees. If you try to resist the pressure with your arms rather than your whole body, you will lose control of your legs on the ball.

# Full Flexion Pattern Development

Trunk flexion exercises provoke controversy, with some opinions going so far as to suggest that they are dangerous and should never be performed for fear of back injury. The reality is that some athletes need to be able to flex their trunks powerfully. Dancers also need to be able to do this as they must be able to meet the diverse movement demands of their choreographers. They are more likely to be injured if they are not properly prepared. Avoiding the issue is not the solution.

The line between useful and risky is marked by the foundations that a person has developed. If they have a well-functioning deep support system in the trunk, these activities do not pose a risk. However, for those who start at this end of the programme without adequate preparation, some of the concerns may hold true.

These exercises work on coordination of the trunk and hip flexor group. Until Phase 4, the focus has been on developing a neutral trunk that can support the hip flexion action. This is because the trunk flexors such as rectus abdominis are often overactive, and the deep stabilisers such as transversus abdominis (TrA) which maintain a neutral trunk, are often underactive. For activities such as running or cross-country skiing, this pattern will provide inadequate support for the pelvis and spine against hip flexion, so establishing a more-effective strategy has to be a priority.

For activities that require a trunk and hip flexion combination movement (e.g. diving or gymnastics), a lack of TrA activity creates a flexion pattern where the movement muscles are not acting on a stable foundation. The flexion pattern is not complete as a component is missing, so activating TrA has therefore been a priority in order to construct a complete flexion pattern.

The following exercises now integrate TrA, rectus abdominis and the hip flexor muscles into the full flexion pattern. They have been used as "core" exercises for many years, but having followed Phases 1–3, you will see that these movements represent only one pattern of several which need to be addressed in a balanced stability programme. If powerful trunk flexion is not a component of your sport, the time you spend on stability training should not be overly biased towards movements of this type at the expense of other more relevant positions.

These are not priority movements for athletes with lower back pain. People with back pain often mistakenly interpret the advice to strengthen their abdominals to mean sit-ups. However, these flexion pattern exercises should only be performed on a foundation of deep trunk control. If you are suffering from lower back pain, seek the advice of a trained therapist before adding these exercises to your programme.

The following exercises can be made far more effective if you focus on keeping your lower abdomen in throughout the movement and use equal focus on the up and the down phase of the movement.

## ○ Curl-ups

Lie on your back with your knees bent and feet flat on the floor. Your hands rest on the front of your hips. Nod your chin slightly and sink your lower abdominals towards your spine as you slide your hands up your thighs to curl your trunk from the floor. Maintain the abdominals in their sunken position to fold your spine back to the floor.

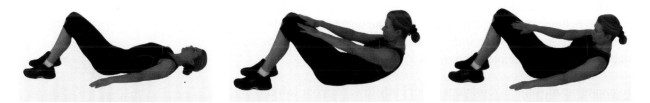

To add an oblique element, slide your hand up your opposite thigh as you curl. To increase the loading of the exercise, place your hands level with your ears. It is easier to have your elbows pointing forward and harder to have them pointing sideways.

## ○ Toe Touch Sit-ups

Begin as for the exercise above. As you curl up, lift one leg and reach with your opposite hand to touch it. Replace your foot on the floor as you fold your spine back to the start position, controlling your trunk at each level by tucking your abdominals inwards.

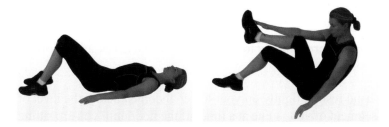

## ○ Ball Bounce Sit-ups

Lie down facing a wall with a Swiss Ball in both hands and your knees bent. Take the ball over your head, lengthening your spine along the floor so that your abdomen drops towards your spine.

Keeping your lower abdominals in, rapidly pull the ball forward and throw it hard against the wall. Catch it as it rebounds and continue to move back to the floor again, controlling the motion by keeping your lower abdominals in.

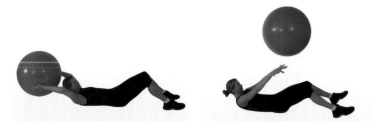

## ○ Extended Lever Swiss Ball Sit-ups

The sit-up movement is often performed from the floor which only allows development of trunk curling control from neutral. Sports such as cricket and gymnastics require an athlete to use the abdominals through a larger range of movement.

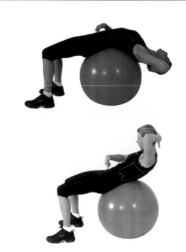

Sit on a Swiss Ball and walk yourself out until your spine is curved over the ball. Your head and shoulders will be supported by your arm which is folded behind your neck. Place the other hand on your lower abdomen to make sure that you keep it drawn in towards your spine to create a stable platform for the movement.

To create the movement, curl your upper body towards your lower body. Make sure that your spine peels off the ball, joint by joint, on the way up, and reconnects with it, joint by joint, on the way back down.

## ○ Straight Leg Curl-ups

The Straight Leg Curl-up trains a higher level of spinal flexion control than the basic Curl-up. Straight Leg Curl-ups have been frowned upon for many years and there is a prevailing belief that they are dangerous for the lower back. This belief is certainly well-founded if the movement is performed without a well-functioning TrA at speeds that exceed your control capabilities. However, as you have worked your way to this point, you should have the necessary spinal control to perform this exercise without difficulty.

### Should I do this exercise if I have a back problem?

If you are currently experiencing lower back pain, you are unlikely to possess the control necessary. Prioritise exercises from Phases 1–3 to develop this control.

Lie flat on the floor with the fingertips of one hand resting lightly on your lower abdomen below the level of your navel. Starting from your head, curl one segment of your spine at a time off the floor until you are sitting up. Your lower abdomen should have remained flat throughout the motion.

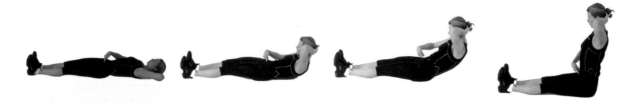

To reverse the action, focus on controlling the movement from your lower abdomen, placing one segment at a time back on the floor until you are lying flat again. The movement should be very smooth and you should not miss any segment as you curl and uncurl.

If you can perform the Straight Leg Curl-up, go on to try the Double Toe Touch.

## ○ Double Toe Touch

Lie with your knees bent and your feet flat on the floor. Your hands are on the front of your hips. Keeping your lower abdominals in and your head and neck relaxed, curl up as you lift both feet from the floor. Touch your toes and uncurl as you place your feet back on the floor.

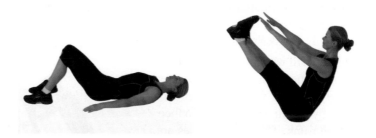

A diver or gymnast will be able to perform this exercise as a V-sit with straight legs and straight arms throughout the entire movement.

This is not an exercise for beginners. You need to have securely established your TrA in the previous 3 Phases before attempting this exercise.

**Should I do this exercise if I have a back problem?**

If you are currently experiencing lower back pain, you are unlikely to possess the control necessary. Prioritise exercises from Phases 1–3 to develop this control.

# Stability Reactions

## ○ Ball Follow

In Chapter 3, the Ball Follow was introduced as a method for assessing whole-body movement. The exercise stimulates the need to react accurately with good mobility and whole-body stability. It can be varied by increasing the pressure between the two athletes.

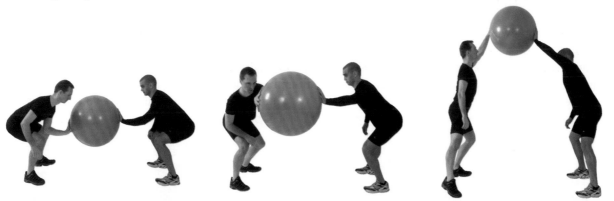

Hold a Swiss Ball between you using one hand each. Your feet will be apart. Increase the pressure on the ball. One of you will lead the movement and the other will follow. The leader will attempt to throw the follower off balance, varying the movement and forcing the follower to react. Use the widest range and the most creative combinations of movement that you can. Progress with increased speed and increased pressure.

## ○ Wrestle Walking

Wrestle Walking stimulates neuromuscular bracing responses from the trunk and pelvis.

### Variation 1: Trunk Pressures

One athlete will walk or jog in a straight line. This is the focus athlete. A partner will apply varying pressure at random intervals by pushing sideways into their pelvis and trunk. The pressure does not have to be heavy. The focus athlete tries to maintain a straight line of movement.

### Variation 2: Arm Pressures

This variation is for sports like football where a player needs to keep another player away from their trunk as they move. The focus athlete will bend his elbow and lift his arm to just below shoulder height. His focus is to keep pushing his elbow away from him. The partner will deliver pressure through the arm, trying to push the elbow towards the focus athlete's body, thus pushing him off balance easily.

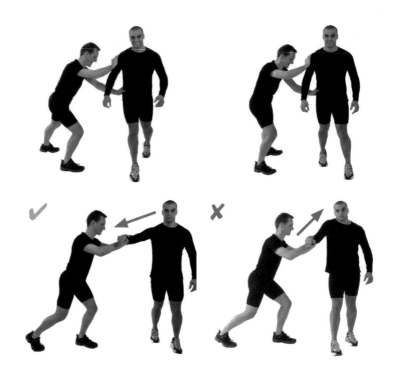

## ○ Push Jumps

Athletes in sports where jumping is involved need to be adaptable in their landings. Basketball players and footballers are often contacted in the air. Landing awkwardly may increase their injury risk or influence their ability to move off quickly after landing. Push Jumps should be started off both legs. The focus athlete will jump and try to land in the same spot. The partner will apply a sideways pressure through the hips or trunk when the focus athlete is in the air. It is harder for the focus athlete to control a trunk push than a pelvic push, so you may choose to mix these up. If landing on a single leg, push from the opposite side.

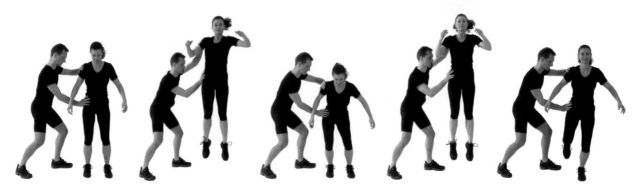

**Variation 1:** Jump and Go

Increase the complexity of the task by asking the focus athlete to move quickly to a marker directly after the Push Jump. He must control his landing and immediately move to a target or new task so there is an element of distraction for the landing task as he thinks about the next movement. Drills can be constructed where the Push Jump starts a sequence that may involve acceleration, change of direction, catching or kicking.

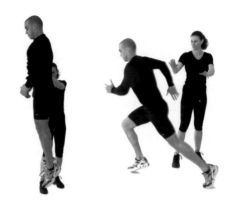

**Variation 2:** Catch and Go

A handball or basketball player can be pushed further by performing the Push Jump while catching a ball. The greater distraction requires greater landing control. Vary the direction of the throw to vary the task.

## ○ Change of Direction

This drill ensures that you are equally happy moving off both legs and turning in both directions. If you can overcome a strong dominance in turning coordination, you can minimise the twisting knee stress caused by a poor turn in your non-dominant direction. Phase 3 introduced the relationship between foot movement and body movement. This drill further develops that relationship.

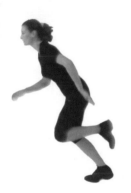
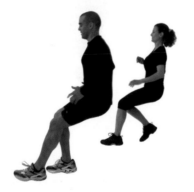
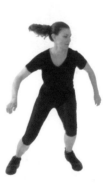

Sprint forward until commanded to brake and back pedal as quickly as possible. To brake well, you will keep your knees elastic and drop your hips quickly and smoothly. If you are trying to counter a strong forward force, the quickest route is to drop it down. Trying to fight your forward momentum is not effective at speed.

As you backpedal, you will receive a command to turn to your right and sprint towards a target. On the next run through, turn to your left and sprint towards a target.

You may need to run through these drills slowly at first to feel the difference between left and right. Is there a difference in footwork or the turning of your pelvis? Try to make them as similar as you can and then increase the speed.

# Mobility

## ○ Corkscrew — Chest Opening Spinal Twist

As Phase 4 has introduced higher-level arm loading and greater global stabiliser activity in the trunk, this exercise lengthens the muscular chain from the shoulder to the hip.

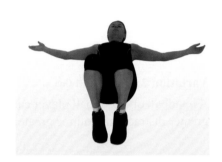

Lie on your back with your knees bent and feet flat on the floor. Your arms will be flat on the floor level with your shoulders, with the palms turned upwards. Cross your right knee over your left knee. Move your left foot slightly to the right. Keeping your right shoulder on the floor, slowly allow your knees to fall to the left.

Focus on breathing into your lower ribs so that you gain maximum lengthening. If you allow your right shoulder to lift, you will lose the benefit of the stretch.

Once you have relaxed into this position for several breaths, slide your right arm up towards your head and let it rest on the floor. Continue to breathe into your lower ribs for several breath cycles before releasing the stretch and returning to the start position.

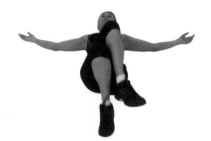
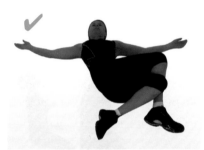
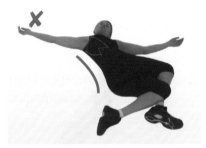

Correctly rotating around a secure spine.        Spine incorrectly allowed to sag.

## ○ Chicken Wings — Chest Opening with Internal Shoulder Rotation

Stand in your balloon posture and put both hands behind your back with one hand resting on the palm of the other. Maintaining a neutral lumbar spine by drawing your lower abdomen in a little, open your chest and press your elbows back. If this is easy, grasp your elbows. Maintain your neutral spine and open your chest. Hold this position for a few breath cycles and reverse your arm position so that the other arm is on top.

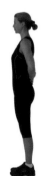
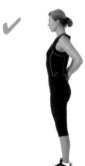
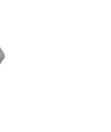
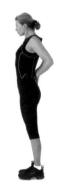

Maintain a neutral spine and head position.        Incorrect spinal position.

## ○ Tail-up

This exercise lengthens the hamstrings in partnership with pelvic mobility.

Stand with your feet no more than hip-width apart in front of a chair. Place both hands on the seat of the chair. Imagine where your tailbone is and tilt it upwards towards the ceiling so that the inwards curve of your lower back deepens. Repeat this movement several times and sustain the final movement for several breaths.

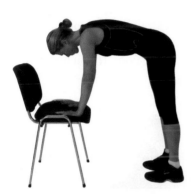 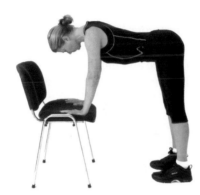

If you have good hamstring flexibility, you will need to place your hands on a lower support in order to achieve a stretch.

### Variation

You can add pelvic rotation to the Tail-up stretch. Start in the basic Tail-up position. Keeping your tailbone tilted to the ceiling, soften one knee which will drop the pelvis on that side. This will intensify the feeling in your straight leg. Straighten the bent knee and repeat on the other side.

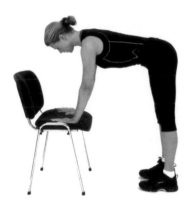 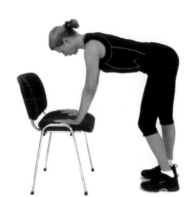 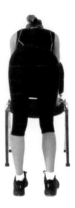

## ○ Hip Ranger

This exercise gently mobilises your hips into flexion and extension. Take your time with this one and let yourself relax into the position.

Start from a kneeling position on the floor. Slide one leg straight out behind you and fold your body down over your front knee. Breathe and allow yourself to sink into your hip joint. Perform 5 breath cycles as your front hip moves further into flexion.

Now work the other hip into extension. Keep your legs in the same position and straighten up through your trunk. If you can keep your balance, place both hands on your front knee to help you to straighten. If you need more support, keep one hand on your knee and the fingertips of the other on the floor. If you need more support, use a book to prop yourself up. Perform 5 breath cycles and swap legs.

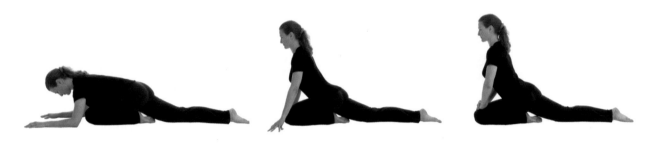

### Programme Summary

The four Phases are intended to provide a sensible progression for increasingly dynamic control. The proportion of each Phase that you eventually use in your programme will depend upon the demands of your sport.

A balanced programme is likely to incorporate elements from each phase. Phase 1 elements can be retained for pre-activation prior to training or in the cool-down period for maintenance. Some sports will have very few Phase 4 exercises in their programme as Phase 2 and 3 elements are more relevant to their needs, but dynamic, multidirectional sports will incorporate many of the Phase 4 elements.

# 10 | Stability Across the Training Programme

Stability Principles for Warm-ups and Mobility
Body Weight Training
Elastic Resistance Exercises
Stability in the Gym Environment
Static Stretches

Stability in combination with balance, functional mobility, proprioception and symmetry fosters and maintains ideal joint mechanics and movement patterns. Specific stability exercises are designed to trigger and reinforce stabiliser muscle activation. They also help to reduce the limitation of mobility and alteration of joint mechanics that occur through overactivity and excess tension in the global muscle groups.

This focused work is beneficial but only if it transfers into efficient functional movement. Specific stability exercises can therefore only have an impact if the principles of effective movement are applied and reinforced in all areas of training.

The rules outlined for stability training are the same for any other aspect of the training programme:

- Maintaining the balloon posture establishes the critical head-on-neck position no matter whether you are standing, running, squatting or performing press-ups. Allowing your neck to collapse so that your head is pulled back or your chin pulled upward or forward will compromise your shoulder mechanics, decrease the effectiveness of your hip muscles, and make it difficult to switch on your deep abdominal muscles.

- Relax your face and jaw.

- Breathe normally.

- Keep the back of your neck long to ensure that your shoulders are not pulled towards your ears.

- Keep your chest open to prevent shoulder stress and over-dependence upon the pectoral muscles for support.

- Maintain a firm central axis: don't let your trunk collapse.

- Maintain a listening foot. If it becomes rigid, it indicates poor body orientation over the foot and poor balance.

- Keep your pelvis level and your knee in line with your hip and ankle.

- Release any tension you don't need.

- Aim for purity of movement. Know what you are trying to achieve with any exercise you are engaged in and make sure that you commit to quality performance.

This chapter highlights some of the common errors and misunderstandings that can occur in other areas of the training programme.

## Stability Principles for Warm-ups and Mobility

A good warm-up will incorporate several elements in order to prepare the body for action. One of these is to take the joints and muscles through their full range with rhythmic, repeated movements. This is not just a muscular activity but an opportunity to warm up the neuromuscular patterns that will be needed for sporting activity, thereby reinforcing the sequencing of the muscles and joints in the kinetic chain.

If you don't pay attention to your movement at this time, you can reinforce poor movement habits and miss some of the benefits of the warm-up. Even if you aren't paying attention, your nervous system is – and it is recording the way you move. Don't feed your nervous system a poor movement when you warm-up if you are trying to improve your technique in other areas of training.

The following exercises commonly appear in warm-up or cool-down routines but are usually performed incorrectly. Once you start to apply the stability principles to these movements, it is easy to recognise the errors and identify them in other movements that you may use in your warm-up.

### ○ High Knee Lifts

This movement combines ankle mobility with hip mobility and provides the opportunity to wake up the neuromuscular patterns for clean hip flexion on the movement side and stability on the support side. It also encourages balance and precise body weight placement over the forefoot.

Step forward onto your left heel and roll up onto your toes, driving the right knee upwards. Your balloon posture is your best focus for this motion as it reminds you to bring your knee up to your trunk instead of your trunk collapsing towards your knee. This reinforces a sound hip flexion pattern on a stable trunk.

At the top of the movement, aim for a straight line in your supporting leg from your toe through your knee and hip to your shoulder. Pause in this balanced position for a moment and then continue.

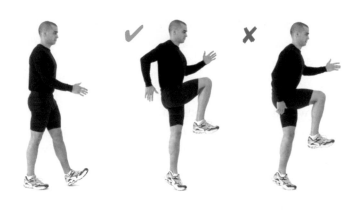

To further reinforce balance and symmetry, perform this as a walking drill with both arms stretched over your head. You should be able to maintain a straight horizontal line between your armpits and a vertical central axis. You should feel as though you are perfectly aligned over your forefoot.

## Variation 1

Perform the High Knee Lift, and as you balance on your supporting leg, straighten out your other knee before stepping forward. Focus on really stretching your arms and trunk out of your pelvis.

## Variation 2

Perform the High Knee Lift with a trunk twist. Place your hands behind your head, and maintaining a light, tall posture, turn your upper body in the direction of the lifting leg, i.e. as you lift your left knee, turn your chest and head to the left.

## What would a poor performance look like?

- The trunk collapses towards the leg.

- If you collapse slightly to one side, shortening the side of your trunk or moving your hands to one side, this usually indicates that you are trying to use your latissimus dorsi to help stabilise your trunk. This will throw off you off balance and make you overuse your groin muscles to maintain control. This problem is quite common and often associated with groin injuries and poor gluteal activation on the support side.

## ○ Heel Flicks

Maintaining your balloon posture, flick your heels up at the back to lengthen your quadriceps. You are aiming to maintain a straight line down the front of your body when you perform this exercise. Remember to lengthen through the back of your neck to help your trunk to straighten and your lower abdominals to draw inwards.

## What would a poor performance look like?

Hip bending.

The most common error for this motion is allowing your spine to arch into extension. When you do this, you allow your pelvis to tip forward, losing your neutral trunk position, bending your hips and failing to properly lengthen the quadriceps.

## ○ Side Skips

Side Skips address adduction-abduction mobility in the hips and also trigger GMed to push-off effectively. Keep your central axis straight and firm as you reach with one leg and push with the other.

**What would a poor performance look like?**

- Using the trunk to generate the movement which makes the trunk seem to rock from side to side. This decreases the exercise's effect on mobility and activation.

- Initiating the movement from the shoulders, raising them towards the ears.

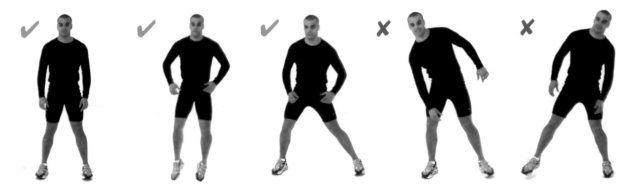

## ○ Progressive Lunges

The correct form for lunges still applies in the warm-up. Maintain a firm vertical central axis throughout the movement, and pay attention to GMax as you push out of your lunge.

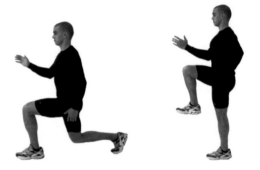

**What would a poor performance look like?**

- Allowing yourself to collapse your lumbar spine into extension, and allowing your knee to drift inside your ankle, fails to activate correct neuromuscular patterns and does not fully lengthen the hip flexor muscles.

- Allowing your trunk to tip forward and backwards as you move indicates that you are not using your GMax adequately.

---

### ○ Variation: Progressive Lunges with a Twist

Start with both arms out to the side. As you step forward onto your left leg, turn your upper body to the left. Your arms should stay parallel.

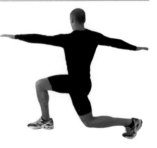

## ○ Stride Openers

This movement aims to mobilise both the front and back of the hips and give a sensation of length to the hip motion.

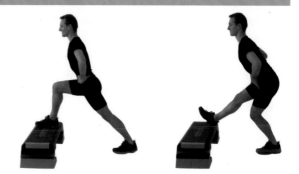

For the basic movement, place one foot on a bench and perform a deep lunge onto it, keeping your back foot facing forward and your trunk neutral. Then push your hips back, keeping your chest up and focusing on pressing your tailbone backwards.

**What would a poor performance look like?**

• Collapsing the trunk into extension on the way forward.

• Collapsing the trunk into flexion on the way back.

## ○ Wood Chops and Spiral Movements

These movements involve the joints from the feet to the shoulders, activating rotational mobility and control.

A basic Spiral is the less complex movement and is helpful to establish rotation of the pelvis over a fixed foot as well as a sense of rotating around a firm central axis. It also plays a kinaesthetic role in differentiating between the pelvis and the thorax. Once the pelvis has reached its limit, the thorax continues to move into its full available range: you should be aware of your pelvis and shoulders moving at slightly different times.

To benefit from this exercise, start with balloon posture to establish your central axis and draw your lower belly inwards. Turn your body to one side, transferring the weight onto this foot. Allow your other foot to turn in the direction of movement so that the pelvis is free to continue moving over the fixed foot. Allow your shoulders to keep turning freely and let your arms swing. As you reverse the movement, be aware that it is your abdominals that are maintaining the central axis for rotation.

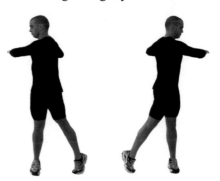

**What would a poor performance look like?**

• Deepening of the lumbar curve, indicating loss of control of the spine.

• Insufficient pelvic rotation.

The Wood Chop adds another dimension to this movement by incorporating an up and down element. The same factors apply as for the Spiral, but this time as you turn, you will bend your hips and knees, keeping your body upright. As you reverse the movement, you will straighten your legs and move your arms up and across.

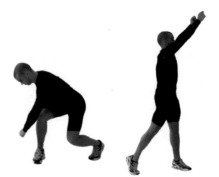

**What would a poor performance look like?**

The most common error is to bend your back instead of your hips and knees.

## ○ Leg Swings

Stand on one leg and lift your body up over your supporting hip to activate GMed. Stay tall and swing the other leg fully back and forth, allowing your arms to move normally. Your trunk should stay vertical and your leg should swing in a straight line. Your pelvis should remain in a constant position throughout the movement.

**What would a poor performance look like?**

The common error associated with this exercise is movement of the lower back. It should stay in a constant position throughout the exercise.

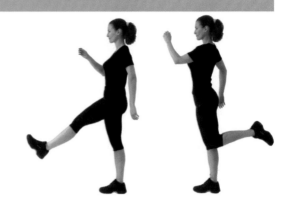

The movements included in a warm-up depend upon the sport and its demands. A warm-up will become increasingly specific to the sport, starting with general movements and activation exercises, and ending with sport-specific drills.

Examples of this include:

- an elite Olympic weight lifter who performs Balance Board Squats prior to warming up her lifts with the bar, in order to optimise her symmetry of weight bearing and lower zone activation.

- an international sprinter who incorporates wobble cushion balance exercises, Greyhound and Superman prior to his walking drills and dynamic movements to fine tune his central alignment and coordinate his anterior and posterior chains before his track session.

- the coach of a junior ski squad who finds that his athletes show more control on their early runs on the slopes if they add neuromuscular challenges like Swiss Ball kneeling drills to their warm-up.

- a world-class triathlete who finds that she runs technically better if she performs pre-activation exercises that trigger the balloon posture and pelvic muscle timing as part of the warm-up prior to a running session.

# Body Weight Training

Body weight exercises are perceived to be safe, simple and effective elements to include in circuit training. For this reason, they are often given to young athletes or make up part of a circuit for adult athletes to perform with intensity and speed. Once you start to recognise the fundamentals of good form, you realise as you observe the performance of these exercises that often they are not reinforcing desired functional patterns but simply reinforcing poor ones.

Junior athletes performing full body weight press-ups rarely demonstrate scapular stability or even trunk stability. They do become stronger at press-ups with practise, but may develop muscle imbalances and poor patterning to achieve this. If the total pattern is poor, i.e. the contribution of stabilisers and mobilisers is unbalanced, transfer of improved press-up strength to a specific sporting activity is diminished. You may need to start on a low-load exercise like the Wall Press to develop the stable pattern and use other more supported exercises for strength. As you master the pattern, you can progressively load the movement so that the entire pattern strengthens safely and effectively.

A sensible progression route for press-ups would be: Wall Press $\longrightarrow$ Single Leg Wall Press $\longrightarrow$ OTT Press-ups $\longrightarrow$ Press-ups: Levels 1, 2 and 3.

Repetitive lunges or step-ups may be a low load relative to weight training, but speed and number of repetitions can accentuate poor mechanics. The initial objective is not how many repetitions you can do, but how well you do them. You want to condition the pattern – not just the muscles. Once you have consolidated this form, you can increase speed or endurance.

Body weight exercises can be very effective as long as you understand the form with which they should be performed. There is no doubt that you are likely to have the strength in your mobility muscles to perform a movement, and that body weight may be a fraction of what these muscles are capable of lifting, but if the smaller stabilisers cannot withstand the load and maintain a stable pattern, you will create a situation of increasing imbalance.

# Elastic Resistance Exercises

Stretch band exercises are often given by coaches to young athletes for arm strengthening, particularly with the aim of improving rotator cuff performance. This is so seldom challenged that it has become standard practice, especially in sports such as tennis. However, without a good appreciation of correct shoulder mechanics, these exercises are more likely to cause problems than solve them.

As we learned in Chapter 3, shoulder mechanics depend on a variety of factors. The shoulder joint should be able to rotate around a stable axis. That is, the head of the humerus (the ball of the ball-and-socket joint) should not drift back and forth in response to rotational movement. In order to have a stable axis, the scapula (which provides the socket of the ball-and-socket joint) must be securely positioned throughout the movement. This often depends upon having an independently stable trunk and pelvis so that the shoulder is not pulled into a poor position due to body positioning errors.

Unfortunately, stretch band exercises are often given to young children with none of these elements in place. The amount of resistance at the hand end is greater than their ability to stabilise, causing them to recruit alternative muscles in order to perform the movement. The most common of these is pectoralis major which pulls the shoulder forward. The axis for shoulder rotation is lost and athletes learn to stabilise their arms superficially from the front surface of their chests rather than effectively training the rotator cuff. This pattern is reinforced with repetition and can lead to loss of mobility and a weak, ineffective rotator cuff.

The argument from a tennis point of view is that the amount of resistance is less than that which is applied when they hit a tennis ball. The answer to this is that a ground stroke in tennis is generated by the sum of all moving body parts from the feet through the trunk to the arm. It is not merely a function of upper body strength. The situation is worsened by individuals who believe that tying the stretch band to a tennis racket and performing arm movements makes the exercise sports specific. It is more likely to break down the coordination pattern throughout the kinetic chain as the young athlete engages the resistance at the hand before moving the body, a reversal of the normal movement pattern.

Regardless of varying opinions on their benefits, stretch band exercises will continue to be used for shoulder training by many coaches in many sports. Because of this, a simple process is provided below for commonly used exercises to make sure that future biomechanical problems are not caused.

1 Basic tests such as Wall Press, Superman and Diamond should be performed to gain an impression of basic stability around the trunk and scapula. Also test shoulder internal rotation.

2 Basic pelvic and trunk stability should be established.

3 Basic isolated scapular stability and rotator cuff activation should be in place. Exercises like Diamond, Superman and OTT should improve scapular control. Exercises that load the arms such as Wall Press and OTT also help to activate the rotator cuff muscles.

4 Practising shoulder internal rotation (see Chapter 3) helps to establish the rotational axis.

With this foundation established, resistance from the hand can be introduced.

## ○ Internal Shoulder Rotation in Neutral

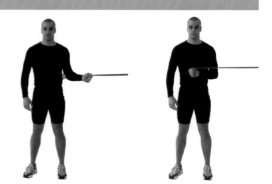

The athlete should start in the balloon posture to activate the trunk stabilisers, place the shoulder in neutral and open the chest. For active internal rotation in a neutral, position, the elbow should be bent to 90 degrees so that the forearm is horizontal and the wrist is straight. A tennis ball can be held lightly between the elbow and the body to prevent the arm drifting out of position. Step away from the stretch band's fixed point until the working arm rotates outwards to its limit. This is the start position.

Athletes can place their free hand over the front of their shoulder to ensure that it does not drift forward during the movement. Keeping the wrist straight, use the lightest resistance to train the pattern and only progress within the limits of the athlete's ability to maintain the pattern.

## ○ External Shoulder Rotation in Neutral

For external rotation in neutral, the first four steps should be in place. The athlete will hold the stretch band between his hands and start in the balloon posture with the forearms horizontal, wrists straight, and palms facing the floor. Again, a tennis ball can be held lightly between the elbow and the body.

Keeping the wrists parallel with the floor, move one away from the other. The shoulder itself should not move and the wrists should not turn upwards. As the wrist returns to the start position, the shoulder should not be dragged forward.

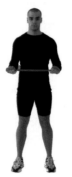
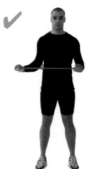
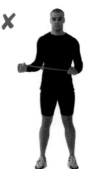

Poor form: wrist turning.

## ○ External Shoulder Rotation in Abduction

Rotational exercises are often taken from neutral into 90 degrees at the shoulder for greater relevance to sporting movements. This is far more difficult to control and in young athletes should only be done under supervision.

The first four steps should be in place. The pattern should be practised first without resistance. The athlete abducts his shoulder to 90 degrees with the elbow bent. He places his other hand across the front of his shoulder to the underside of his arm. This will help to keep the shoulder and arm in place.

The athlete then rotates his arm fully from external to internal rotation, maintaining a consistent shoulder position. The shoulder should not drift forward into his hand. It is common practice to rest the arm on a table to maintain a consistent elbow position, but this can allow the athlete to overuse latissimus dorsi by pulling down into the table. This is a common patterning dysfunction that can be avoided by having the athlete self-monitor his arm position.

Athletes can progress their control with a low load but higher speed by throwing and catching a tennis ball in this position. They can also progress at higher load and low speed by introducing light elastic resistance.

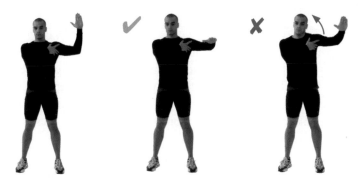

Loss of the shoulder as a fixed point.

## Elastic Resistance for the Lower Limb

Similar principles apply for exercises prescribed for the lower limb. With the band around their ankles, athletes are asked to pull the band in a variety of directions. However, the usefulness of these exercises depends entirely on the set-up and maintenance of pelvic and trunk stability throughout the movement.

The basic principles are:

1. Test the Standing Knee Lift and Static Lunge to gain an impression of the athlete's pelvic stability and body alignment.

2. If these are poor, start with Phase 1 activation exercises such as String of Pearls Bridge, Greyhound and Clam to build foundation stability.

3. Once the athlete has gained some basic pelvic control, resistance can be added.

### ○ Lower Limb Abduction in Neutral

Stand with feet together, using the balloon posture to increase stabiliser activation in the trunk. Shift the weight onto one leg, lift and position the body over the supporting hip to make sure that GMed will activate appropriately. Move your leg out against the stretch band resistance. Keep a straight line down the body to the foot.

It may be helpful to keep the arms above the head to prevent collapse of the trunk. The pelvis should remain in a secure position and shouldn't tip forward, backward or sideways.

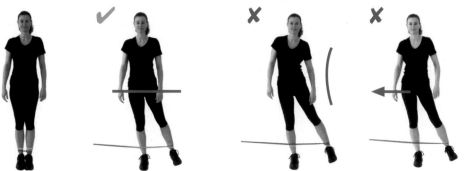

Loss of trunk control.          Loss of pelvic control.

## Stability in the Gym Environment

This book focuses on establishing effective neuromuscular patterns for stability and freedom of movement. These patterns should provide a foundation for strength and power training, but fundamental errors in exercise selection and performance can lead to imbalance and poor transfer of strength gains to performance.

### Single Leg Vs Double Leg Activities in the Weights Room

There is a tendency to assume that weights performed on a single leg will develop more stability than performing the same exercise on two legs. This is not always the case. If an athlete uses excessive foot, ankle and lower leg muscle activity to maintain single leg balance, performing weights on a single leg will amplify the problem and create a rigid, non-listening foot. The specific exercise may seem to improve, but that improvement will not transfer into a functional change. They are more likely to become increasingly functionally rigid instead of dynamically stable.

If you are planning to add single leg weights exercises to your programme, make sure that you focus on maintaining a relaxed foot and ankle, and that you draw your body up over your hip to activate your GMax and GMed effectively.

---

**Clipboard Notes**

A 27-year-old professional golfer presented with both technical and injury problems. She had pain in her lower back and shins that was not resolving. She also lacked power and was trying to address this by increasing her time in the weights room.

The striking thing about this player was the high degree of tension in superficial muscles like her back extensors and rectus abdominis, as well as in distal muscle groups such as those of her lower legs and feet. She had correspondingly low tone in more central muscles such as GMax and TrA. This level of imbalance required even higher total body tension to control her golf swing. This made it impossible for her to achieve the sequential rotation from her feet through her pelvis and trunk that was necessary to generate power in her swing.

The player had been given single leg bicep and deltoid exercises by her trainer with the aim of improving stability and balance. The degree of muscle tension in her feet and lower legs as she performed these exercises demonstrated a primary and habitual poor stabilising strategy. Selecting the position that most amplified this poor strategy and then loading it could only worsen the problem.

The player's strength and conditioning coach was very receptive to this information and adjusted the gym programme so that central stability could be developed as well as effective weight transference. All initial exercises were done in bilateral weightbearing. Her remedial programme involved listening foot exercises to improve ankle and foot dissociation as well as rotation mobility drills to improve her movement sequencing. The shin and lower back pain resolved and the player was able to make technical adjustments more easily.

Conversely, if a sport requires powerful alternating leg movement, limiting the gym programme to bilateral activities may be missing a key component. If you are a cyclist, for example, the amount of effective force that you are able to exert through the pedal is dependent upon the stability of your pelvis to support your leg muscles in alternating patterns. A cyclist with strong leg muscles but poor pelvic and trunk stability can only access a proportion of his strength as some of it will be dissipated through loss of a fixed point for muscles to pull from.

Bilateral squats can build muscular strength in sports-relevant muscles but they do not address the accessibility of this strength when stability is challenged. Unilateral activities such as Lunges, Step-ups and Single Leg Squats should be included in the programme to ensure that a sports-relevant pattern is trained.

## Purity and Purpose of Movement

The effectiveness of an exercise is easily lost if the essential movement is not well understood. Among the most common offenders against this principle are calf raises and squats.

### Calf raises

These should be performed with a stable, well-aligned ankle, but athletes with a poor pattern will allow the ankle to collapse outwards as they push upwards, displacing their weight onto the outer joints of the forefoot. A pattern like this in a runner or jumper can give rise to posterior shin splints (a painful sensation on the inner aspect of the tibia).

### Squats

Athletes are sometimes taught to over-emphasise their lumbar curve when they squat. This cue can be misinterpreted and as they focus on keeping the lumbar curve, they move their

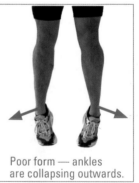

Good form — straight ankles.

Poor form — ankles are collapsing outwards.

hips backwards as they squat instead of focusing on lowering their hips towards the floor. Their trunk continues to move downwards with a deep curve after the hips have stopped bending. This has the effect of loading the back extensors, proximal hamstrings and quadriceps, but the GMax can become underactive.

Squats should target strength in the knee and hip extensors in a coordinated pattern. It is common to see athletes missing out on transferable strength because they are strengthening the knee extensors and back extensors instead.

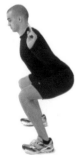

The spine is maintained in a neutral position.

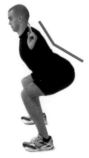

The athlete is over-accentuating his lumbar curve.

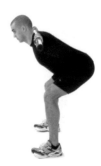

The athlete is moving his spine instead of bending at the hips.

## ○ Power Cleans

The Power Clean movement should be a smooth, coordinated, multi-joint movement. Two common problems occur:

1. The first is a sequencing problem. Athletes are so focused on driving up onto their toes and moving the bar upwards quickly, that they have achieved this position before the hips have fully straightened. If this is the case, an important hip extension element of the pattern has been missed. An athlete who does this looks as if they are slightly bent at the hip when the bar reaches shoulder height.

2. The second common error is a conceptual problem. Because you start with your hips and knees bent, the hips seem to need to move forward in order to straighten and your head seems to need to move backwards. While this is true in a sense, working from this conceptual framework can lead you to drive your head back and displace your whole pelvis forward, causing you to overextend your lower back. The athlete who does this looks to be bending backwards excessively as they raise the bar.

A Power Clean is like releasing the lid from a jack-in-the-box. As you drop into your start position, it is like someone closing the lid and compressing your springs. As you drive upwards, your "springs" release so that your hips, knees and ankles all unfold and straighten with coordinated timing. If you are lifting a heavy weight, your shoulders may move slightly backwards as you drive upwards, but there is no sudden backwards bending movement concentrated in the lower back. The movement impulse is upwards.

If this coordination is difficult, try it without the bar first. Focus on compressing your springs by bending your hips, knees and ankles. Release explosively by launching yourself straight up like an arrow, making sure that your trunk doesn't lose balance forward, backwards or sideways.

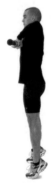 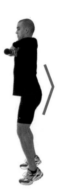 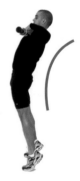

The athlete is driving straight up.      The bar has been pulled up before the legs have straightened.      The athlete is over-bending the spine.

## ○ Forward Plate Raises

Use of momentum and poor patterning lead to a trunk stability problem with this exercise. When performed poorly, athletes start with too heavy a weight, so they initiate the movement with legs and trunk in order to start the plate moving. Athletes who do this end up in a position where the back is deeply bent backwards and the arms do not reach their full range of motion.

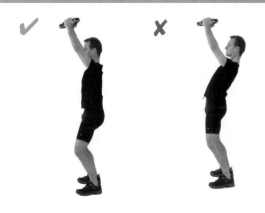

The movement should be simple. Hold a weight plate in both hands in front of you. Stand with hips and knees soft and your trunk upright. Raise the plate above your head and bring it back down again. Your trunk should remain in a constant position throughout the movement.

## ○ Bicep Curls

This exercise falls victim to use of momentum instead of strength. You see the athlete's body shifting forward and backward with the movement, or the shoulder rolling forward every time the weight is lifted.

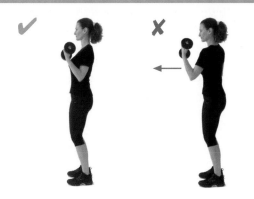

To avoid this error, start in an upright posture. Neither your body nor your shoulder should move. The only movement should be elbow bending as you raise the weight to your shoulder. The same system can apply to many resistance exercises. Work out what should be moving first. Eliminate movement from all other body parts.

## ○ Upright Row

Although the target muscle for this exercise is the lateral deltoid of the shoulder, a poorly performed Upright Row will tend instead to work upper trapezius, the muscle running across the top of your shoulder and up the side of your neck.

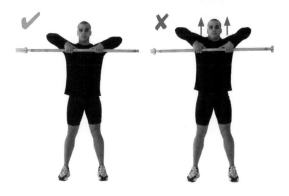

Using the same system as you did in Bicep Curls, start in an upright position with your arms straight in front of you. Make sure that the shoulder movement remains isolated and that the shoulders remain fixed points. The only movement should be your elbow moving upwards to shoulder height. You should not see your shoulders moving towards your ears.

There are many other examples of exercises performed poorly in the gym setting. However, if you adhere to the principle of a neutral spinal position, a neutral shoulder posture, and precise movement at the joints directly involved for the muscles you are targeting, you will avoid most of the problems that occur.

## Stability and the Periodised Training Programme

A periodised training programme precisely outlines the timing of strength, power and speed development to best prepare the athlete for competition. Rigid adherence to set programmes can have a detrimental effect, however. The power phase presents the most trouble as athletes may be asked to perform explosive movements that exceed their ability to compensate. If their control is inadequately developed for the task, injury is inevitable. Bounding drills are common offenders because they are perceived as body weight exercises, which are not considered to be potentially harmful.

As previously discussed, poorly controlled body weight exercises at speed or high repetition are as potentially problematic as any weights exercise. If you are prepared to be flexible however, periodisation targets can be met while still developing optimal patterns.

---

### Clipboard Notes

A 15-year-old sprinter showing exceptional potential was brought in for screening. He was found to have extremely poor trunk and pelvic stability. Due to his age, his coach was programming body weight exercises, and according to the periodised programme, the athlete was due to begin a power development phase. This athlete did not have sufficient pelvic stability to control a Static Lunge, and a Dynamic Lunge amplified his poor trunk control.

Among the exercises proposed by his coach were alternating deep split jumps (jumping on the spot from a deep lunge on the left to a deep lunge on the right). When it was explained that the athlete could not perform the simplest version of this without collapse, the coach interpreted this as him not being able to start the power development phase. This was not true. It simply required thinking about it in a structured way with movement quality as the key design component.

The modified programme was designed to meet competitive and developmental needs. Power work was done bilaterally (with both legs together). Broad jumping, box jumping and Medicine Ball Cleans all addressed power development. While this was happening, control of unilateral activities was being trained in order to lay down the stability foundations for strength and eventually power work that would safely and effectively support the athlete's physical and technical development.

Activation of the trunk and pelvic stabilisers followed by controlled weightbearing activities such as the Supported Single Leg Squat, Lunges, Step-ups, Wall Press and OTT on the Swiss Ball established control patterns. Once these patterns were established, the athlete could confidently progress into more dynamic tasks without fear of later breakdown or a technical plateau.

# Static Stretches

Static stretches may be used as part of a flexibility development and maintenance programme. As a general principle, long, sustained static stretches should not be performed directly prior to competition or dynamic training, so they do not appear as part of the warm-up. As with the dynamic flexibility exercises used in a warm-up, they are susceptible to performance errors. The following commonly performed stretches are regular offenders.

## ○ Quadricep Stretch

The key concept for any stretch is to take one end of the muscle away from the other end. That is, the origin and insertion move away from each other. The common error in this popular stretch is to allow the origin of the muscle to move towards the insertion by letting the pelvis tilt forward. This collapses the lumbar spine into extension and allows the hip to bend, decreasing the stretch on the muscle.

For an effective stretch, use balloon posture with your lower belly drawn in, keep your knees together and squeeze your GMax.

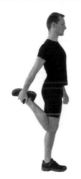
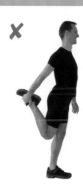

## ○ Hip Flexor Stretch

This stretch often suffers a similar fate to the Quadricep Stretch: the pelvis is allowed to tip forward and the lumbar spine to sag into extension.

To perform it well, start in a half-kneeling position, draw your body up into a balloon posture, and tilt your pelvis as if you are tucking your tail under. For a greater lengthening effect through the whole side, maintain this pelvic position and stretch the arm up, allowing the ribs to lift on the supporting side.

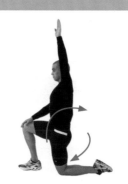

## ○ Hamstring Stretch

There are many ways to lengthen the hamstrings but the effectiveness of the stretch is often lost through inaccurate movement. The effectiveness of lying on your back with one leg straightening towards the ceiling is greatly reduced if you have the other leg bent as this allows the pelvis to tip backwards, taking the origin towards the insertion of the muscle.

To correct this, press one leg straight into the floor and press the other one to the ceiling (or the wall behind you if you are very flexible).

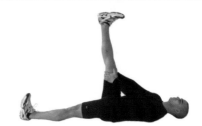

If you are trying to stretch hamstrings by putting your foot on a bench, do not try to touch your toes or put your head on your knee: this will stress the spine more than the hamstring muscles. Instead, make sure that your feet and pelvis are facing forward and simply move your tailbone backwards while keeping your head and chest up. This tilts the pelvis so that the origin of the hamstring muscle is moved away from the insertion without stressing the spine.

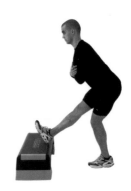

## Supine Buttock Stretches

Athletes can often be seen repetitively manipulating their backs as they attempt to stretch the muscles in their buttocks. Regardless of which buttock muscle you are trying to stretch, focus on the hip, not the spine.

### ○ Piriformis Stretch

Piriformis is a deep muscle that links the femur with the sacrum, the triangular bone at the base of your spine. It is quite specific to stretch but can bring relief from stiffness in the lower back as well as the hip.

Lie on your back with both legs straight. Raise one knee until your hip is at 90 degrees. Move it across your body until it is in line with your navel. Grasp your shin with your opposite hand and place your other hand on the outside of your knee. Gently guide the whole leg in the direction of your opposite shoulder. Both sides of your pelvis should stay on the floor.

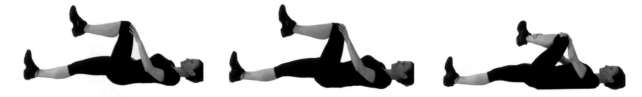

### ○ General Buttock Stretch

Lie on your back with your knees bent. Rest the ankle of your left leg on your right thigh. This creates a hole for you to reach your left arm through. Raise your legs and clasp your fingers behind your right thigh, continuing to draw the legs gently towards you. Focus on keeping your pelvis on the floor so that your hips are able to stretch more effectively.

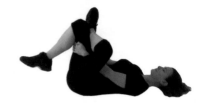

## ○ Shoulder Stretch

Stretches for the front of the shoulder can be difficult to perform safely and effectively. Swimmers in particular can be seen performing a risky version that involves bracing a hand on a doorway or wall and turning the body away from it. This tends to force the ball of the shoulder forward in its socket, stressing the deep structures that help to control the shoulder joint and not providing a productive muscular stretch. The risks outweigh the benefits in this stretch.

The following three-stage bilateral stretch is safe and effective if performed with trunk stability.

### ○ Stage 1: Pectoralis Minor

Stand with one foot in front of the other in a doorway with your hands level with your shoulders. Tuck your elbows into your sides and do not let them move backwards. Keep your trunk neutral by drawing in your lower belly and shift your weight towards your front foot. Keep the elbows forward and allow the chest to open. Do not allow your elbows to drift backwards.

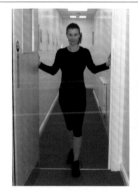 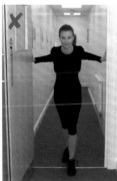

### ○ Stage 2: Pectoralis Major

Move your arms up the doorway so that your elbows are level with your shoulders. Keep your lower belly in to prevent your spine from sagging into extension and shift your weight onto your front foot.

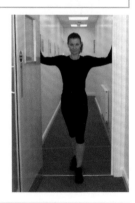

### ○ Stage 3: Pectoralis Major

Slide your arms up the doorway so that your elbows are at head level. Repeat the same movement.

If you do not have a doorway, you can modify this stretch as follows:

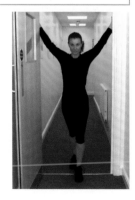

## Step 1

Stretch both arms up above your head and turn your palms away from each other. Keeping your lower belly drawn in to maintain your spinal position, pull both elbows down and back, opening the chest.

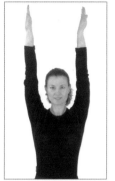
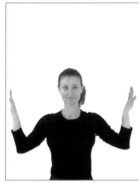

## Step 2

Place the whole forearm against a wall or other available surface. Make sure that your body is positioned level with the arm and then turn your head and trunk away from the arm without leaning forward. The stretch can be repeated with the arm positioned slightly higher.

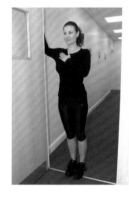
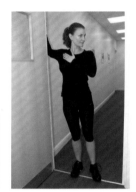

## ○ Latissimus Dorsi Stretch

The common error for this stretch is allowing the pelvis to slide out sideways as you bend your trunk in the opposite direction. This fails to fulfil the origin and insertion rule of stretching, as it takes the muscle off load by making the origin mobile instead of fixed.

To avoid this, stand with both arms over your head and a neutral spine. Grasp one of your wrists and pull that arm upwards towards the ceiling. Maintaining this position, move the arm towards your head and allow yourself to tip into the stretch, feeling the ribs of that side lifting and opening.

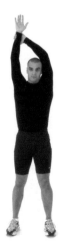
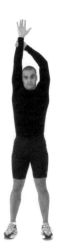
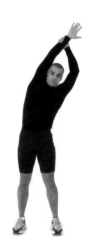

## ○ Latissimus Dorsi Stretch with the Swiss Ball

### Step 1

Kneel on the floor with both hands on a Swiss Ball. Sit back onto your heels and push the ball as far from you as possible. Relax your chest down towards the floor.

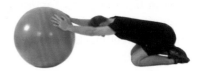

### Step 2

Kneel on the floor with your hands on the Swiss Ball. Move your right hand so that it crosses over your left hand. Sit back onto your heels and make sure that your hips stay central. Push the ball away from you and roll it to the left, feeling your right side lengthen. Maintain your pelvis as a fixed point and do not allow it to drift sideways by allowing your hips to move out to the right.

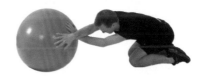

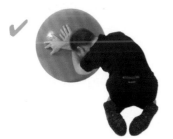

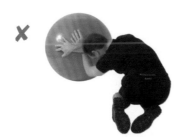

Correct pelvic positioning.

Loss of a fixed point: the pelvis has drifted sideways.

## ○ Posterior Shoulder Stretch

Start in balloon posture and raise one arm in front of you with the elbow bent and hand pointing to the ceiling. Keeping your shoulder relaxed down, move the arm across your body, guiding it with your other hand. Repeat the movement but this time start with your forearm horizontal to the floor. Focus on keeping your shoulder down.

Athletes can often be seen performing these stretches with the shoulder collapsed upwards towards the ear. This means that the shoulder can no longer function as a fixed point. When this happens, they miss the tight muscles on the back of their shoulder and pull their scapula around instead.

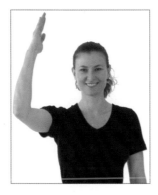

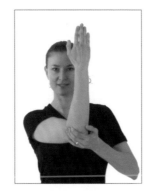

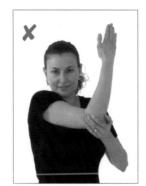

## ○ Tricep Stretch

Start in balloon posture with your lower belly drawn in and maintain this spinal position throughout the exercise. Lift your arm to the ceiling and drop your hand so that it contacts the scapula of the same side. Using your other hand to help, aim to point your elbow directly upwards towards the ceiling.

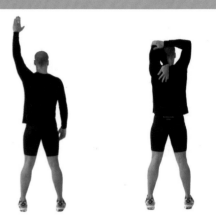

The key to good performance of this exercise is the position of the lumbar spine. The common error is to collapse the trunk into extension in an attempt to pull the elbow back further. Athletes also try to pull the arm behind the head and miss the tricep stretch altogether.

### Chapter Summary

Stability concepts should be maintained throughout the training programme. In order to do this you will need:

**1** An understanding of the correct muscular patterns and actions for the exercise.

**2** An ability to detect a movement dysfunction or error.

**3** An understanding that stability principles apply to all types of training and are necessary for correct performance of any movement.

**4** An appreciation that a stability programme should be multi-modal (use a variety of exercises, movements and equipment); multi-planar (use a variety of movement directions); proprioceptive (use a variety of high- and low-level exercises to stimulate awareness and control) and diversified (challenge your body with unfamiliar movements and different objectives).

# 11 | Sample Programmes

The four Phases of Part Two set out a collection of broadly applicable exercises. For convenience, a collection of exercises relevant to a variety of sports is provided below as a guideline to streamlining a programme. This does not mean that these are the only exercises from the four Phases that are relevant to the sport; they have simply been prioritised for clarity.

These programmes are complementary and intended to be performed alongside the rest of the training and testing programme. For each sport, there are additional specific muscle length tests and joint mobility tests that sports medicine professionals can apply.

# Running

For efficiency and speed, runners need to eliminate any excessive sideways or up and down movements. Their bodies need to be able to smoothly and symmetrically counter-rotate around a secure central longitudinal axis (CLA). This will require balance and mobility as well as trunk and pelvic stability. The runner must be trained to maintain a neutral spinal position with low effort so as not to interfere with their breathing pattern and spinal rotational mobility.

The runner is aiming for short foot contact times on the ground, and this will require good pelvic stability to prevent coronal or sideways collapse of the hip. Ineffective gluteal action can also cause collapse in the sagittal plane where the hip and knee bend too much on impact, dropping the runner's body on each step and increasing muscular load. In sprinters, this problem makes them appear as though their body is always behind their feet rather than their feet propelling their body forward. In any runner it can predispose the knee, Achilles tendon, hip flexors and lower back to injury.

## Priority Tests

- SSCT (with Eyes Open and Eyes Closed to check the sensory feedback from each foot and that the CLA is maintained centrally in Single Leg Stance)
- Static Lunge (to check support behaviour of mid- to inner-range GMax, lateral pelvic stability and trunk control)
- Lunge Drive (for propulsion behaviour)
- Standing Knee Lift (for hip and pelvic stability)
- Standing Leg Swing (for a secure CLA, pelvic stability and functional mobility)
- Thigh Slides (for thoracic rotation capability)

## Priority Exercises

**Phase 1**
- All trunk and lower limb activation exercises
- Breathing Technique (Chapter 4)
- Listening Foot (Chapter 4)
- Counter Body Rotation (Around the CLA), or Thigh Slides and Knee Creepers

**Phase 2**
- Single Leg Bounce
- OTT
- Lunges
- Step-ups
- Space Invaders
- Sway
- Balance

**Phase 3**
- Medicine Ball Sweep
- Medicine Ball Spiral
- Pulley Pull Drive
- Cross Body Pull
- Standing Stretch Band Leg Drive
- Standing Knee Lift Drive
- Aeroplane Sequence
- Walking Drills

**Phase 4**
- Side Squat Tosses
- Follow Through Rotations
- Stair Bounding
- Side Leaps

# Golf

The golfer needs to ensure that he or she has no blocks to joint rotation from the foot all the way through the spine and shoulder. A firm CLA to support trunk rotation, good stabilisers of the pelvis and dynamic balance are also necessary. If any of these factors are compromised, a golfer can be vulnerable to lower back, wrist, knee or shoulder injuries.

## Priority Tests

- SSCT (for sensory feedback from the feet)

- Static Lunge (for hip support from GMax and a centrally balanced trunk)

- Standing Knee Lift (for pelvic and trunk alignment and control)

- Seated Hamstring Test (for spinal proprioception and hamstring length)

- Total Body Rotation (for hip and spinal rotation)

- Seated Thoracic Mobility

- Seated Lumbopelvic Mobility

- Listening Foot (for lower leg mobility)

- Diamond (for external rotation at the shoulder)

- Superman (for integration of upper, central and lower control zones)

## Priority Exercises

**Phase 1**
- Listening Foot

- All Phase 1 exercises

**Phase 2**
- OTT Twisting Squat Thrust

- Lunges

- Sway

- Ski Jumper

- Balance

- All Phase 2 mobility poses

**Phase 3**
- Medicine Ball Clean

- Medicine Ball Sweep

- Medicine Ball Spiral

- Straight Pulley Push

- Trunk Rotation Pulley Push

- Progressive Lunge

- Swiss Ball Pendulum

- Swiss Ball Body Spin

- Aeroplane Sequence

**Phase 4**
- Side Squat Tosses

- Follow Through Rotations

- Kneeling Ball Balance (with arm movements and trunk rotation)

- Swiss Ball Side Raises

- Pendulum Lunges

- Corkscrew

## Equestrian

The equestrian athlete requires a secure CLA through effective stability, symmetry, lumbopelvic and hip mobility and balance. When not on the horse, movement and posture habits influence and reinforce a sense of body orientation and weight distribution, and this affects rider position when mounted. Testing on the ground can therefore identify habits that may be affecting the riding position. Training off the horse to correct these imbalances can improve the position, posture and mobility of the rider.

### Priority Tests
- SSCT
- Static Lunge
- Seated Knee Lift on a Ball
- Standing Knee Press
- Superman
- Seated Lumbopelvic Mobility (all directions)
- Seated Forward Trunk Tilt (to assess control of the neutral spine)
- Vertical Hip Release (to assess the trunk's response to hip bending)

### Priority Exercises
**Phase 1**
- Any Phase 1 exercise
- Seated Lumbopelvic Mobility
- Listening Foot

**Phase 2**
- Single Leg Bounce
- OTT
- Pull Backs
- Sway
- Ski Jumper

**Phase 3**
- Medicine Ball Sweep
- Medicine Ball Spiral
- Straight Pulley Push
- Pulley Pull

**Phase 4**
- Kneeling Ball Balance
- Curl-ups
- Tail-up
- Corkscrew
- Hip Ranger

## Football, Handball and Basketball

Dynamic multidirectional sports require good control of momentum in all directions; the ability to drive powerfully from the lower body, the ability to withstand contact from other players, and well controlled jumps and landings. These types of sport sustain high rates of knee, ankle and back injuries if dynamic balance and stability are inadequate.

### Priority Tests
- Capsule Assessment
- Jump Landings
- Leap and Return
- Rotational Jumps

### Priority Exercises
**Phase 1**
- Any Phase 1 exercise

**Phase 2**
- OTT
- Pull Backs
- Lunges
- Step-ups

- Space Invaders
- Suspension Bridge
- Ski Jumper
- Balance
- Any of the mobility poses
- Standing Leg Swing Balance
- Lunge Progressions (with catching tasks)
- Windscreen Wipers

**Phase 3**
- Any Phase 3 exercise

**Phase 4**
- Any Phase 4 exercise

## Cross-Country Skiing

These athletes require a strong neutral trunk position combined with powerful hip drive. Without attention to detail in their dynamic posture, they can easily overuse their back muscles to keep their pelvis secure, increasing their risk of lower back pain and decreasing their hip drive.

### Priority Tests
- Capsule Assessment
- Seated Forward Trunk Tilt
- Standing Leg Swing
- Priority Exercises

**Phase 1**
- Any Phase 1 exercise
- Seated Lumbopelvic Mobility

**Phase 2**
- OTT
- Pull Backs
- Lunges
- Step-ups
- Space Invaders

- Suspension Bridge
- Ski Jumper
- Balance

**Phase 3**
- Straight Pulley Push
- Pulley Pull
- Medicine Ball Clean
- Medicine Ball Sweep
- Trunk Incline Pulley Push
- Pulley Pull Drive

**Phase 4**
- Side Squat Tosses
- Overhead Tosses
- Stair Bounding
- Side Leaps

## Cycling

Small asymmetries and deviations out of the sagittal plane can affect efficiency and power in cyclists. They should be trained to keep the pelvis in a consistent position by accessing the gluteal group, and learn to flex the hip without side-bending the spine. They should also learn how to keep the knee aligned with their hip.

A secure trunk using low-effort abdominal activity will allow these athletes to breathe normally as they cycle. Compressing the body in a sprint situation will give a short-term blast of power, but the same strategy cannot be sustained in long road races. Road racers and triathletes should develop independent trunk control so that they are not over-dependent upon their arms for stability and so that they do not restrict their rib cage expansion by overusing the abdominal oblique muscles.

### Priority Tests
- Capsule Assessment
- Step-ups

## Priority Exercises

**Phase 1**
- Seated Knee Lift
- Greyhound
- String of Pearls Bridge
- Clam
- Superman

**Phase 2**
- Ski Shifts
- Step-ups
- OTT
- Ski Jumper
- Space Invaders
- Suspension Bridge
- Lunges

**Phase 3**
- Medicine Ball Sweep
- Straight Pulley Push
- Progressive Lunge
- Incline Plank Knee Drive

**Phase 4**
- Swiss Ball Elbow Circles
- Elbow Support Knee Drive
- Hip Ranger

## Rowing

Three common complaints associated with rowing are lower back pain, knee pain and stress fractures of the ribs [60]. Full and coordinated joint motion throughout the kinetic chain is necessary to prevent over-stress in some areas due to poor mobility in others. For example, poor hip bending mobility can cause rowers to compensate by bending excessively in the spine and knees to reach their catch position, or they may over-reach with their arms to strain for a little extra range. If these body parts are repetitively loaded in positions just beyond their safe zone, the whole kinetic chain is compromised and injury is likely to occur.

Rowers will often be told to "keep their chest up" in order to avoid collapse of this kind, but if they do not have sufficient hip joint mobility or lack sufficient trunk and pelvic control, this will not be achievable. The ability to control the relationship between the pelvis and the spine is critical in order to achieve an effective drive but is also essential to minimise lower back stress.

## Priority Tests
- Capsule Assessment
- Seated Forward Trunk Tilt
- Supine Hip Flexion

## Priority Exercises

**Phase 1**
- Ball Bouncing
- Greyhound and progressions
- Seated Knee Lift
- String of Pearls Bridge
- Hip Pops
- Hip Swivels
- Diamond
- The Sphinx
- Wall Press
- Straight-up Hamstring Mobility
- Wind-up Stretch
- Total Body Rotation (Although not a feature of the rowing movement, its role in removing myofascial restrictions may influence joint mobility.)

**Phase 2**
- Single Leg Bounce
- OTT and OTT Squat Thrust
- Upper Zone Stabiliser

- Pull Backs

- Lunges

- Ski Jumper

- Step-ups

- Any Phase 2 mobility exercise

**Phase 3**
- Medicine Ball Clean

- Medicine Ball Sweep

- Trunk Incline Pulley Push

- Pulley Pull

- Pulley Pull Drive

- Progressive Lunge

- Incline Plank Knee Drive

**Phase 4**
- Tail-up

- Hip Ranger

- Side Squat Tosses

- Toss and Stretch

- Overhead Tosses

- Quick Rotations

- Stair Bounding

- Swiss Ball Side Raises

- Swiss Ball Full Press-ups

- Swiss Ball Elbow Circles

- Elbow Support Knee Drive

- Single Leg Squat

- Swiss Ball Hamstring Curl

- Toe Touch Sit-ups

- Ball Bounce Sit-ups

# Swimming

Lower back and shoulder pain are frequent complaints among swimmers. Swimmers with lower back pain often demonstrate over-active erector spinae (superficial back extensor muscles), inadequate control of the lumbopelvic junction and poor trunk and pelvic stabiliser activation.

Shoulder problems can come from a variety of sources but there are some common features. The trunk is often not stable enough to provide a foundation to support the pull; the scapula is often not dynamically stable and the glenohumeral joint is subject to muscle imbalances.

The other important thing to remember is that you are testing both for swimming and for dry land training. It is not unusual for a swimmer to be uninjured until he or she takes up strength training in the gym.

## Priority Tests

- Double Arm Raise

- Seated Hamstring Test

- Static Lunge

- Standing Knee Lift

- Seated Knee Lift on a Ball

- Total Body Rotation

- Diamond

- Wall Press

- Superman

- Double Arm Floor Press

- Standing Leg Swing

- Windscreen Wipers

## Priority Exercises

**Phase 1**
- Ball Bouncing

- Greyhound and progressions

- Seated Knee Lift

- String of Pearls Bridge
- Hip Pops
- Hand Slides
- Diamond
- Windscreen Wipers
- The Sphinx
- Wall Press
- Superman
- Star Hold
- Straight-up Hamstring Mobility
- Floor Press
- Standing Leg Swing

**Phase 2**
- OTT
- OTT Circles
- OTT Press-ups
- Upper Zone Stabiliser
- Pull Backs
- Supported Lunge
- Supported Single Leg Squat
- Static Lunge and progressions
- Sway
- Ski Jumper
- Floor Bridge
- Press-ups (Levels 1–3)
- Triangle Pose
- Extended Warrior Pose
- Revolving Lunge
- Hip and Spine Twist

**Phase 3**
- Medicine Ball Sweep
- Straight Pulley Push
- Pulley Pull
- Swiss Ball Body Spin

- Swiss Ball Press-ups
- Handstand (all levels)
- Star Sequence

**Phase 4**
- Side Squat Tosses
- Toss and Stretch
- Overhead Tosses
- Plyometric Press-ups (Levels 1–3)
- Swiss Ball Side Raises
- Swiss Ball Full Press-ups
- Curl-ups
- Toe Touch Sit-ups
- Ball Bounce Sit-ups
- Corkscrew
- Chicken Wings
- Tail-up

## Tennis

For effective stroke production, the tennis player needs great integration from the feet through the legs, pelvis, trunk and arms. Rotational mobility of the pelvis over the hips and the shoulders over the pelvis should be unrestricted. Pelvic and trunk control needs to be dynamic to allow that rotation mobility to provide a foundation for power. Without pelvic and trunk stability, the shoulder becomes vulnerable as explained in Chapter 3, but the shoulder is also prone to its own muscle imbalances. To prevent injury and maximise technical proficiency, the lower, central and upper control zones must all be managed.

### Priority Tests
- Capsule Assessment
- Jump Landings
- Hop and Return
- Lunge Progressions (with catching tasks)
- Windscreen Wipers

- Diamond
- Double Arm Floor Press
- Momentum Control

## Priority Exercises

**Phase 1**
- Any Phase 1 exercise

**Phase 2**
- OTT
- OTT Circles
- OTT Twisting Squat Thrust
- OTT Scissors
- Upper Zone Stabiliser
- Pull Backs
- Dynamic Lunge and progressions
- Step-ups
- Space Invaders
- Pullover
- Sway
- Ski Jumper
- Floor Bridge
- Press-ups (Levels 1–3)
- Wobble Cushion Steps
- Compass Balance
- Single Leg Balance with Medicine Ball Movements
- Triangle Pose
- Extended Warrior Pose
- Revolving Lunge
- Hip and Spine Twist

**Phase 3**
- Medicine Ball Clean
- Medicine Ball Sweep
- Medicine Ball Spiral
- Straight Pulley Push
- Trunk Rotation Pulley Push

- Pulley Pull
- Compass Lunges
- Swiss Ball Body Spin
- Handstand (all levels)
- Aeroplane Sequence
- Star Sequence

**Phase 4**
- Any Phase 4 exercise

## Flatwater or Sprint Kayak

This is a sport where accurate, symmetrical repetition of a skill at speed is challenged by the changing elements of wind and water. It requires sensory perception and rapid neuromuscular adjustments in order to maintain efficient, powerful form.

The paddler needs good central control, shoulder stability and mobility through hamstrings, pelvis and thorax. Training regimens that focus solely on core strengthening can restrict rotation if the paddler does not have sufficient mobility through the legs, spine and shoulders. Rotational restriction, whether caused by actual muscular tightness or secondary mobility loss due to bracing in order to cope with loss of control on the water, will cause unwelcome movements as the body tries to compensate, especially around the shoulder and lower back.

The list below shows how you can adapt relevant exercises into tests in order to gain insight into paddling-specific movement potential.

## Priority Tests
- Seated Thoracic Mobility
- Seated Lumbopelvic Mobility
- Seated Forward Trunk Tilt
- Straight-up Hamstring Mobility
- Seated Knee Lift on a Ball (for coronal plane spinal control)
- Diamond (for scapular and shoulder stability)

All tests of lumbopelvic movements sitting on the ball are relevant. Test 5.1 examines whether you can move your spine into the correct sitting position, 5.2 tests whether you give more to one side than the other, and 5.3 looks at the available motion for the actual paddling action.

For the test of Straight-up Hamstring Mobility, press your foot out to the point that corresponds to maximum knee extension in your kayak. Rotate into the Wind-up Stretch. If this can be performed well, move into Straight-up Hamstring Mobility and add Seated Forward Trunk Tilt. Finally, rotate in this position.

## Priority Exercises

The exercises are aimed at creating a secure CLA and the mobility needed to rotate the thorax and pelvis around this axis; the anterior chain patterning to enable rotational torque generation without bracing and a relaxed, effective shoulder position. Phase 3 exercises emphasise coordination from legs through to arms.

**Phase 1**
- Knee Creepers
- Thigh Slides
- Diamond (for scapular awareness and mobility)
- Ball Bouncing (with side arm movements)
- Seated Knee Lift
- Straight-up Hamstring Mobility (progressing to Wind-up Stretch)
- Greyhound
- Floor Press

**Phase 2**
- OTT Circles (to prevent sideways trunk bending)
- Single Leg Bounce
- Pull Backs (modification: as the arm pulls back, the whole chest turns with it keeping the pelvis facing forward)
- Step-ups
- Compass Balance
- Lunges (with thoracic rotation)
- Upper Zone Stabiliser
- Revolving Lunge
- Hip and Spine Twist

**Phase 3**
- Pulley Pull
- Medicine Ball Sweep
- Medicine Ball Clean
- Medicine Ball Spiral
- Swiss Ball Pendulum

**Phase 4**
- Corkscrew
- Kneeling Ball Balance (with thoracic rotation)
- Quick Rotations
- Swiss Ball Side Raises
- Tail-up
- Toss and Stretch
- Side Squat Tosses

# Sample Group Session for a Professional Football Club

This is an example of a training session provided for a professional football team. Initially the players found even simple exercises challenging and quite a few experienced post-exercise soreness in the first week or so. However, as their stability and movement patterns improved, the injury rate in the team significantly reduced, and players reported feeling more confident about their bodies.

**Warm-up**
- Ball Follow
- Star Sequence
- Total Body Rotation

**Dynamic stability**
- Static Lunge
- Lunge with added rotation and eyes closed
- Multidirectional Catching Lunges

**Jumping**
- Single Leg Landings
- Leap sideways onto one leg and balance
- Push Jumps
- Single Leg Push Jumps

**Medicine ball**
- Medicine Ball Clean
- Medicine Ball Sweep
- Toss and Stretch
- Follow Through Rotations
- Overhead Tosses

**Stretch band**
- Space Invaders
- Stretch Band Lunge with partner resistance

**Swiss Ball**
- Ski Jumper
- OTT
- Wall Squat (with diagonal medicine ball movement)
- Sway
- Twisted Floor Bridge (with side-bend, rotation and forward tilt)
- Aeroplane Sequence

**Focused stability-mobility**
- Greyhound
- Clam
- Counter Body Rotation
- Hip and Spine Twist
- Triangle Pose
- Extended Warrior Pose
- Revolving Lunge

# 12 | Rehabilitation Pathways

Working with athletes is an art as well as a science. We have to appreciate not only their movement but also their motivation, attitudes and beliefs. We also need to understand the context and environment within which they work and very often the culture of the sport, its development and attitudes.

Integration of sports medicine principles into the coaching environment can be met with resistance if the sports medicine professional doesn't communicate in a way that is meaningful to the coach and the athlete. Taking time to understand the sport and its demands often saves time in the long run.

The following list of good working principles is the result of many years of experience troubleshooting for athletes and sporting organisations.

- Assume nothing and therefore consider everything.

- Apply absolute attention to detail, both structurally and functionally.

- Technical problems are not caused by personal style just because the athlete is a high flyer.

- The best performer is not necessarily the one with the least issues. He/she is the one who compensates most effectively for them. When the ability to compensate is exceeded by the demands on body and mind, a cycle of injury often ensues. Assess accurately without prejudice.

- The issues that predispose to injury are usually the same as those that influence performance. Assess the movements and control that the athlete will require or encounter in his sport, even those that seem too obvious to examine.

- In order to develop self-awareness and responsibility, actively engage the athlete by asking for direct feedback during exercises. The ability to give high-quality feedback may never have been developed in the athlete but it can be learned. Acquiring this skill and providing opportunities to use it increases confidence and internal motivation.

- Keep it relevant. An athlete who has never been injured doesn't prioritise prevention but if the programme might improve performance they will more readily engage with it.

- The art of applying science to sport is in making potentially complex concepts seem simple and accessible. Know the rocket science but teach it as though it is simple common sense.

- A common error in athletic development is to randomly add variety and complexity without attending to quality. Adding variety to training drills can enhance motor skill acquisition but will not automatically foster ideal movement habits if sound movement foundations are not already in place. The experience of this author is that talented athletes find a way to manage a task using their own particular patterns and attributes. These patterns may not however be the best strategies for continued improvement or injury resistance. Progress athletic development by building secure foundations and challenging them in a systematic manner.

- Perform everything with excellence, from the warm-up across the whole programme. The mind and body note every movement pattern whether it is good or bad, so feed only the most efficient messages into the nervous system.

- Performance plateaus and chronic injuries relate to training that only asks "how many?", "how much?", "how far?" and "how fast?" without insisting on "how well?".

- Aim for effortless control. It trims away inefficiency, facilitates balance and stimulates the most-effective muscle patterns.

- Train for confidence, adaptability and creativity. Athletes with these qualities work out how to solve problems and exploit opportunities.

- Communicate and integrate. The multidisciplinary team needs to be on board. Although individual priorities may be different between professional personnel, the overall goal should be the same. Gaps in the programme emerge if one professional's findings do not influence the planning of other team members.

- Keep the big picture in mind: long-range planning creates the basis for long-term success rather than short-term achievement.

- Professional athletes should enjoy their movement in training and performing. They should also understand that the best of the best know how to make it look easy even when it isn't.

## Treatment Pathways

The following stories outline the rehabilitation pathways taken for athletes with a variety of injuries. They are not intended to be comprehensive case studies. Their purpose is to illustrate the relevance of functional tests and the application of the principles set out in this book to specific presentations. Each of the athletes described had chronic or recurrent injuries. They had previously received standard local treatment for their pain but this approach had been unable to resolve their problem. For all of these athletes there was a fundamental functional movement issue causing a structural breakdown.

## The Tennis Player with Shin Pain

A 23-year-old tennis player presented to the clinic with bilateral inner shin pain of six months duration. She was palpably tender over her tibialis posterior muscle but had no other musculoskeletal pain.

The player was relatively slow off the mark and unstable when trying to control her momentum on court. When questioned, she said she had noticed that her knees tended to collapse inwards when training. She had been practising exercises in the gym and trying to gain knee control for five months.

The outline below describes a 30-minute session aimed at changing her patterns. The player was observed with her shoes off during testing.

## Main Findings for Function-related Testing

### SSCT

The entire leg rotated medially from the hip, turning the knee inwards and flattening the foot. This movement was amplified by adding a simple arm movement. The greater the balance challenge, the more deeply the leg would rotate.

Several points should be considered from this result. The inability to maintain the femur in neutral indicates that further investigation of hip control and GMax–GMed activity will be necessary. The tendency to depend on the inner part of the foot for balance and control will lead us to investigate sensory awareness in the sole of the foot. The response to simple arm movements with eyes open implies dissociation problems.

### Natural Squat

The athlete was unable to drop her centre of gravity in balance. Her foot pressure rolled medially on both sides, drawing her knees inwards. She therefore lacked vertical force management, which will be necessary for momentum control and change of direction.

There was no marked restriction in ankle dorsiflexion range of motion, nor in hip or knee flexion, so the athlete had the motion available, but was unable to use it functionally.

### Static Lunge

The athlete's knees collapsed inwards immediately in the movement. She moved her hips backwards instead of downwards, indicating a lack of eccentric control in GMax. She therefore lacked a support behaviour in her lower control zone. Without a support response in each leg, propulsive potential will be diminished.

### Listening Foot

Performing this test indicated that the athlete had very poor awareness of the central forefoot area and very little control of her foot and ankle, other than in the collapsed position, where the medial border of her foot was contacting the floor. She was over-using tibialis anterior and posterior to control her foot pressure even in a reduced weightbearing position. She was unable to activate popliteus.

## Likely Mechanism of Injury

The athlete would push off her stance limb with her foot and leg in an inwardly collapsed position causing tibialis posterior to repetitively contract while on stretch.

## Treatment Approach

### Proprioception–Dissociation at the Foot and Ankle

The athlete first worked on her plantar surface connection with the Listening Foot exercise. After being shown how to feel how her fibula moved in response to her foot pressure, she was able to decrease her excessive peripheral muscle activity and increase the sensitivity of her foot control.

The same technique was applied in standing with the athlete feeling movement in her hip joint in response to changes in foot pressure. This helped her to make a sensory connection between her foot and her hip.

### Activation

The Clam was used to increase awareness and basic muscle function in the area of the lateral hip.

The String of Pearls Bridge enabled the athlete to differentiate between hip extension and back extension. The athlete was then able to initiate GMax as a primary extensor, rather than initiating the motion with her erector spinae. This was quickly progressed to Hip Swivels in the bridge position to introduce alternating GMax responses.

Some simple Ball Bouncing with arms stretched above the head increased the athlete's central tone and stimulated trunk stabiliser responses. It also provided a dynamic neuromuscular task for her to learn to maintain knee control and a neutral foot position without full loading.

### Balance

Having increased the plantar surface's sensory connection and established activation of the gluteal group, Basic Balance was reintroduced, with the athlete focusing on the feeling under her foot. She was quickly able to recognise the feeling of her limb collapsing and was able to correct it.

### Increasing Functional Loading

The athlete was taught a Wall Squat with the Swiss Ball in order to develop an awareness of her spinal position, knee and foot position and eccentric control of her GMax. In testing, we learned that this athlete shifted her pelvis backwards when performing the Static Lunge to compensate for inadequate eccentric GMax control. Using the ball decreases the complexity of the movement compared to a Natural Squat by limiting the number of possible compensations in the kinetic chain from the foot to the spine. By maintaining a consistent trunk and ankle position, it was easy for the athlete to detect errors in her hip movement.

Once the athlete felt secure in her hip, foot and knee control, she was progressed to a Supported Lunge. The ball version slightly decreases the loading on the limb, making it an ideal intermediate step towards full body weight control.

### Re-testing at the End of the Session

The Static Lunge was re-tested. Foot, knee and hip control was achieved to 95 degrees of knee flexion. On Basic Balance testing, the athlete could detect control problems early and correct them.

A foundation like this can then be built upon at increasing functional levels. The key was establishing awareness links between the foot and the hip, and increasing sensory awareness around the foot and ankle. With this in place, the positive support reflex could be accessed to improve hip, knee and pelvic control.

The programme will progress a variety of elements. Variations upon the Static Lunge will be included, ensuring that the control zones can move independently while maintaining connection. Agility and momentum control will benefit from Natural Squat variations to develop speed and accuracy in vertical force management. Lower limb propulsion will be developed, beginning with Lunge Drives for timing at the hip alongside Walking Drills to coordinate ankle and foot action.

# The Rower with Lower Back Pain

This athlete presented with severe recurrent episodes of lower back pain which failed to respond to standard treatment regimens. He was unable to continue with his sport due to this problem.

## Main Findings for Function-related Testing

- **Seated Lumbopelvic Mobility**: Poor mobility and dissociation.

- **Seated Hamstring Test:** Poor trunk proprioception and postural control.

- **Supine Hip Flexion:** Pelvis rotated posteriorly at 80 degrees of hip flexion.

- **Seated Forward Trunk Tilt:** Trunk folded into flexion early in the motion.

- **Static Lunge:** Poor lateral pelvic control, overuse of latissimus dorsi.

- **Vertical Hip Release:** Lack of hip flexion.

- **Basic Balance:** Poor trunk orientation over each foot.

## Likely Mechanism of Injury

This athlete was relatively more flexible in his spine than in his hips and had poor awareness and control of his lumbopelvic region. In the recovery phase of his stroke, his spine bent into flexion very early, partly because he had greater mobility in it than in his hips, and partly because he lacked the proprioception and control in his spine to prevent it. This placed him in a poor position for engaging the water resistance on his catch and placed maximum stress on his back at the beginning of his pull.

## Treatment Approach

Proprioception and activation were high priorities for this athlete. He started with some gentle Ball Bouncing, trying to land accurately in the same place each time. This addressed several issues: trunk orientation, trunk stabiliser activation and proprioception.

Following this, he practised basic lumbopelvic movements, smoothly tilting the pelvis is each direction and recovering to a neutral position after each one. This task combined controlled mobility with proprioception. Lateral pelvic tilts with recovery to neutral during Ball Bouncing was then added, in order to increase trunk activation and the neuromuscular aspect of the task. The athlete became far more confident about his spine in response to this activity.

For the hip to lumbar spine relationship, manual therapy to restore hip mobility, followed by a sustained positional hold in the new range, allowed the athlete to improve his hip mobility and relax his back. The athlete maintained this as part of his home programme.

For basic TrA activation and integration, the athlete learned the Greyhound and the Wall Press. He was accustomed to collapsing his trunk into a flexed position, so these two exercises introduced the concept of activating stabilisers to maintain a neutral trunk position. Once he could achieve this, he performed the Seated Forward Trunk Tilt to combine the neutral trunk control with hip flexion.

The String of Pearls Bridge was introduced to enable initiation of the rower's GMax. This awareness was then applied to the Wall Squat. This movement had several purposes. The rower had a primary movement dysfunction involving his hips and lumbar spine. He would flex his lumbar spine rather than flex his hips. The Wall Squat altered his movement pattern by teaching him how to flex his hips and knees while maintaining a consistent spinal position. In this manner it worked on kinaesthetic, proprioceptive and stabilising elements while also training eccentric and concentric GMax activity.

Once the Wall Squat had been mastered, the rower was progressed to the Natural Squat.

Once these Phase 1 elements were established, the rower was able to progress to OTT. The basic OTT increased trunk control in the neutral position, and then the OTT Squat Thrust was added in this position to further train the relationship between the neutral trunk and the flexing hip.

The Pelvic BLT was progressed to the single-leg position sitting on the ball. This required higher-level movement control and dynamic lumbopelvic stability.

Ski Jumper was added to coordinate sustained hip and back extensor activity with neutral trunk control. To coordinate dynamic hip and trunk motion, Medicine Ball Cleans and lunge variations were introduced, with rotation added when the basic movement was achieved.

For low-load dynamic trunk control and endurance, the rower was asked to sit on the ergo machine (ergometer) with his hands on his head and a neutral trunk. He was asked to maintain his trunk position as he moved forward and backwards on the ergo machine. Pulley exercises and general gym exercises were finally added to restore confidence in a training environment.

The outcome for the athlete was increased confidence, decreased pain and a return to sporting activity.

# The Sprinter with Recurrent Groin and Hamstring Strains

This athlete had a two-year history of recurrent injury. He complained of chronic tightness around his hips, a loss of technical proficiency and restricted movement in his right shoulder. Prior to these problems emerging, he had sustained a minor right knee injury.

## Main Findings for Function-related Testing

- **SSCT:** Extremely poor balance on both legs with the right leg slightly worse. Foot rigidity evident on the right foot.

- **Walking drills**: Loss of CLA when stepping onto the left foot. Trunk collapsed to the right.

- **Standing Leg Swing:** The athlete was unable to perform a Standing Leg Swing on either leg. He lacked sufficient balance and support through his stance leg to achieve the movement.

- **Standing Knee Lift**: The athlete pulled down with his right latissimus dorsi if asked to lift his right knee. He was compensating through his posterior oblique myofascial sling.

- **Static Lunge:** Pelvis tipped laterally and anteriorly; lumbar spine collapsed into extension; right knee deviated medially. The athlete therefore demonstrated a lack of support in the lower control zone.

- **Lunge Drive:** Strong hamstring dominance, with the pelvis pulled into posterior tilt and the stance knee flexed. The athlete therefore demonstrated a poor propulsive strategy.

## Likely Mechanism of Injury

This athlete was unable to maintain a vertical CLA. When stepping onto his left foot, his trunk would collapse to the right, which biased his left adductors to increase their role in extending his hip and maintaining balance. His GMax did not activate spontaneously in any position or movement, so his adductor group and his hamstrings were overloaded to compensate. By pulling his right shoulder down, the athlete was unable to move his elbow backwards, giving him the perception of shoulder stiffness where there was none present.

This athlete was highly dominant in his hamstrings and erector spinae. He also lacked the awareness to detect that he consistently moved his lumbar spine instead of his hip. His poor trunk stabilising strategy depended upon his erector spinae and his hip flexors, as his TrA was not active. This amplified his feelings of hip stiffness. The absence of a listening foot on the right was linked to poor pelvic control on the right side, again causing overuse of his hamstrings.

Because the athlete could not productively move his hips up and forward with hip extension, he ran in a "sitting down" position, pulling his body over his fixed foot with his hamstrings instead of pushing his hips forward over his fixed foot. He therefore lacked an effective propulsive strategy.

## Treatment Approach

This athlete required a classic progression through the four Phases.

In Phase 1, all the exercises were used to increase lumbopelvic awareness and activate the athlete's GMax, GMed and TrA. To create a supportive lower control zone, the Listening Foot exercise was introduced immediately, and this was critical in improving his balance and for encouraging normal support responses in his right leg. Seated Lumbopelvic Mobility movements and Ball Bouncing were used to increase the athlete's awareness and control of his pelvic position relative to his spine.

Wall Press worked on symmetry and trunk control in a position that established a secure CLA. This began the development of zone stacking control. Superman worked on dissociation of lower limb movement from the trunk by requiring the athlete to flex and extend his hip with consistent control of his spine. Along with Greyhound, this began to establish the elastic support strategy. Both are necessary for a sprinter.

The athlete then worked through Phase 2, aiming for a long body shape with low effort. Lunges and Ski Jumper developed posterior chain coordination with trunk control, and Single Leg Bounce challenged his body orientation over the fixed foot. His OTT was eventually progressed through to OTT Single Leg Squat Thrusts for high-level hip flexion patterning as he had a tendency to let his right knee drift medially on flexion.

Phase 3 was important in establishing correct timing between the athlete's knees and hips. The Medicine Ball Cleans and Medicine Ball Sweeps trained full-range coordinated extension of the lower limb from the floor and continued to train the CLA at a higher level. Because the athlete needed to resume a strength training programme in the gym, this pattern needed to be firmly established. Pulley exercises trained global control with a lengthened trunk position. The Standing Stretch Band Leg Drive focused the athlete on actively moving his body over his stance hip.

Phase 4 introduced speed and load demands to the athlete's control as well as adding variability to his stability challenges. Stair Bounding ensured that full propulsion was generated from the athlete's lower body without the trunk posture being affected.

Once this athlete achieved a secure CLA, the strain on his groin decreased. Previous treatment approaches had tried to activate the major stabilising groups, but in order to be successful, they had to be combined with proprioceptive and kinaesthetic awareness work. This tied in nicely with the athlete's technical work on the track as it made sense of his movement problems and increased his motivation to comply with the programme.

# The Golfer with Lower Back Pain

This athlete presented to the clinic with a history of increasing lower back problems and a persistent barrier to technical improvement. She was attempting to increase her power with a gym-based resistance programme but was seeing no improvement.

## Main Findings for Function-related Testing

- **SSCT:** Extremely poor balance, with particular rigidity in the right foot and ankle.

- **Basic standing position:** The athlete displayed excessive muscle activity in her tibialis anterior and quadriceps in quiet standing. She had poor tone in her lower abdominal region and high tone in her upper abdominal region.

- **Pelvic rotation over the fixed foot in standing:** limited mobility in the hips, with a tendency to extend the lower back and over-rotate the upper trunk to compensate.

- **Medicine Ball Square Rotation:** The athlete tended to move as a block, displaying difficulty in separating the shoulders from the hips. She therefore was unable to access her elastic spiral support mechanism.

- **Seated Forward Trunk Tilt:** The athlete displayed a tendency towards spinal extension, and the end position provoked strong erector spinae activity.

## Likely Mechanism of Injury

There were several contributing factors. The player's habitual address position placed her in lumbar extension, which was sustained with high erector spinae tension. As she moved into her backswing, her inability to separate her thorax from her pelvis caused her to shift her hips excessively sideways and disengage her control zones to achieve movement. As she began her swing through from this position, her right lower leg was unable to rotate adequately, causing her to "jump" into her swing and try to force her pelvis into a poorly timed extreme rotation. Without adequate available hip mobility, her spine was forced into excessive extension and side-bending, putting a compression force through her lumbar facet joints.

## Treatment Approach

Stability, mobility and awareness needed to be worked on simultaneously. The first step was achieving a listening foot on the right side which would permit the lower leg to rotate normally in the swing. This was combined with standing pelvic rotation awareness and hip mobility to reduce the excessive sideways weight shift in her backswing, and provide a basis for maintaining the tensile relationship between the upper and lower trunk that would allow her to generate more power.

As this movement vocabulary was being developed, the player was taught Greyhound to lay foundations for elastic support, along with Wall Press and Ball Bouncing to activate TrA and train awareness and control of a neutral trunk position. She was also taught Wall Squats to learn how to control her hip without using her back extensors, and to increase the proportion of control coming from her hip region rather than her back and lower legs.

Once these elements were in place, it was possible to progress into Phase 2 and 3 exercises such as Ski Jumper, OTT and the Swiss Ball Body Spin, as well as integrating the yoga-based mobility sequences for control and flexibility.

As for the sprinter (see page 346), the player's rehabilitation was strongly connected to analysis of her stroke problems. Addressing the movement barriers in addition to the stability problems increased the specificity of the treatment and targeted prevention of further problems. She was able to resume playing at a professional level with an increase in technical proficiency and minimal discomfort.

# The Tennis Player with Shoulder Pain

This left-handed player came to the clinic with increasing anterior shoulder pain, particularly on open forehands and slice backhands. Her playing tolerance had dropped to 30 minutes before pain stopped her.

## Main Findings for Function-related Testing

- **Postural observation:** The player had an over-developed upper trapezius and pectoralis major on her left side.

- In normal gait, the player did not rotate her upper trunk effectively.

- **Static Lunge:** The player showed a tendency to tip forward on the lunge and an unwillingness to move into full range of motion at the hip and knee.

- **Windscreen Wipers**: The head of the humerus would slide forward as the player rotated her arm.

- **Seated Thoracic Mobility:** The player rotated poorly in both directions.

- Scapular and trunk stability was normal on formal testing.

## Likely Mechanism of Injury

When playing a forehand, the player rotated herself as a block rather than separating her pelvic and thoracic rotation. Without this rotation dissociation, she did not transfer force effectively through her body during the stroke, and did not access potential elastic energy in her trunk to generate power. This caused her to overuse her arm to deliver power in her stroke.

On the slice backhand, the player kept her front knee relatively straight and tipped her body forward instead, placing her shoulder at a difficult angle for withstanding and creating force. She had trained her scapula to "set", so it did not move in response to her arm action to decrease the loading on the shoulder joint. Instead, the head of her humerus was driven forward in the socket, interrupting the axis of rotation and showing up as a shoulder control issue. The player's perception of muscular effort was on the anterior surface of the shoulder instead of the posterior surface.

## Treatment Approach

In standing, the player was introduced to Total Body Rotation (Chapter 6) in order to increase her awareness of pelvic and thoracic rotation as well as optimise her available mobility. Performing it rhythmically while allowing the arms to swing with the movement helped her to feel the elastic spiral effect as the thorax followed the pelvis into the motion. Medicine Ball Square Rotation (Chapter 7) was used to enable rotation of the thorax over the pelvis, and Pelvic Rotation Over a Fixed Foot (Chapter 6) established the sensation of movement initiating from the pelvis, while allowing the shoulders to follow. This movement was progressed to a forehand action, integrating the arm into the movement.

Hand Slides (Chapter 6) was performed to increase the player's appreciation of scapular protraction and retraction. Although her scapular control was quite good in overhead positions, her scapular mobility at less abducted positions was poor.

The player's trunk, pelvic and scapular control were fundamentally sound, and her shoulder control problems were a response to a global movement error. She could actually be considered to be too stable, to the point where motion throughout the body has been compromised, thereby amplifying the forces on the shoulder. Her problem was global functional mobility, coordination and timing. Once the mobility awareness had been restored and assimilated into her movement, the shoulder loading was reduced.

This entire session took place on court so that the new movement awareness could immediately be integrated into the tennis stroke. The player continued to play for two hours with no onset of pain, and no return of it later.

## The Footballer with Knee Pain

This player had undergone reconstructive surgery for the anterior cruciate ligament (ACL) in his right knee one year previously. He continued to experience increasing pain and a feeling of instability in his knee, despite the ligament showing no signs of insufficiency on testing. The player had undergone standard rehabilitation for his knee but was now no longer able to train or play.

## Main Findings for Function-related Testing

- **SSCT:** Extremely poor balance on the right leg with visible rigidity in the foot and ankle.

- **Standing Knee Lift:** The player tipped his trunk to the right when lifting his left knee and collapsed his trunk to the right when he lifted his right knee.

- **Static Lunge:** The pelvis tipped laterally and tilted forward with loss of knee alignment on both left and right knees. The support strategy was therefore poor.

- **Jump Landings:** Loss of normal shock absorbing motion in the knee and hip. The player landed with stiff joints, causing more pain than was necessary. His neuromuscular strategy was therefore poor.

## Mechanism of Continuing Pain

The rigidity observed in the right foot was confirmed with the Listening Foot exercise. The player had no active tibial rotation, which affected the self-locking mechanism of the knee.

With foot rigidity comes a faulty positive support mechanism. The player's quadricep and gluteal muscle coordination and timing was impaired. He used maladaptive strategies such as stiffening his joints to cope with impact and momentum control. With poor GMed and GMax support, the player's pelvic stability was inadequate to cope with change of direction activities. The poor pelvic platform led to a loss of trunk control which increased the gravitational forces acting on his knee.

## Treatment Approach

All of the Phase 1 exercises were used as this player was initially unable to activate trunk or pelvic stabilisers. The tibial rotation and sensory feedback from the right foot needed to be established to enable the pelvic stabilisers to activate. The player performed active Listening Foot exercises to improve this. This was backed up with Clam and String of Pearls Bridge exercises to encourage activation of the pelvic stabilisers, and unlock his lumbopelvic region to enable GMax firing. Superman trained the player to support his weightbearing hip and establish his CLA.

The Phase 2 exercises were added to the programme with emphasis on maintaining a vertical CLA as the player tended to support his trunk tipped to the right through habit. Step-ups and Lunges were priority movements to establish the support strategy. Space Invaders integrated trunk control with the pelvis and hip. He needed to focus on his Vertical Hip Release to avoid tipping his trunk excessively forward during this exercise.

In Phase 3 most of the medicine ball exercises were used in order to coordinate and sequence the hip and knee movement.

In Phase 4, the player's strategies for controlling momentum were addressed, because he required up to six steps to control his momentum, whereas only two steps were necessary. This was the result of failing to drop his centre of gravity effectively to check his speed. Particular care was taken to address landing from jumps, especially if contacted in the air.

Having taken an approach that restored neurosensory elements as well as stability and strength, the player reported feeling stronger, his pain diminished and his speed and agility improved. He was able to return to Premier League play.

# The Dressage Rider with Lower Back Pain and Performance Problems

This rider was experiencing ongoing spinal pain as well as persistent performance barriers. When observed, she rode with her weight predominantly down her right side. As with many riders, she had a history of falls from horses since childhood.

## Main Findings for Function-related Testing

- **Pelvic Side Tilts:** Poor to the left.

- **Standing Knee Lift:** Poor when lifting the right knee.

- **Seated Knee Lift on a Swiss Ball:** Poor when lifting the right knee.

- **SSCT:** Poor balance on the left leg.

- **Listening Foot:** Poor on left side.

## Likely Mechanism of Injury

The relationship between this rider's left foot, left side of the body, sense of body orientation and balance mechanisms was impaired. Her testing results are common in riders who sustain blows to the pelvis and back through falls, and sometimes being kicked by horses. These blows can interrupt normal pelvic mechanics and the effect can continue to influence a rider's movement and control despite the original pain of injury subsiding.

The rider's sensory feedback was most consistent through her right side. She was unable to evenly weightbear in the saddle, not due to pain, but because she perceived that her weight was evenly distributed when her CLA collapsed over her right side. This was her "normal" position.

## Treatment Approach

The main aim for this rider was to achieve symmetry in order to relieve the stress on her spine, restore normal lumbopelvic mobility, and allow her to use weight and leg aids effectively. To enable the rider to start establishing a firm CLA, the left foot was stimulated with the Listening Foot exercise, followed by Pelvic Side Tilts to release her left side.

Once she could sit with weight through both sides of her pelvis, she was introduced to Ball Bouncing with her arms stretched above her head in order to practice a neutral, centred trunk position. Placing a broomstick in her hands as she sat with her arms above her head, she practised bouncing with lateral pelvic tilt, landing on one side of the pelvis, bouncing in the centre, and then bouncing on the other side, while keeping the broomstick horizontal.

The Greyhound and the Wall Press further encouraged trunk symmetry and TrA activation. Hip Swivels started to establish GMax activity and lumbopelvic mobility. The rider practised standing balance exercises to encourage pelvic stability, stable central orientation over both sides of the body and increased sensory feedback from her left side.

As she progressed, forward and backward lumbopelvic tilting and Thigh Slides for pelvic rotation were introduced to enable better movement in response to the horse's motion. The rider could progress into Phase 2 with OTT, Static Lunge and Ski Jumper to increase anterior and posterior chain balance and stability.

Ball bouncing exercises proved to be very effective in assisting the rider to find a new position when on her horse. She imagined the feeling of sitting on the ball as she rode and she found that this helped her to find a central position. The horse was able to strike off into a canter equally on both sides as a result. A central, balanced position decreased the stress on the rider's spine, and allowed her to respond to the horse's movement, improving the security of her seat.

# The Triathlete with Chronic Achilles Tendonitis

This athlete had been struggling with left Achilles tendon pain for three months. She had undergone an eccentric loading programme and conservative treatment including electrotherapy and soft tissue massage. This had not helped and she was unable to continue running.

## Main Findings for Function-related Testing

- **Gait assessment:** The athlete demonstrated asymmetry in pelvic rotation. She did not advance the right side of her pelvis as she pushed off her left foot, causing her to push harder with her left calf. Lack of pelvic rotation also made it impossible to extend the left hip, and affected gluteal timing. The athlete therefore had a propulsion dysfunction.

- **Standing Knee Lift:** The athlete was unable to maintain a straight supporting left hip as she raised her right knee.

- **Static Lunge:** Poor pelvic control and unwillingness to adequately bend the left hip was observed.

- **Listening Foot:** The athlete was unable to alter her foot pressure on the floor. Both feet were functionally rigid and unable to provide accurate sensory feedback.

- **SSCT:** The athlete's body rotated to the left when standing on her left leg.

## Likely Mechanism of Injury

This athlete had a combination of stability and mobility issues. Her poor GMed and GMax performance caused her pelvis to collapse on impact with the ground, increasing foot contact times and lower limb loading. She also had a fundamental locomotion dysfunction in that she lacked symmetry of pelvic rotation as she ran, causing her to over-push with her calf muscle.

## Treatment Approach

In order to directly address the biomechanical aspects of the problem, the athlete was taught Counter Body Rotation while lying on her side (Chapter 6). She was surprised to find the marked difference in her mobility from one side to the other. Once she had experienced this, she was asked to apply the feeling to her normal walking, simply noticing pelvic rotation as she moved.

Basic Phase 1 GMax and GMed exercises were learned in order to experience activation. This was progressed into weightbearing with the Static Lunge and Step-ups to gain hip control through outer-, mid- and inner ranges and establish the support strategy. The Standing Stretch Band Leg Drive from the lunge position was used to address her propulsive strategy, giving the athlete the feeling of moving her hip forward over her fixed foot using GMax instead of overusing her calf. The Step-up was progressed by adding a high knee lift from the trail leg, aiming to increase the speed of hip extension on the supporting leg.

Once the athlete could establish a balanced position of the pelvis over the leg, calf raises were added, ensuring that the athlete's body could maintain its alignment.

The biggest factor in this athlete's recovery was treatment of her faulty movement patterns rather than focusing exclusively on regimens for the Achilles tendon. Once the counter body rotation was re-established, along with the ability to support her body weight on impact with the ground and then to extend her hip, the athlete's symptoms began to diminish. She was able to return to running without further problems.

# The Golfer with Shoulder Pain

This athlete had a two-year history of pain across his right upper trapezius, right scapula, and right thoracolumbar area. He had invested a great deal of money on treatment with no improvement in his symptoms. Despite the amount of treatment this athlete had received, no one had ever looked at his swing. All of his prior treatment had been directed to the area of pain, not the cause of the tissue stress.

On observation, it was found that the player tended to swing the club around his body on the back swing, disconnecting the arm motion from his body.

## Main Findings for Function-related Testing

- **Total body rotation:** Extremely poor to the right.

- **Total body rotation with hips and knees bent:** this provoked the right hip to shoot backwards, dropping the left shoulder.

- **Thoracic rotation:** Normal.

- **Cervical rotation:** Normal.

- **External rotation of the right shoulder:** Moderately restricted.

## Likely Mechanism of Injury

Due to pelvic rotation restrictions, the player was shifting his right hip backwards. This caused him to drop his left shoulder as he swung the club backwards, making it necessary for him to over-pull with the muscles of his neck and posterior shoulder on the right side.

## Treatment Approach

The main priority for this athlete was to restore the pelvic rotation necessary to correct his swing. He performed the Total Body Rotation exercise to start restoring mobility in his hip, followed by Pelvic Rotation Over a Fixed Foot to raise his awareness of the pelvic rotation movement and establish it as part of his movement vocabulary. The athlete was also taught the Piriformis Stretch to address his basic mobility restriction.

At the end of the first session, the athlete re-evaluated his swing and found that he could swing without discomfort and with an increased sensation of free rotation.

The athlete's programme was expanded to include the Phase 1 exercises: Greyhound to increase elastic support, String of Pearls Bridge to unlock his lumbar spine, Hip Pops and Clam as well as Diamond to address his shoulder external rotation. He added Phase 2 exercises: Ski Jumper, OTT, and Suspension Bridge. Finally, the yoga-based mobility sequences from Phases 2 and 3 were added.

The athlete continued to travel and play at competition level and so was unavailable for actual treatment; however, after two months of regular, independent practice, he reported greatly improved performance with minimal discomfort.

# The Professional Footballer with Lower Back Pain and Groin Pain

This player was referred by his club with a history of lower back pain and acute right groin pain which stopped him playing. Hernia had been eliminated as a possible diagnosis.

## Main Findings for Function-Related Testing

- **Static Lunge:** Very poor control of pelvis, knee and trunk; decreased hip flexion and a forward-inclined trunk.

- **Double Arm Raise:** Poor trunk control; no evidence of abdominal activity in response to arm raise and forward pelvic shift.

- **Standing Knee Lift:** Loss of control over the right stance leg; dependence on right latissimus dorsi; right side-bending of the trunk on lifting the right knee and overactive feet.

- Palpable insufficiency of multifidus in the lower lumbar spine.

## Likely Mechanism of Injury

Global control problems amplifying forces in the groin.

## Treatment Approach

After manual therapy treatment to the pelvis, the player was taught Counter Body Rotation in sidelying to establish better muscle patterns around his lumbar spine. He performed these along with Greyhound, String of Pearls Bridge and Superman as his first programme.

Initially the player had difficulty with very simple movements. He was unable to sit on a Swiss Ball with his arms above his head, or move his right arm down to his side without losing control of his trunk. He was also unable to perform a simple Wall Press. This underlines the importance of assessment without prejudice: international-level athletes would be expected to be able to perform such simple movements, but they are seldom evaluated.

To overcome these problems, the player needed to be taught correct breathing patterns. He was unable to stabilise his trunk using an efficient muscle pattern, and his over-dependence on his abdominal oblique muscles had forced him to use an upper chest breathing pattern. Once he learned how to breathe and how to use the balloon cue to correct his posture, his control pattern changed and his progress was swift.

Once the basic TrA contraction was established and integrated with OTT, hip flexion was added with the OTT Squat Thrust and eventually the OTT Single Leg Squat Thrust. Spinal rotation control was added by OTT Twisting Squat Thrust.

The collapse of the player's trunk and difficulty maintaining a strong vertical axis were addressed with Pelvic BLT, progressing to a Single Leg BLT.

The Supported Lunge helped the player to deepen his hip movement with control which then transferred over to normal body weight lunges. The player's lower back pain was resolved in one session and the groin pain resolved in three sessions. Recommendations were made for continued progression of the player's dynamic stability to develop it to an acceptable level for the demands of his sport.

# The Long Jumper with Chronic Bilateral Anterior Compartment Syndrome

This athlete had struggled since her early teenage years with shin pain associated with running and jumping. This had eventually escalated into a compartment syndrome involving her tibialis anterior on both sides, for which she received a bilateral fasciotomy.

This had failed to correct the problem and the athlete pursued physiotherapy. However despite stabilising exercises being prescribed, there was no improvement in the athlete's symptoms.

She had not been able to run for three years and even walking could provoke her symptoms. She also suffered from pelvic and hip pain and right shoulder pain.

## Main Findings for Function-related Testing

- **SSCT:** Extremely poor with a functionally rigid foot on both sides.

- **Static and Dynamic Lunges:** Both poor with tipping of the trunk to the right. The hips moved backwards rather than downwards, indicating unwillingness to use GMax eccentrically.

- **Double Arm Raise:** Pelvis drifted forward markedly, indicating poor trunk control and postural habits.

- **Standing Knee Lift:** Overdependence on latissimus dorsi on both left and right stance.

- **Lunge Drive:** Poor propulsive pattern, with the trunk tipped backwards causing the quads and tibialis anterior to work hard to maintain an upright position.

## Likely Mechanism of Injury

This athlete's primary balance strategy was to overuse her tibialis anterior muscle. She also attempted to pull her tibia over her foot to move forward, instead of using her larger posterior leg muscles to push her body over the foot. In normal stance, she was unable to straighten her knees or hips, and stood with her pelvis shifted forward.

Instead of running with her trunk supported by her pelvis, she collapsed her spine into a deep extension arch so that her pelvis was carried behind her spine with her hips very flexed. To counteract this she tried to pull her shoulders back in an attempt to improve her posture as instructed by her coach. This combination put her pelvic muscles at a disadvantage and increased her dependence upon tibialis anterior. The area of the athlete's lower legs was congested, hard and lacked normal pliable muscle quality.

## Treatment Approach

In the initial stages, this athlete required myofascial release to the scarred areas of her shins in addition to soft tissue mobilisation and manual lymphatic drainage. This was necessary to establish a healing environment through reducing congestion and increasing normal circulation. Retraining of movement patterns was the key element to recovery for the athlete however, as her natural pattern of locomotion aggravated the area of her pain.

*Step 1* was activation of the pelvic and trunk stabilisers. Although the athlete had been performing stabilising exercises, she was not using the muscles that they were designed to address. She started with the String of Pearls Bridge to release her lumbar lock, Hip Pops and Hip Swivels to restore hip/pelvis mobility, as well as Clam and the Standing Knee Press for hip abductor strength. She performed Greyhound exercises, Superman and Wall Press to learn to coordinate her three control zones and achieve a neutral spinal position. In order to prepare for weightbearing exercise, she performed Listening Foot exercises followed by Basic Balance.

*Step 2* established restoration of counter body rotation and progressed CLA control by adding OTT, Ski Jumper and Suspension Bridge. The Supported Lunge enabled the athlete to develop a sound support strategy, and to work her hips through range.

*Step 3* focused on teaching the athlete to move her hip forward over the supporting foot, so the Lunge Drive and then Standing Stretch Band Leg Drive were added. A Static Lunge with lateral elastic resistance to the ribs proved to be extremely effective in coordinating the trunk with the pelvis.

This was not a quick fix and it took some time for the tissues in the local area to normalise. However, the athlete was eventually able to return to running several times a week.

# Appendix 1: Commonly Used Terms

## Positional Relationships

### Anterior (or ventral)
The front surface of the body or structure within the body. It can also describe a relationship between body parts, e.g. the sternum is anterior to the lungs, so anterior also means towards the front. The lungs as a structure will have an anterior surface.

### Posterior (or dorsal)
The back surface of the body or structure within the body, e.g. your back is your posterior surface and your spine is posterior to your lungs.

### Superior
The structure is higher on the body with respect to another structure, e.g. your head is superior to your shoulders.

### Inferior
The structure is lower on the body with respect to another structure, e.g. your feet are inferior to your knees.

### Proximal
The part of a body structure that is closest to your body's centre, e.g. your femur is more proximal than your tibia.

### Distal
The part of a body structure which is furthest from your body's centre, e.g. your hand is more distal than your elbow.

## Movement Terms

### Spine
**Flexion:** bending forward.
**Extension:** bending backward.
**Lateral flexion:** side-bending.

### Knee
**Flexion:** bending the knee.
**Extension:** straightening the knee.

### Hip
**Flexion:** moving the thigh forwards to bend the hip.

**Extension:** moving the thigh backwards to straighten the hip.

**Abduction:** moving the thigh away from the midline of the body.

**Adduction:** moving the thigh towards or across the midline of the body.

**Lateral rotation:** the thigh turns outwards.
**Medial rotation:** the thigh turns inwards.

### Shoulder
**Flexion:** moving the arm forward and up in a straight line.

**Extension:** moving the arm back in a straight line.

**Abduction:** moving the arm away from the body.

**Adduction:** moving the arm in the direction of or across the midline of the body.

**Lateral rotation:** moving the arm so that the inside surface faces relatively forwards.

**Medial rotation:** the inside surface of the arm faces relatively backwards.

## Planes of Movement

### Sagittal
The plane of flexion and extension, or forward and backward motion, e.g. cycling.

### Coronal
Sideways motions such as abduction and adduction, e.g. performing a cartwheel.

### Transverse
The plane of rotation within the body, e.g. striking a baseball.

## Muscle Contraction Terms

### Inner range

The muscle is acting when it is shortest, e.g. if your elbow is fully bent and you try to actively bend it further, the bicep is contracting at its shortest.

### Outer range

The muscle is contracting at its longest, e.g. in a pull-up, starting with your elbows straight would be starting in the outer range as the bicep is at its longest.

### Mid range

The point between these two extremes, and usually the strongest position for a muscle, e.g. a pull-up is easier if you start with your elbows bent.

### Concentric

As the muscle generates force it shortens, e.g. the biceps in a bicep curl.

### Eccentric

As the muscle contracts it lengthens, e.g. the quadriceps as you move into a deep squat.

### Isometric

The muscle does not change length as it contracts, e.g. the weightlifter holding a bar over her head is clearly working her muscles but they are sustaining a position and therefore not changing length.

## Motor Control Terms

### Base of support

The total area contained between surface contact points of the body, e.g. standing on one foot offers a small base of support. Supporting your body on hands and knees offers a large base of support. A larger base is generally more stable.

### Postural control

The body's ability to act automatically to control its equilibrium in response to feedback from visual, vestibular (inner ear) and somatosensory (muscles, tendons, skin and ligaments) sources. It is also the body's ability to prepare for movement in response to the impulse to move, a response that triggers weight shift and stabiliser activity to produce a foundation for movement. This preparation is called a **feedforward** response.

### Dissociation

The ability to move a body part smoothly and independently of other parts. If you fix with global muscle groups it will make it difficult to move freely due to excessive muscle tension.

### Proprioception

Awareness of joint position or joint motion generated by sensory feedback from the body.

### Positive support response

The response of hip and knee extensors to stimulation to the sole of the foot, usually weightbearing.

### Open chain

Movement where the distal end of the movement segment is not fixed, e.g. throwing a ball.

### Closed chain

Movement where the distal movement segment is fixed, e.g. leg press.

# Appendix 2: List of Common Patterns

Throughout this book, many muscle action relationships have been discussed. This table summarises these relationships. The directional relationship simply refers to the position of the overactive groups with respect to the underactive groups.

| Directional relationship | Anatomical relationship | Overactive muscles | Action of overactive muscles | Underactive/poorly timed muscles |
|---|---|---|---|---|
| Vertical | Proportion of upper to lower body used for force production. Overuse of arms | Pectoralis major Pectoralis minor Anterior deltoid | Creating and controlling force | TrA/multifidus/ internal obliques. Poor force transfer through trunk to pelvis |
| Vertical | Lower leg activity with respect to hip activity | Tibialis anterior | Pulling leg forward over fixed foot | GMax/hamstrings failing to push hip forward over fixed foot |
| Vertical | Lower leg activity with respect to pelvis-hip control | Gastrocnemius/ soleus/flexor hallucis | Stabilising the leg peripherally | Poor GMed/GMax, unstable CLA |
| Vertical posterior | Lumbopelvic region to hip | Hamstrings Erector spinae | Controlling extensor forces at lumbopelvic and hip regions | GMax/multifidus |
| Vertical anterior | Pelvis to hip | Superficial abdominals (rectus abdominis, external obliques) and hip flexors (iliopsoas and rectus femoris) | Controlling the pelvis/ hip relationship | Transversus abdominis |
| Diagonal | Pelvis to contralateral shoulder | Latissimus dorsi | Maintaining the posterior oblique myofascial sling | GMax opposite side |
| Lateral | Trunk to unilateral pelvis | Quadratus lumborum | Managing the position of the trunk on the pelvis | GMed |
| Lateral | Medial to lateral hip | Adductor group | Controlling the hip | GMax/GMed/deep rotators of the hip |
| Anteroposterior | Upper limb to trunk | Pectoralis major Pectoralis minor Anterior deltoid | Supporting and transferring the load between the upper limb and trunk | Serratus anterior/ lower trapezius/ rotator cuff |
| Anteroposterior cross pattern | Lumbar spine to pelvis | Hip flexors Erector spinae | Stabilising the lumbopelvic relationship | Transversus abdominis/GMax |

# Appendix 3: Scoring Charts for the Capsule Functional Assessment

The capsule functional assessment is a general array of tests that can be applied to anyone involved in sport. It is not intended to be sports specific but covers the main areas involved in basic control. For more information on sports-specific testing, refer to Chapter 11.

The following charts can be used to record a baseline impression of physical competence. Functional movements are difficult to measure objectively as there are many variables to consider throughout the kinetic chain. The intention of this test procedure is to quickly and simply highlight control problems that should be considered when planning training programmes.

If any of the tests scores two or more, it qualifies as a high-priority area. If the sum of all the totals in the capsule functional assessment exceeds five, the overall rating for the athlete is remedial high priority (RHP). If the score is between three and five, the rating will be remedial priority (RP). If the score is less than two, the athlete is rated as competent (C).

Once you have done this, formulate an action plan. Work out your priority areas and refer to the book for a plan to address them. Look at your training programme and make sure that it addresses your priority areas. For example, if you have poor lower and central control, hopping and bounding will increase your risk of injury. Prioritise improvement in your control while working on explosive power off both legs instead of alternate legs in order to satisfy training goals while developing the movement patterns to support them.

Finally, work out whether your findings can be linked to your technique. The concepts presented in Chapters 1 and 2 can help you to link test findings to movement issues.

# Capsule Functional Assessment Charts

**Name:** _____

**Date of birth:** _____

**Date of testing:** _____

## ❶ Balance

**Scoring:** Select only the highest scoring error that you observe, i.e. select only one of the first three options. Add a point each if foot or face fixing are observed.

| SSCT (Balance) | | Eyes Open (Balance) | | Eyes Closed (Balance) | |
|---|---|---|---|---|---|
| | | R | L | R | L |
| Wobbles | 1 | | | | |
| Foot shifts | 2 | | | | |
| Toe touch | 3 | | | | |
| Foot rigid | 1 | | | | |
| Face fix | 1 | | | | |
| **Total:** | | | | | |

**Balance subtotal:** _____

## ❷ Mobility Relationships

**Scoring:** Circle the relevant score.

| Double Arm Raise | | Seated Hamstring Test | R | L | Total Body Rotation | R | L |
|---|---|---|---|---|---|---|---|
| Pelvis rotated forward/ spinal curve deepens | 3 | Spinal position is lost | 3 | 3 | Turn limit is a third of a semicircle | 2 | 2 |
| Pelvis/weight shifted forward | 3 | Knee does not fully straighten | 2 | 2 | Turn limit is two-thirds of a semicircle | 1 | 1 |
| Shoulders less than 180 degrees | 3 | | | | Incorrect foot pressure response | 1 | 1 |
| **Total:** | | **Total:** | | | **Total:** | | |

**Mobility relationships subtotal:** _____

### ❸ Lower and Central Control Zone Stability

| Static Lunge (Eyes Open) | | R leg forward | L leg forward | Static Lunge (Eyes Closed) | | R leg forward | L leg forward | Dynamic Lunge | | R leg forward | L leg forward |
|---|---|---|---|---|---|---|---|---|---|---|---|
| Knee moves inwards | 3 | | | Knee moves inwards | 3 | | | Knee moves inwards | 3 | | |
| Pelvis tips sideways | 3 | | | Pelvis tips sideways | 3 | | | Pelvis tips sideways | 3 | | |
| Hips move backward (lumbar curve deepens) | 3 | | | Hips move backward (lumbar curve deepens) | 3 | | | Hips move backward (lumbar curve deepens) | 3 | | |
| Trunk tips sideways | 3 | | | Trunk tips sideways | 3 | | | Trunk tips sideways | 3 | | |
| One arm drops lower than the other | 3 | | | One arm drops lower than the other | 3 | | | Trunk collapses forwards | 3 | | |
| | | | | | | | | Front heel lifts from floor | 3 | | |
| Lip biting or facial fixing | 1 | | | Lip biting or facial fixing | 1 | | | Moving shoulders back initiates return to start position | 3 | | |
| Rigid front foot | 1 | | | Rigid front foot | 1 | | | Lip biting or facial fixing | 1 | | |
| | | | | | | | | Rigid front foot | 1 | | |
| **Total:** | | | | **Total:** | | | | **Total:** | | | |

| Lunge Drive | | R lift | L lift | Natural Squat | | R lift | L lift |
|---|---|---|---|---|---|---|---|
| Pelvis is tucked under in posterior tilt | 3 | | | Thigh does not reach a horizontal position | 3 | | |
| Stance knee is bent | 3 | | | Knees and ankles collapse inwards or outwards | 3 | | |
| Trunk is shorter at the front than at the back | 3 | | | Angle of trunk tilts too far forward | 3 | | |
| Trunk is longer at the front than at the back | 3 | | | Change in trunk shape, either into flexion or extension | 3 | | |
| Trunk is tilted sideways | 3 | | | The pelvis does not sit centrally between the legs | 3 | | |
| Lip biting or facial fixing | 1 | | | Balance point is in heels | 3 | | |
| Foot fixing | 1 | | | Facial fixing | 1 | | |
| **Total:** | | | | **Total:** | | | |

| Standing Knee Lift | | R lift | L lift | Seated Knee Lift | | R lift | L lift |
|---|---|---|---|---|---|---|---|
| Hip hitches up on the lifting side/trunk shortens on that side | 3 | | | Hip hitches up on the lifting side/trunk shortens on that side | 3 | | |
| Stance hip moves out to the side | 3 | | | Pelvis moves out to the side | 3 | | |
| One arm moves lower | 2 | | | One arm moves lower | 3 | | |
| Trunk tips sideways | 3 | | | Trunk tips sideways | 3 | | |
| Leg does not lift straight | 2 | | | Leg does not lift straight | 3 | | |
| Spine extends | 3 | | | Facial fixing | 1 | | |
| Spine flexes | 3 | | | Foot fixing | 1 | | |
| Facial fixing | 1 | | | | | | |
| Foot fixing | 1 | | | | | | |
| **Total:** | | | | **Total:** | | | |

## Lower and central control zone stability subtotal: _____

④ Upper Control Zone Stability

| Diamond | R | L | Wall Press | R | L |
|---------|---|---|------------|---|---|
| Hands turn palms upwards instead of wrists amd forearms lifting | 3 | | Chin tilts upward | 3 | |
| Shoulders move towards ears | 3 | | Shoulders move up, or scapulae wing off the rib cage | 3 | |
| Hands lift less than 10 cm | 3 | | Pelvis drifts forward | 3 | |
| Shoulder sinks to the floor | 3 | | Stomach protrudes | 3 | |
| | | | Upper body bends forward | 3 | |
| **Total:** | | | **Total:** | | |

**Upper control zone stability subtotal:** _____

⑤ Basic Global Control

| Superman | | R arm/L leg raised | L arm/R leg raised |
|----------|---|--------------------|--------------------|
| Head position is lost | 2 | | |
| Shoulders move up, or scapula wings off rib cage | 3 | | |
| Chest drops on unsupported side | 3 | | |
| Pelvis rotates upwards or downwards on unsupported side | 3 | | |
| Stomach protrudes-spinal curve deepens | 3 | | |
| Facial fixing | 1 | | |
| **Total:** | | | |

**Basic global control subtotal:** _____

## Score Summary

| | |
|---|---|
| **1. Balance** | |
| **2. Mobility relationships** | |
| **3. Lower and central control zone stability** | |
| **4. Upper control zone stability** | |
| **5. Basic global control** | |

**Overall total score:** _____

## Action Plan

**1** Priority areas: _____

_____

**2** Strength and conditioning programme implications: _____

_____

**3** Technique implications: _____

_____

# Bibliography and References

1 Abt, J.P., Smoglia, J.M., Bricj, M.J., Jolly, J., Lephart, S., & Fu, F.: 2007. Relationship between cycling mechanics and core stability. *J. of Strength and Conditioning Research*, **21**(4): 1300–1304.

2 Alon, R.: 1996. *Mindful Spontaneity: Returning to Natural Movement*. North Atlantic Books, Berkeley, CA.

3 Anderson, T.: 1996. Biomechanics and running economy. *Sports Medicine*, **22**(2): 76–89.

4 Barlow, W.: 1973. *The Alexander Principle: How to Use Your Body Without Stress*. Victor Gollancz, London.

5 Bergmark, A.: 1989. Stability of the lumbar spine: a study in mechanical engineering. *Acta Orthopedica Scandinavica*, **230**: 20–24.

6 Besier, T.F., Lloyd, D.G., Ackland, T.R. & Cochrane, J.L.: 2001. Anticipatory effects on knee joint loading during running and cutting manoeuvres. *Medicine and Science in Sports and Exercise*, **33**(7): 1176–81.

7 Bolgla, L.A. & Keskula, D.R.: 2000. A review of the relationship among knee effusion, quadriceps inhibition and knee function. *J. of Sport Rehabilitation*, **9**(2): 160–168.

8 Bosch, F.: 2012. The Mechanics of Sprinting. Lecture delivered at "Running" Conference, UK.

9 Bullock-Saxton, J.E., Janda, V. & Bullock, M.I.: 1994. The influence of ankle sprain injury on muscle activation during hip extension. *Int. J. of Sports Medicine*, **15**(6): 330–334.

10 Burden, A.M., Grimshaw, P.N. & Wallace, E.S.: 1998. Hip and shoulder rotations during the golf swing of sub-10 handicap players. *J. Sports Sci*ence, **16**(2):165–176.

11 Burnett, A., Cornelius, M., Dankaerts, W. & O'Sullivan, P.: 2004. Spinal kinematics and trunk muscle activity in cyclists: a comparison between healthy controls and non-specific chronic low back pain subjects: a pilot investigation. *J. of Manual Therapy*, **9**(4): 211–219.

12 Cairns, M.C., Foster, N.E., & Wright, C.: 2006. Randomized controlled trial of specific spinal stabilization exercises and conventional physiotherapy for recurrent low back pain. *Spine*, **1**:31(19): E670–681.

13 Chappell, J.D., Yu, B., Kirkendall, D.T. & Garrett, W.E.: 2002. A comparison of knee kinetics between male and female recreational athletes in stop-jump tasks. *Am. J. of Sports Medicine*, **30**(2): 261–267.

14 Christina, R.W.: 1996. Major determinants of the transfer of training: Implications for enhancing sport performance. In: Kim, K.W. (ed.) *Human Performance Determinants in Sport*. Korean Society of Sport Psychology, Seoul, pp. 25–52.

15 Comerford, M.J. & Mottram, S.L.: 2001. Movement and stability dysfunction: contemporary developments. *J. of Manual Therapy*, **6**(1): 15–26.

16 Cortes, N., Quammen, D., Lucci, S., Greska, E., & Onate, J.: 2012. A functional agility short-term fatigue protocol changes lower extremity mechanics. *J. Sports Sci*. **30**(8): 797-805.

17 Cowan, S.M., Hodges, P.W., Bennell, K.L., & Crossley, K.M.: 2002. Altered vastii recruitment when people with patellofemoral pain syndrome complete a postural task. *Arch. Phys. Med. Rehabil.*, **83**(7): 989–995.

18 Cowan, S.M., Schache, A.G., Brukner, P., Bennell, K.L., Hodges, P.W., Coburn, P. & Crossley, K.M.: 2004. Delayed onset of transversus abdominus in long-standing groin pain. *Med. Sci. Sports Exerc.*, **36**(12): 2040–2045.

19 Decker, M., Torry, M., Noonan, T., Riviere, A. & Strerett, W.: 2002. Landing adaptations after ACL reconstruction. *Medicine and Science in Sport and Exercise*, **34**(9): 1408–1413.

20 De Luca, L., Di Giorgio, P., Signoriello, G., Sorrentino, E., Rivellini, G., D'Amore, E., De Luca, B. & Murray, J.A.: 2004. Relationship between hiatal hernia and inguinal hernia. *Digestive Diseases and Sciences*, **49**(2): 243–247.

21 Diallo, O., Dore, E., Duche, P. & Van Praagh, E.: 2001. Effects of plyometric training followed by a reduced training programme on physical performance in prepubescent soccer players. *J. of Sports Medicine and Physical Fitness*, **4**(3): 342–348.

22 Dickerman, R.D., Smith, A. & Stevens, Q.E.: 2004. Umbilical and bilateral inguinal hernias in a veteran powerlifter: is it a pressure-overload syndrome? *Clinical J. of Sport Medicine*, **14**(2): 95–96.

23 Don Tigny, R.: 2005. Critical analysis of the functional dynamics of the sacroiliac joints as they pertain to normal gait. *J. of Orthopaedic Medicine*, **27**(1): 3–10.

24 Dufek, J. & Bates, B.: 1990. The evaluation and prediction of impact forces during landings. *Medicine and Science in Sports and Exercise*, **22**(2): 370–377.

25 Ellenbecker, T.S., Roetert, E.P., Piorkowski, P.A. & Schulz, D.A.: 1996. Glenohumeral joint internal and external rotation range of motion in elite junior tennis players. *J. of Orthopaedic and Sports Physical Therapy*, **24**(6): 336–341.

26 Elphinston, J. & Pook, P.: 2000. *The Core Workout: The Definitive Guide To Swiss Ball Training for Athletes, Coaches and Fitness Professionals*. Lotus Publishing, Chichester.

27 Elphinston, J. & Hardman, S.L.: 2006. Effect of an integrated functional stability program on injury rates in an international netball squad. *J. Sci. Med. Sport*, **9**(1–2): 169–176.

28 Elphinston, J.: 2006. *Total Stabilitets-Traning: Prestationsutvecklande, Skadeforebyggande, Ovingar Och Teori*. SISU Idrottsbocker, Stockholm.

29 Escorsell, A., Gines, A., Llach, J., Garcia-Pagan, J.C., Bordas, J.M., Bosch, J. & Rodes, J.: 2002. Increasing intra-abdominal pressure increases pressure, volume, and wall tension in esophageal varices. H*epatology*, **36**(4): 936–940.

30 Feldenkrais, M.: 1972. *Awareness through Movement*. Harper and Row, New York.

31 Fleisig, G.S., Barrentine, S.W., Escamilla, R.F. & Andrews, J.R.: 1996. Biomechanics of overhand throwing with implications for injuries. *J. of Sports Medicine*, **21**(6): 421–437.

32 Garrick, J.G. & Requa, R.: 2005. Structured exercises to prevent lower limb injuries in young handball players. *Clinical J. of Sport Medicine*, **15**(5): 398.

33 Gibbons, S.: 2001. Biomechanics and stability mechanisms of psoas major. In: Conference Proceedings 4th Interdisciplinary World Congress on Low Back and Pelvic Pain, pp. 246–247.

34 Gracovetsky, S.A.: 1997. Linking the spinal engine with the legs: a theory of human gait. In: Vleeming, A., Mooney, V., Dorman, T., Snijders, C. & Stoeckart, R. (eds.). *Movement, Stability and Low Back Pain: The Essential Role of the Pelvis*. Churchill Livingstone, Edinburgh, pp. 243–251.

35 Grenier, S.G. & McGill, S.M.: 2007. Quantification of lumbar stability by using two different abdominal activation strategies. *Arch. Phys. Med. Rehabil.*, **88**(1): 54–62.

36 Grimstone, S.K. & Hodges, P.W.: 2003. Impaired postural compensation for respiration in people with recurrent low back pain. *Experimental Brain Research*, **151**(2): 218–224.

37 Hagins, M. & Lamberg, E.M.: 2006. Natural breath control during lifting tasks: effect of load. *European J. of Applied Physiology*, **96**(4): 453–458.

38 Hall, K.G., Domingues, D.A. & Cavazos, R.: 1994. Contextual interference effects with skilled baseball players. *Perceptual and Motor Skills*, **78**(3): 835–841.

39 Hamlyn, N., Behm, D.G. & Young, W.B.: 2007. Trunk muscle activation during dynamic weight training exercises and isometric instability exercises. *J. of Strength and Conditioning Research*, **21**(4): 1108–1112.

40 Hassanlouei, H., Arendt-Nielsen, L., Kersting, U.G., Falla, D.: 2012. Effect of exercise-induced fatigue on postural control of the knee. *J. Electromyogr Kinesiol.* **22**(3): 342–347.

41 Hewett, T.E., Myer, G.D., Ford, K.R., Heidt, R.S. Jr., Colosimo, A.J., McLean, S.G., van den Bogert, A.J., Paterno, M.V. & Succop, P.: 2005. Biomechanical measures of neuromuscular control and valgus loading of the knee predict anterior cruciate ligament injury risk in female athletes: a prospective study. *Am. J. of Sports Medicine*, **33**(4): 492–501.

42 Hides, J.A., Richardson, C.A. & Jull, G.A.: 1996. Multifidus recovery is not automatic following resolution of acute first-episode low back pain. *Spine*, **21**(23): 2763–2769.

43 Hintermeister, R.A., O'Connor, D.D., Lange, G.W., Dillman, C.J. & Steadman, J.R.: 1997. Muscle activity in wedge, parallel, and giant slalom skiing. *Medicine and Science in Sports and Exercise*, **29**(4): 548–553.

44 Hodges, P. & Richardson, C.A.: 1997. Feedforward contraction of transversus abdominis is not influenced by the direction of arm movement. *Experimental Brain Research*, **114**(2): 362–370.

45 Hodges, P. & Gandieva, S.C.: 2000. Changes in intra-abdominal pressure during postural and respiratory activation of the human diaphragm. *J. Appl. Physiol.*, Sept. **89**(3): 967–976.

46 Hodges, P.: 2001. Changes in motor planning of feedforward postural responses of the trunk muscles in low back pain. *Experimental Brain Research*, **141**(2): 261–266.

47 Hodges, P.W., Heijnen, I. & Gandevia, S.C.: 2001. Postural activity of the diaphragm is reduced in humans when respiratory demand increases. *J. of Physiology*, **537**(3): 999–1008.

48 Hodges, P.W., Gurfinkel, V.S., Brumagne, S., Smith, T.C. & Cordo, P.C.: 2002. Coexistence of stability and mobility in postural control: evidence from postural compensation for respiration. *Experimental Brain Research*, **144**(3): 293–302.

49 Hodges, P.W., Eriksson, A.E., Shirley, D. & Gandevia, S.C.: 2005. Intra-abdominal pressure increases stiffness of the lumbar spine. *J. of Biomechanics*, **38**(9): 1873–1880.

50 Hodges, P.W., Sapsford, R., & Pengel, L.H.: 2007. Postural and respiratory functions of the pelvic floor muscles. *Neurourol Urodyn.* **26**(3): 362–371.

51 Hudson, J.L.: 1986. Coordination of segments in the vertical jump. *Medicine and Science in Sports and Exercise*, **18**(2): 242–251.

52 Hungerford, B., Gilleard, W. & Hodges, P.W.: 2003. Evidence of altered lumbo-pelvic muscle recruitment in the presence of sacroiliac joint pain. *Spine*, **28**(14): 1593–1600.

53 Hurd, W.J., Chmielewski, T.L., Axe, M.J., Davis, I. & Snyder-Mackler, L.: 2004. Differences in normal and perturbed walking kinematics between male and female athletes. *Clinical Biomechanics*, 19(5): 465–472.

54 Huxel, K.C., Swanik, C.B., Swanik, K.A., Bartolozzi, A.R., Hillstrom, H.J., Sitler, M.R. & Moffit, D.M.: 2008. Stiffness regulation and muscle-recruitment strategies of the shoulder in response to external rotation perturbations. *J. Bone Joint Surg. Am.*, **90**(1): 154–162.

55 Irmischer, B.S., Harris, C., Pfeiffer, R.P., DeBeliso, M.A., Adams, K.J. & Shea, K.G.: 2004. Effects of a knee ligament injury prevention exercise program on impact forces in women. *J. of Strength and Conditioning Research*, **18**(4): 703–707.

56 Ishikawa, M., Komi, P.V., Grey, M.J., Lepola, V. & Bruggemann, G.P.: 2005. Muscle-tendon interaction and elastic energy usage in human walking. *J. of Applied Physiology*, **99**(2): 603–608.

57 Itoi, E., Kuechle, D.K., Newman, S.R., Morrey, B.F., & An, K.N.: 1993. Stabilising function of the biceps in stable and unstable shoulders. *J. Bone Joint Surg. Br.*, **75**(4): 546–550.

58 Itoi, E., Newman, S.R., Kuechle, D.K., Morrey, B.F. & An, K.N.: 1994. Dynamic anterior stabilisers of the shoulder with the arm in abduction. *J. Bone Joint Surg. Br.*, **76**(5): 834–836.

59 Jackson, O.: 1999. Neuro-orthopaedics and geriatric rehabilitation: balance, flexibility, coordination: improving function for older persons, using the Feldenkrais method. *Northeast Seminars*, East Hampstead, NH.

60 Janda, V.: 1983. On the concept of postural muscles and posture in man. *Aus. J. Physioth.*, **29**(3): 83–84.

61 Jull, G., Kristjansson, E. & Dall'Alba, P.: 2004. Impairment in the cervical flexors: a comparison of whiplash and insidious onset neck pain patients. *J. of Manual Therapy*, **9**(2): 89–94.

62 Jung, A.P.: 2003. The impact of resistance training on distance running performance. *J. of Sports Med.*, **33**(7): 539–552.

63 Karlson, K.: 2000. Rowing injuries. Identifying and treating musculoskeletal and non-musculoskeletal conditions. *The Physician and Sports Medicine*, **28**(4): 40–50.

64 Khayambashi, K., Mohammadkhani, Z., Ghaznavi, K., Lyle, M.A., Powers, C.M.: 2012. The effects of isolated hip abductor and external rotator muscle strengthening on pain, health status, and hip strength in females with patellofemoral pain: a randomized controlled trial. J. Orthop. Sports Phys. Ther., **42**(1): 22–29

65 Kibler, W.B., McMullen, J. & Uhl, T.: 2001. Shoulder rehabilitation strategies, guidelines and practice. *Orthopedic Clinics of North America*, **32**(3): 527–538.

66 Kolar, P.: 1999. The sensomotor nature of postural functions: its fundamental role in rehabilitation of the motor system. *J. of Orthopaedic Medicine*, **21**(2): 40–45.

67 Kornecki, S.: 1992. Mechanism of muscular stabilisation process in joints. *J. of Biomechanics*, **25**(3): 235–245.

68 Kristjansson, E.: 2004. Reliability of ultrasonography for the cervical multifidus muscle in asymptomatic and symptomatic patients. *J. of Manual Therapy*, 9(2): 83–88.

69 Kulig, K., Loudon, J.K., Popovich, J.M. Jr., Pollard, C.D. & Winder, B.R.: 2011. Dancers with Achilles tendinopathy demonstrate altered lower extremity takeoff kinematics. *J. Orthop. Sports Phys. Ther.*, **41**(8): 606–613.

70 LaBella, C.R., Huxford, M.R., Grissom, J., Kim, K.Y., Peng,J., Christoffel, K.K.: 2011 Effect of neuromuscular warm-up on injuries in female soccer and basketball athletes in urban public high schools: cluster randomized controlled trial. *Arch. Pediatr. Adolesc. Med.* **165**(11): 1033–1040.

71 Lee, D.G.: 2005. The thorax: an integrated approach for restoring function, relieving pain. *Physiotherapist Corporation*, Canada.

72 Lee, D. & Vleeming, A.: 2000. Diagnostic tools for the impaired pelvis. *American Back Society Annual Meeting*, December 7–9, Vancouver, Canada.

73 Leetun, D.T., Ireland, M.L., Willson, J.D., Ballantyne, B.T., & Davis, I.M.: 2004. Core stability measures as risk factors for lower extremity injury in athletes. *Med. Sci. Sports Exerc.* **36**(6): 926–934.

74 Lephart, S.: 2003. Sensorimotor system: performance and protection. Paper presented at the Seventh Olympic Conference in Sports Sciences, Athens, 7–11 October.

75 Lewit, K.: 1999. Chain reactions in the locomotor system in the light of coactivation patterns based on developmental neurology. *J. of Orthopaedic Medicine*, **21**(2): 52–57.

76 Li, L. & Caldwell, G.E.: 1998. Muscle coordination in cycling: effect of surface incline and posture. *J. of Applied Physiology*, **85**(3): 927–934.

77 Loudon, J. & Reiman, M.: 2012. Lower Extremity Kinematics in Running Athletes With and Without a History of Medial Shin Pain. *Int. J. of Sp. and Phys. Therapy*, Vol.7, No.4, p.356.

78 Louw, Q., Grimmer, K. & Vaughan, C.: 2006. Biomechanical outcomes of a knee neuromuscular exercise programme among adolescent basketball players: a pilot study. *Physical Therapy in Sport*, 7: 65–73.

79 Magarey, M.E. & Jones, M.A.: 2003. Dynamic evaluation and early management of altered motor control around the shoulder complex. Manual Therapy, **8**(4): 195–206.

80 Malinzak, R.A, Colby, S.M., Kirkendall, D.T., Yu, B. & Garrett, W.E.: 2001. A comparison of knee joint motion patterns between men and women in selected athletic tasks. *Clinical Biomechanics*, **16**(5): 438–445.

81 Mascal, C.L., Landel, R. & Powers, C.: 2003. Management of patellofemoral pain targeting hip, pelvis, and trunk muscle function: two case reports. *J. of Orthopaedic and Sports Physical Therapy*, **33**(11): 647–660.

82 McLean, S.G., Felin, R.E., Suedekum, N., Calabrese, G., Passerallo, A., & Joy, S.: 2007. Impact of fatigue on gender-based high-risk landing strategies. *J. of Med. Sci. Sports Exerc.*, **39**(3): 502–514.

83 McNair, P.J., Prapavessis, H. & Callender, K.: 2000. Decreasing landing forces: effect of instruction. *Br. J. of Sports Medicine*, **34**(4): 293–296.

84 McNitt-Gray, J.L., Hester, D.M., Mathiyakom, W. & Munkasy, B.A.: 2001. Mechanical demand and multijoint control during landing depend on orientation of the body segments relative to the reaction force. *J. of Biomechanics*, **34**(11): 1471–1482.

85 Mellor, R., & Hodges, P.W.: 2006. Effect of knee joint angle on motor unit synchronization. *J. Orthop. Res.*, **24**(7): 1420–1426.

86 Mens, J., Inklaar, H., Koes, B.W., & Stam, H.J.: 2006. Anew view on adduction-related groin pain. *Clin. J. Sport Med.* 16(1): 15–19.

87 Mok, N.W., Brauer, S.G. & Hodges, P.W.: 2004. Hip strategy for balance control in quiet standing is reduced in people with low back pain. *Spine*, **29**(6): E107–112.

88 Moraes, G.F., Faria, C.D. & Teixeira-Salmela, L.F.: 2008. Scapular muscle recruitment patterns and isokinetic strength ratios of the shoulder rotator muscles in individuals with and without impingement syndrome. *J. Shoulder Elbow Sur.*, **17**(1): 48S–53S.

89 Moseley, G.L., Nicholas, M.K. & Hodges, P.W.: 2004. Pain differs from non-painful attention-demanding or stressful tasks in its effect on postural control patterns of trunk muscles. *Experimental Brain Research*, **156**(1): 64–71.

90 Moseley, G.L., Nicholas, M.K. & Hodges, P.W.: 2004. Does anticipation of back pain predispose to back trouble? Brain, **127**(10): 2339–2347.

91 Mottram, S. & Comerford, M.: 1998. Stability dysfunction and low back pain. *J. of Orthopaedic Medicine*, **20**(2): 13–19.

92 Myer, G.D., Ford, K.R., Brent, J.L. & Hewett, T.E.: 2006. Te effects of plyometric vs. dynamic stabilization and balance training on power, balance, and landing force in female athletes. *J. Strength Cond. Res.*, **20**(2): 345–353.

93 Myer, G.D., Ford, K.R., McLean, S.G. & Hewett, T.E.: 2006. The effects of plyometric versus dynamic stabilization and balance training on lower extremity biomechanics. *Am. J. Sports Med.*, **34**(3): 445–455.

94 Myers, T.: 2008. *Anatomy Trains: Myofascial Meridians for Manual and Movement Therapists, 2e.* Churchill Livingstone, Edinburgh, (Chapter 2).

95 Myklebust, G., Engebretsen, L., Braekken, I.H., Skjolberg, A, Olsen, O.E. & Bahr, R.: 2007. Prevention of noncontact anterior cruciate ligament injuries in elite and adolescent female team handball athletes. *Instr. Course Lect.* 3:56: 407–418.

96 Neptune, R.R., Zajac, F.E. & Kautz, S.A.: 2004. Muscle force redistributes segmental power for body progression during walking. *Gait and Posture*, **19**(2): 194–205.

97 Newcomer, K.L., Laskowski, E.R., Yu, B., Johnson, J.C. & An, K.N.: 2000. Differences in repositioning error among patients with low back pain compared with control subjects. *Spine*, **25**(19): 2488–2493.

98 Nuzzo, J.L., McCaulley, G.O., Cormie, P. & Cavill, M.J.: 2008. Trunk muscle activity during stability ball and free weight exercises. *J. of Strength and Conditioning Research,* **22**(1): 95–102.

99 Nyland, J.A., Caborn, D.N., Shapiro, R. & Johnson, D.L.: 1997. Fatigue after eccentric quadriceps femoris work produces earlier gastrocnemius and delayed quadriceps femoris activation during crossover cutting among normal athletic women. *Knee Surg. Sports Traumatol. Arthrosc.* **5**(3): 162-167.

100 Nyland, J, Lachman, N., Kocabey, Y., Brosky, J., Altun, R. & Caborn, D.: 2005. Anatomy, function, and rehabilitation of the popliteus musculotendinous complex. *J. Orthop. Sports Phys. Ther.* **35**(3): 165–179.

101 Oberländer, K.D., Brüggemann, G.P., Höher, J. & Karamanidis, K.: 2012. Altered landing mechanics in ACL-reconstructed patients. *Med. Sci. Sports Exerc.* [E-pub ahead of print].

102 Olsen, O.E., Myklebust, G., Engebretsen, L., Holme, I. & Bahr, R.: 2005. Exercises to prevent lower limb injuries in youth sports: cluster randomised controlled trial. *British Medical Journal*, **330**(7489): 449.

103 Onate, J.A., Guskiewicz, K.M. & Sullivan, R.J.: 2001. Augmented feedback reduces jump-landing forces. *J. of Orthopaedic and Sports Physical Therapy*, **31**(9): 511–517.

104 O'Sullivan, P.B., Burnett, A., Floyd, A.N., Gadson, K., Logiudice, J., Miller, D. & Quirke, H.: 2003. Lumbar repositioning deficit in a specific low back pain population. *Spine*, **28**(10): 1074–1079.

105 O'Sullivan, P.B., Phyty, G.D., Twomey, L.T. & Allison, G.T.: 1997. Evaluation of specific stabilizing exercise in the treatment of chronic low back pain with radiologic diagnosis of spondylolysis or spondylolisthesis. *Spine*. Dec. 15, **22**(24): 2959–2967.

106 Paoletti,S.: 2006. *The Fasciae: Anatomy, Dysfunction and Treatment*. (Chapter 2). Eastland Press, Seattle.

107 Park, E., Schöner, G. & Scholz, J.P.: 2012. Functional synergies underlying control of upright posture during changes in head orientation. *PLoS One*. **7**(8): e41583.

108 Pfeiffer, R.P., Shea, K.G., Roberts, D., Grandstrand, S., & Bond, L.: 2006. Lack of effect of a knee ligament injury prevention program on the incidence of non-contact anterior cruciate ligament injury. *J. Bone Joint Surg. Am.*, **88**(8): 1769–1774.

109 Pirouzi, S., Hides, J., Richardson, C., Darnell, R. & Toppenberg, R.: 2006. Low back pain patients demonstrate increased hip extensor muscle activity during submaximal rotation efforts. *Spine*, **15**:31(26): E999–E1005.

110 Podraza, J.T. & White, S.C.: 2010. Effect of knee flexion angle on ground reaction forces, knee moments and muscle co-contraction during an impact-like deceleration landing: implications for the non-contact mechanism of ACL injury. *J. Orthop Res*. **17**(4): 291-5°.

111 Reed, C.A., Ford, K.R., Myer, G.D., Hewett, T.E.: 2012. The effects of isolated and integrated 'core stability' training on athletic performance measures: a systematic review. *Sports Med.*, **1**:42(8): 697–706.

112 Renkawitz, T., Boluki, D. & Grifka, J.: 2006. The association of low back pain, neuromuscular imbalance, and trunk extension strength in athletes. *Spine*, **6**(6): 673–683.

113 Roll, R., Kavounoudias, A. & Roll, J.P.: 2002. Cutaneous afferents from human plantar sole contribute to body posture awareness. *Neuroreport*, **13**(15): 1957–1961.

114 Rose, D.J.: 2003. *Fallproof! A Comprehensive Balance and Mobility Training Programme*. Human Kinetics, Champaign, IL.

115 Ross, A.L. & Hudson, J.L.: 1997. Efficacy of a mini-trampoline program for improving the vertical jump. In: Wilkerson, J.D., Ludwig, K.M. & Zimmermann, W.J. (eds.) *Biomechanics in Sports XV*, Texas Women's University, Denton, pp.63–69.

116 Sahrmann, S.: 2002. *Diagnosis and Treatment of Movement Impairment Syndromes*. Mosby, St. Louis, pp.30–31.

117 Santello, M., McDonagh, M.J. & Challis, J.H.: 2001. Visual and non-visual control of landing movements in humans. *J. of Physiology*, **537**(1): 313–327.

118 Saunders, S.W., Rath, D., & Hodges, P.W.: 2004. Postural and respiratory activation of the trunk muscles changes with mode and speed of locomotion. *Gait Posture*, **20**(3): 280–290.

119 Sell, T., Tsai, Y., Smoglia, J., Myers, J. & Lephart, S.: 2007. Strength, flexibility and balance characteristics of highly proficient golfers. *J. Strength and Conditioning Research*, **21**(4): 1166–1171.

120 Sigward, S. & Powers, C.M.: 2006. The influence of experience on knee mechanics during side-step cutting in females. *Clin Biomech.*, **21**(7): 740–747.

121 So, R.C.H., Ng, J.K.F. & Ng, G.Y.F.: 2005. Muscle recruitment pattern in cycling: a review. *Physical Therapy in Sport*, **6**(2): 89–96.

122 Stanton, R., Reaburn, P.R., & Humphries, B.: 2004. The effect of short-term Swiss ball training on core stability and running economy. *J. Strength Cond. Res.*, **18**(3): 522–528.

123 Tateuchi, H., Taniguchi, M., Mori, N. & Ichihashi, N.: 2012. Balance of hip and trunk muscle activity is associated with increased anterior pelvic tilt during prone hip extension. *J. Electromyogr Kinesiol.*, **22**(3): 391–397.

124 Thompson, C.J., Cobb, K.M., & Blackwell, J.: 2007. Functional training improves club head speed and functional fitness in older golfers. *J. Strength Cond. Res.*, **21**(1): 131–137.

125 Tsai, L.C., McLean, S., Colletti, P.M. & Powers, C.M.: 2012. Greater muscle co-contraction results in increased tibiofemoral compressive forces in females who have undergone anterior cruciate ligament reconstruction. *J. Orthop. Surg.*, Online Early View edition, 22 JUNE, 2012.DOI: 10.1002/jor.22176).

126 Umphred, D.A.: 2001. The limbic system: influence over motor control and learning. In: *Neurological Rehabilitation 4th Ed.*, Mosby, St Louis, pp. 148–177.

127 Urquhart, D.M., Hodges, P.W. & Story, I.H.: 2005. Postural activity of the abdominal muscles varies between regions of these muscles and between body positions. *Gait Posture*, **22**(4): 295–301.

128 Vad, V., Gebeth, A., Dinas, D., Altcheck, D. & Norris, B.: 2003. Hip and shoulder rotation range of motion deficits in professional tennis players. *J. of Science and Medicine in Sport*, **6**(1): 71–75.

129 Van Schie, C., Carrington, A., Vermigli, C. & Boulton, A.: 2004. *Diabetes Care*, (27)7: 1668 –1673.

130 Van Wingerden, J.P., Vleeming, A., Buyruk, H.M. & Raissadat, K.: 2004. Stabilization of the sacroiliac joint in vivo: verification of muscular contribution to force closure of the pelvis. *European Spine Journal*, **13**(3): 199–205.

131 Vleeming, A., Pool-Goudzwaard, A.L., Stoeckart, R., van Wingerden, J.P. & Snijders, C.J.: 1995. The posterior layer of the thoracolumbar fascia. Its function in load transfer from spine to legs. *Spine*, **20**(7): 753–758.

132 Vleeming, A., Mooney, V., Snidjers, C. & Dorman, T. (eds.): 1997. Movement, Stability and Low Back Pain: the Essential Role of the Pelvis. *Churchill Livingstone, Edinburgh.*

133 Vrbanić, T.S., Ravlić-Gulan, J., Gulan, G. & Matovinović, D.: 2007. Balance index score as a predictive factor for lower sports results or anterior cruciate ligament knee injuries in Croatian female athletes–preliminary study. *Coll Antropol.* **31**(1): 253–258.

134 Walker, M., Rothstein, J., Finucare, S. & Lamb, R.: 1987. Relationship between lumbar lordosis, pelvic tilt and abdominal performance. *Physical Therapy*, **67**(4): 512–516.

135 Young, W.B. & Behm, D.G.: 2003. Effect of running, static stretching and practice jumps on explosive force production and jumping performance. *J. of Sports Medicine and Physical Fitness*, **43**(1): 21–27.

136 Zazulak, B.T., Hewett, T.E., Reeves, N.P., Goldberg, B., & Cholewicki, J.: 2007. Deficits in neuromuscular control of the trunk predict knee injury risk: a prospective biomechanical-epidemiologic study. *Am. J. Sports Med.* **35**(7): 1123–1130.

# Index

# Index of Exercises

## Chapter 3

## Chapter 4

## Chapter 5

### Section 1. Simple sensory communication test

### Section 2: Functional mobility

### Section 3. The lower and central control zones

### Section 4: The upper control zone

### Section 5: Basic global control

### Functional mobility testing and mobility training

### Jumps

### Landings

### Higher level pelvic control testing

### Momentum control

## Chapter 8

## Chapter 9